www.harcourt-international.com

Bringing you products from all Harcourt Health Sciences companies including Baillière Tindall, Churchill Livingstone, Mosby and W.B. Saunders

- ▶ **Browse** for latest information on new books, journals and electronic products

- ▶ **Search** for information on over 20 000 published titles with full product information including tables of contents and sample chapters

- ▶ **Keep up to date** with our extensive publishing programme in your field by registering with **eAlert** or requesting postal updates

- ▶ **Secure online ordering** with prompt delivery, as well as full contact details to order by phone, fax or post

- ▶ **News** of special features and promotions

If you are based in the following countries, please visit the country-specific site to receive full details of product availability and local ordering information

USA: www.harcourthealth.com

Canada: www.harcourtcanada.com

Australia: www.harcourt.com.au

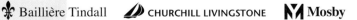 Baillière Tindall CHURCHILL LIVINGSTONE 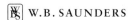 Mosby W.B. SAUNDERS

Endocrine Surgery

2nd Edition

Take a look at the other great titles in the *Companion Series*...

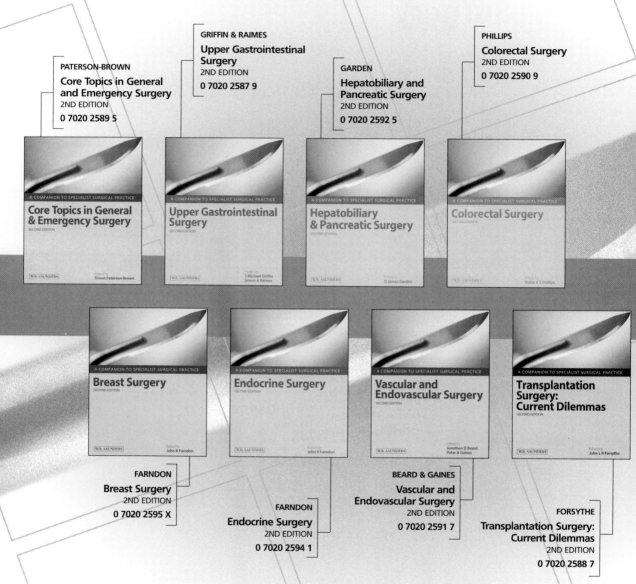
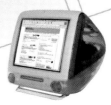
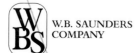

A Companion to Specialist Surgical Practice

Series editors

O. James Garden
Simon Paterson-Brown

Endocrine Surgery

2nd Edition

Edited by

John R. Farndon

Professor and Head of Department
University Department of Surgery
Bristol Royal Infirmary
Bristol

W.B. Saunders Company Limited

London   Edinburgh   New York   Philadelphia   St Louis   Sydney   Toronto 2001

WB SAUNDERS
An imprint of Harcourt Publishers Limited

© Harcourt Publishers Limited 2001

[K] is a registered trademark of Harcourt Publishers Limited

The right of John R. Farndon to be identified as editor of this work has been asserted by him in accordance
with the Copyright, Designs and Patents Act 1988

First edition published in 1997
Second edition 2001

ISBN 0 7020 2594 1

British Library Cataloguing in Publication Data
A catalogue record for this book is available from the British Library

Library of Congress Cataloging in Publication Data
A catalog record for this book is available from the Library of Congress

Note
Medical knowledge is constantly changing. As new information becomes available, changes in treatment,
procedures, equipment and the use of drugs become necessary. The editors and the publishers have taken
care to ensure that the information given in this text is accurate and up to date. However, readers are strongly
advised to confirm that the information, especially with regard to drug usage, complies with the latest
legislation and standards of practice.

Existing UK nomenclature is changing to the system of Recommended International Non-proprietary
Names (rINNs). Until the UK names are no longer in use, these more familiar names are used in this book
in preference to rINNs, details of which may be obtained from the British National Formulary.

Printed in China

Commissioning Editor: Miranda Bromage
Associate Editor: Paul Fam
Project Development Manager: Sheila Black
Project Manager: Cheryl Brant
Production Manager: Mark Sanderson

The
publisher's
policy is to use
**paper manufactured
from sustainable forests**

Contents

Contributors

Nigel D.S. Bax PhD FRCP (London) FRCP (Edinburgh)
Honorary Consultant Physician, Royal Hallamshire Hospital, Central Sheffield University Hospital Trust, Sheffield, UK

John R. Farndon BSc MD FRCS
Professor and Head of Department, University Department of Surgery, Bristol Royal Infirmary, Bristol, UK

Barney J. Harrison MS FRCS
Consultant Surgeon, Northern General Hospital, Sheffield, UK

Jade S. Hiramoto MD
General Surgery Resident, Department of Surgery, University of California, San Francisco, CA, USA

Radu Mihai MD PhD MRCS
Lecturer in Surgery, University of Bristol, UK

Jeffrey A. Norton MD
Professor of surgery, University of California San Francisco; Chief of Surgery, Department of Surgery, San Francisco Veterans Affairs Medical Center, San Francisco, CA, USA

Gary R. Peplinski MD
Assistant Professor of Surgery, Department of Surgery, San Francisco Veterans Affairs Medical Center, San Francisco, CA, USA

Zenon Rayter MS FRCS
Consultant Surgeon, Directorate of Surgery, Bristol Royal Infirmary, Bristol, UK

Gregory P. Sadler MD FRCS
Consultant Surgeon, Department of Endocrine Surgery, University Hospital of Wales, Heath Park, Cardiff, UK

W. James B. Smellie MB MChir FRCS
Consultant Surgeon, Directorate of Surgery, St Thomas' Hospital, London, UK

Malcolm H. Wheeler MD FRCS
Professor and Consultant Surgeon, Department of Endocrine Surgery, University Hospital of Wales, Heath Park, Cardiff, UK

H. Frank Woods DPhil FRCP (London) FRCP (Edinburgh)
Sir George Franklin Professor of Medicine, University of Sheffield;
Honorary Consultant Physician, Royal Hallamshire Hospital, Central Sheffield University Hospital Trust, Sheffield, UK

Anthony E. Young MChir FRCS
Consultant Surgeon, Directorate of Surgery, St Thomas' Hospital, London, UK

Foreword

In their Preface to the first edition, the series editors expressed the hope that the series would meet the needs of the higher surgical trainee and busy practising surgeon, providing up-to-date information on recent developments and succinct coverage of key topics within each specialty area. The outstanding success of the first edition suggests that these ambitions have been fulfilled and that the product is indeed meeting demand and expectations. Throughout the initiative there has been great emphasis on rapid publication, with all of its attendant stresses and strains, so that the reader could be provided with the very latest information. The fact that the second edition is now emerging within three years of the first indicates that O. James Garden and Simon Paterson-Brown and their now established team of volume editors are determined to follow through and maintain the momentum of this excellent series.

Contributors have been hand-picked with great care. They are a widely respected and authoritative group of surgeons and supporting specialists who are at the very forefront of their respective fields. The second edition retains the attractively format of the first, is well illustrated and eminently readable. The needs of the general surgeon are balanced nicely with those of the true surgical subspecialist, and there are significant additions to the range of topics covered. The series has been expanded from seven to eight volumes due to the separation of breast and endocrine surgery. There will be a widespread welcome for the emphasis on evidence-based practice and the highlighting of key references both within the text and the supporting bibliography. I am pleased to see that the authors have endeavoured to use references that are as up-to-date as possible, and readers will welcome their consistent emphasis on recent developments.

A Companion to Specialist Surgical Practice series has filled an important niche in surgical publishing and with the quality and industry of the team now established, it seems destined to continue to do so. I am proud to have been associated with the first edition of the series and feel privileged to have been asked to provide this introduction to its successor. I congratulate all those who have worked so hard to ensure the continued success of the series and wish it well over the years to come. I have no doubt that the second edition will be very well received and recommend it unreservedly.

Sir David Carter MD, Hon DSc, Hon LlD, FRCS (Ed), FRCS (Eng), FRCS (Glas), Hon FRCS (Ire), Hon FACS, Hon FRACS, FAMedSci, FRSE.
Vice Principal, University of Edinburgh, Formerly Chief Medical Officer in Scotland and Regius Professor of Clinical Surgery, Royal Infirmary, Edinburgh, UK

Preface

The Companion to Specialist Surgical Practice series has been designed to meet the needs of the higher surgeon in training and busy practising surgeon who require access to up-to-date information on recent developments in relation to their sub-specialty surgical practice. Many major surgery texts cover the whole of 'general surgery' and may contain information which is not of specific interest to the specialist surgeon. Similarly specialist texts may be outwith the reach of the trainee's finances and, though comprehensive, may fall out-of-date during production or as a consequence of rapid new developments in practice. As for the successful 1st edition, this edition has also been written and produced in a very short time frame, so that the contents are as up-to-date as possible.

Each volume in the *Companion to Specialist Surgical Practice* series provides succinct summaries of all key topics within a specialty and concentrates on the most recent developments and current data. A specialist surgeon, whether in training or in practice, need only refer to the volume relevant to his or her chosen specialist field in addition to the *Core Topics in General and Emergency Surgery.*

We are grateful to our series editors for their perseverance and for their outstanding response to our repeated promptings over the last year. We would like to thank Rachel Stock and Linda Clark from WB Saunders, for their help in getting this project safely launched in the past and would give special thanks to Sue Hodgson, Sheila Black, Paul Fam and Miranda Bromage for piloting this series to it's second edition. We appreciate very much the guidance and assistance of Sir David Carter as a series editor in the 1st series and for writing the foreword to this second series.

We hope that our aim—of providing affordable up-to-date specialist surgical texts—has been met and that all surgeons, in training or in practice, will find the 2nd edition of this series to be a valuable resource.

The addition of new chapters has led to the separation of the *Breast* and *Endocrine* volumes. Although the two specialist subjects are often spoken of at the same time practitioners do not always have specialist expertise in these two areas. A recent survey of members of the British Association of Endocrine Surgeons, for example, showed that only about 50% of endocrine specialists also specialised in breast disease.

Some of the most exciting developments are the chapters on clinical governance and medicolegal aspects of surgical practice. These chapters complement each other, and even if you do not buy both volumes you would be well advised to read the corresponding chapters in the sister textbook.

Within the endocrine volume there is a new chapter on the surgery of salivary glands, and in the breast volume new chapters describe the management of breast cancer in men and infective and inflammatory diseases.

We hope that you are not daunted by the lack of evidence which is beyond reasonable doubt in breast and endocrine disease. We do not think the evidence is present in any greater proportions in any of the other specialist areas. It is interesting to ponder on exactly what types of evidence actually influence innovation and inclusion of new techniques and treatments.

We hope you enjoy these new volumes. We are grateful to previous contributors for bringing their chapters up-to-date and to the new authors for their valuable chapters.

O. James Garden BSc, MB, ChB, MD, FRCS(Glas), FRCS(Ed)
Regius Professor of Clinical Surgery, Department of Clinical and Surgical Sciences (Surgery), Royal Infirmary, Edinburgh

Simon Paterson-Brown MB, BS, MS, MPhil, FRCS(Ed), FRCS(Eng), FCS(HK)
Consultant General and Upper Gastrointestinal Surgeon, Department of Clinical and Surgical Sciences (Surgery), Royal Infirmary, Edinburgh

John R. Farndon BSc MD FRCS
Professor and Head of Department, University Department of Surgery, Bristol Royal Infirmary, Bristol

Evidence-based Practice in Surgery

The second edition of the Companion to Specialist Surgical Practice series has attempted to incorporate, where appropriate, **evidence-based practice in surgery**, which has been highlighted in the text and relevant references. A detailed chapter on evidence-based practice in surgery written by Jonathan Michaels and Kathryn Rigby has been included in the volume on *Core Topics in General and Emergency Surgery* to which the reader is referred for further information on assessing levels of evidence. We are grateful to them for providing this summary for each volume.

Critical appraisal for developing evidence-based practice can be obtained from a number of sources; the most reliable being randomised controlled clinical trials, systematic literature reviews, meta-analysis and observational studies. For practical purposes three grades of evidence can be used, analogous to the levels of 'proof' required in a court of law:

1) **Beyond reasonable doubt**—such evidence is likely to have arisen from high quality randomised controlled trials, systematic reviews, or high quality synthesised evidence such as decision analysis, cost effectiveness analysis or large observational data sets. The studies need to be directly applicable to the population of concern and have clear results. The grade is analogous to burden of proof within a criminal court and may be thought of as corresponding to the usual standard of proof within the medical literature (i.e. $p<0.05$).

2) **On the balance of probabilities**—in many cases a high quality review of literature may fail to reach firm conclusions due to conflicting or inconclusive results, trials of poor methodological quality, or the lack of evidence in the population to which the guidelines apply. In such cases it may still be possible to make a statement as to the best treatment on the 'balance of probabilities'. This is analogous to the decision in a civil court where all the available evidence will be weighed up and the verdict will depend upon the balance of probabilities.

3) **Not proven**—insufficient evidence upon which to base a decision or contradictory evidence.

Depending on the information available three grades of recommendation can be used:

a) strong recommendation, which should be followed unless there are compelling reasons to act otherwise.

b) a recommendation based on evidence of effectiveness, but where there may be other factors to take into account in decision-making, for example the user of the guidelines may be expected to take into account patient preferences, local facilities, local audit results or available resources.

c) a recommendation made where there is no adequate evidence as to the most effective practice, although there may be reasons for making a recommendation in order to minimise cost or reduce the chance of error through a locally agreed protocol. Having highlighted the text and references which are considered to be associated with reasonable evidence in this volume with a "scalpel code", the reader can then reach his or her own conclusion.

1 Parathyroids—primary and secondary disease

Radu Mihai
John R. Farndon

Primary hyperparathyroidism

Primary hyperparathyroidism (1°HPT) is a common endocrine disorder. Because many patients remain asymptomatic, the reported incidence varies according to the means of diagnosis and the population studied and has increased significantly since the use of multichannel biochemical analysers. In the UK the incidence was estimated to be 25 people per 100 000 population[1] but it may reach 1 in 500 in women older than 45 years. The prevalence in older women might be up to 1%.

Aetiology

Monoclonality

Parathyroid adenomas are usually monoclonal, suggesting that one important step in tumour development is a mutation in a progenitor cell. Monoclonality has been demonstrated using X-chromosome inactivation analysis in parathyroid adenomas,[2,3] in sporadic multigland 1°HPT[4] and in parathyroid hyperplasia in patients with familial multiple endocrine neoplasia type 1 (MEN-1).[5,6]

Molecular genetic defects

The molecular events associated with the development of parathyroid neoplasia have not been entirely characterised but several have been implicated. One or more such chromosomal/genetic abnormalities are present in most parathyroid tumours studied, suggesting that parathyroid cells, like many other cell types, require the accumulation of multiple genetic lesions.

1. *Cyclin* D_1 *overexpression* has been demonstrated in parathyroid adenomas, carcinomas and hyperplasia (40%, 90% and 60%, respectively) but not in normal

tissue.[7] Cyclin D_1 oncogene is a cell-cycle regulator of G1/S transition.[8] Its expression is triggered by a clonal chromosomal inversion by which the 5′-regulatory region of the parathyroid hormone (PTH) gene on chromosome 11 is juxtaposed to the *parathyroid adenoma 1 (PRAD1)* gene.[9, 10]

2. *Retinoblastoma (RB) gene deletion* has been found in some aggressive and malignant parathyroid tumours.[11] *RB* is a growth suppressor gene acting as a negative regulator of the G1/S transition in normal cells.[12] The simultaneous deregulation of the RB and cyclin D pathways also described in several other tissues suggests a multicomponent model of tumorigenesis.

3. *Loss of a tumour suppressor gene* is suggested by the loss of heterozygosity in more than 25% of parathyroid adenomas on several chromosome arms,[13, 14] but no such genes have been identified or cloned. Analysis of *p53*, a well studied tumour suppressor gene, shows that none of its characteristic mutations appear in either parathyroid adenomas or carcinomas[15] and that allelic loss of *p53* gene appears in only a minority of carcinomas.[16]

4. *Somatic* MEN-1 *gene mutations* have been identified by several groups in a third of parathyroid adenomas not associated with MEN-1 syndrome,[17–19] confirming previous findings that approximately 30% of parathyroid adenomas show loss of heterozygosity for polymorphic markers on 11q13,[14] the site of the MEN-1 tumour suppressor gene. Interestingly, mutation of the RET proto-oncogene associated with MEN-2 syndrome does not contribute to the pathogenesis of sporadic parathyroid tumours.[20]

Mechanisms involved in parathyroid tumorigenesis in familial syndromes are discussed in Chapter 4.

Radiation-associated HPT

In some series, 15–20% of patients give a history of prior irradiation, but radiation-associated disease rather than radiation-induced disease is a preferred description, because an aetiological link cannot be established. A dose–response relationship exists, with an excess relative risk increased significantly by 0.11/cGy, and this is not influenced by gender or age at first presentation.[21]

Mechanisms

Genetic defects might explain the abnormal growth or proliferation of parathyroid cells but do not account for, or correlate with, the loss of sensitivity to extracellular calcium concentration—the biochemical hallmark of 1°HPT. The recent cloning of a calcium-sensing receptor (CaR) from parathyroid cells[22] has raised the hypothesis that dysfunction of this CaR might explain the abnormal Ca^{2+}-regulated PTH secretion in hyperparathyroidism. It is known that inactivating mutations of CaR causes two autosomal dominant hypercalcaemic disorders:

familial hypocalciuric hypercalcaemia and neonatal severe HPT.[23] No such mutations have been identified in parathyroid tumours,[24,25] and allelic losses on chromosome 3 at the CaR locus appear in less that 10% of tumours.[26] A substantial reduction in the intensity of CaR immunostaining has been described in parathyroid adenomas,[27] and this decreased expression of CaR would be compatible with the functional abnormalities. There is, however, considerable variation in the number of CaR-positive cells in the adenomatous tissues, and expression of the receptor protein does not relate to the set-point error, although it is lower in patients with more increased baseline concentrations of serum PTH.[28] A member of the low density lipoprotein receptor superfamily was reported to be another putative Ca^{2+} sensor on parathyroid cells,[29] with reduced expression in 1°HPT.[30]

PTH binds to specific receptors on the membrane of target cells and induces activation of several intracellular second messengers (cAMP, IP_3, Ca^{2+}). PTH receptors are widely distributed in a variety of cells other than the 'traditional' renal and bone target cells, including fibroblasts, chondrocytes, vascular smooth muscle, fat cells and placental trophoblasts.[31]

Although PTH secretion is still modulated by plasma calcium concentrations, a decreased sensitivity of parathyroid cells to extracellular calcium has been demonstrated. This induces an increased set-point (defined as the calcium level concentration at which PTH secretion is inhibited by 50%) and a shift to the right of the inverse sigmoidal relationship between PTH secretion and calcium concentration. These functional abnormalities explain the maintenance of high plasma PTH concentrations in the face of hypercalcaemia. Furthermore, the frequency and length of pulses of PTH secretion are not abnormal in 1°HPT, but patients have an increased basal secretion and increased amplitude of PTH pulses.[32]

An important regulator of parathyroid cell growth is active vitamin D $(1,25(OH)_2D_3)$, which also inhibits PTH gene transcription by binding to its receptor (VDR) in specific regions of the PTH gene promoter. It is assumed that impaired effects of vitamin D may contribute to the enhanced secretion and proliferation seen in 1°HPT. The VDR *bb* genotype is found in 60% of postmenopausal women with 1°HPT,[33] and since this genotype is linked to decreased transcriptional activity or messenger RNA stability, it accounts for reduced VDR expression and impeded regulatory actions of vitamin D.

Current data suggest that the biochemical severity of 1°HPT is determined by a combination of parameters, such as CaR content, set-point, gland size and secretory output per cell. It remains to be determined whether the pathogenesis of 1°HPT represents a primary abnormality in the control of cell growth with a secondary change in CaR expression and function, a primary alteration in Ca^{2+}-sensing pathways predisposing to somatic mutations in genes controlling growth or a combination of these two mechanisms.

Presentation

Asymptomatic disease

Asymptomatic disease may be found in up to 50% of patients, although definition criteria differ between centres. This contrasts markedly with earlier studies, in which less than 1% of patients did not have identifiable symptoms. It is still unclear whether asymptomatic 1°HPT is a progressive disease because population-based studies are complex and have been conflicting. As many as 95% of asymptomatic patients have manifestations related to 1°HPT and, more importantly, 95% of these patients claimed improvement in symptoms after parathyroidectomy.[34] Others have shown that most asymptomatic patients deteriorate and might require surgery when followed for up to 10 years.

Renal manifestations

Renal manifestations have decreased from 60–70% to 10–20% over the past two decades, but it is unclear what constitutional or environmental factors have affected this incidence as many patients lack renal manifestations despite having had 1°HPT for many years. Polyuria, back pain, colic and haematuria are possible symptoms and signs.

There are two broad categories of kidney lesions: anatomical (nephrolithiasis and nephrocalcinosis) and functional (a spectrum of tubular and glomerular disorders). Functional changes occur in the absence of any demonstrable renal calcification. Reductions in glomerular filtration rate determine increases of blood urea nitrogen and creatinine concentrations. Impairment of bicarbonate transport in the proximal tubule causes proximal tubular acidosis type II. This hyperchloraemic acidosis contrasts with the mild alkalosis accompanying hypercalcaemia of other causes (as in malignancy and vitamin D intoxication). Aminoaciduria, glycosuria and a decreased capacity to concentrate urine (nephrogenous diabetes insipidus) can occur. The pathogenesis of nephrolithiasis remains unclear as there is no correlation with hypercalciuria. The propensity for crystallisation and crystal growth of stone-forming constituents of urine is increased by the urinary acidosis, and excess of vitamin D and/or calcium in the diet provides a positive risk factor.

Skeletal involvement

Osteitis fibrosa cystica has decreased in incidence from more than 50% in 1930–50 to 9% in the 1970s and nearly zero in recent series. Excess PTH initiates bone remodelling, and increased bone resorption is associated with enhanced bone formation. There are region-specific differences in bone mass, with low values in areas with cortical bone (e.g. radius) and normal/high values in vertebrae and iliac crest (trabecular bone).

Figure 1.1
Brown tumour of the mandible in a patient with primary hyperparathyroidism

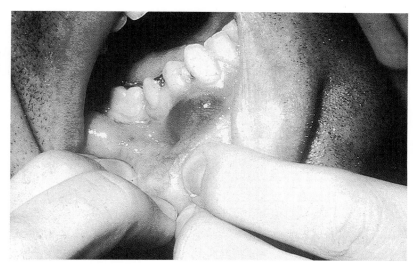

Histological bone markers of excess PTH include reduction in the number of trabeculae, increase in multinucleated osteoclasts, Howship's lacunae on the surface of the bone and replacement of normal cellular and marrow elements by fibrovascular tissue. Fractures are rarely seen today.

Even patients with mild asymptomatic 1°HPT already have major bone loss at diagnosis, and parathyroidectomy has only an initial positive effect on bone mineralisation but no long-term advantage.[35]

Articular manifestations

Chondrocalcinosis with attacks of pseudogout, juxta-articular erosions, traumatic synovitis and periarthritis are recognised complications of 1°HPT.

Neuromuscular and neuropsychiatric manifestations

The real incidence of neuromuscular and neuropsychiatric manifestations is difficult to evaluate because some of the symptoms may be non-specific or reflect degenerative or ageing features. Extreme weakness and fatigue, particularly involving proximal musculature of the lower extremities, can be present and improves after surgery. Many patients with 1°HPT are asymptomatic.

A loss of 'well being' is frequently encounted. Depression, apathy, lethargy, confusion, personality changes, memory impairment and occasionally overt psychosis are the effect of hypercalcaemia and excess PTH concentrations.

Gastrointestinal involvement

Anorexia, nausea, dyspepsia, constipation and abdominal pain are frequent symptoms. Peptic ulcer disease seems to be a true manifestation of symptomatic 1°HPT and not just a coincidental relationship. In a minority of patients, ulcers are due to gastrin-producing tumours that are present as part of the Zollinger–Ellison syndrome of MEN-1 syndrome.

Pancreatitis may occur, but a cause–effect relationship is uncertain. In acute 1°HPT, 25% of patients may have pancreatitis. Normocalcaemia in a patient with severe acute pancreatitis should raise the question of 1°HPT as an aetiological factor, saponification calcium absorption giving a spurious normal calcium concentration.

Hypertension and left ventricular hypertrophy

High blood pressure is often present at the time of diagnosis, but a specific correlation is not easily identified. Plasma renin activity, plasma aldosterone concentration and whole-body exchangeable sodium do not differ between normotensive and hypertensive patients with 1°HPT and are unchanged after surgery. A role of impaired renal function is supported by the inverse relationship between mean arterial pressure and glomerular filtration rate before and after parathyroidectomy. Recently, a parathyroid hypertensive factor (PHF) has been purified from the plasma of spontaneously hypertensive rats and medium derived from organ culture of their parathyroid glands.[36] Furthermore, the presence of PHF is linked with hypertension in patients with 1°HPT, and postparathyroidectomy blood pressure falls in parallel with PHF levels.[37]

A high prevalence of left ventricular hypertrophy has been reported in 1°HPT. Although arterial hypertension is regarded as the principal factor, the pathogenesis of left ventricular hypertrophy is not completely defined. In a recent study, multiple regression analysis demonstrated that serum PTH concentrations were associated with left ventricular mass index values as the strongest predicting variable. Furthermore, 6 months after parathyroidectomy left ventricular mass index values decreased without changes in mean blood pressure.[38]

Increased risk of premature death

Although an overall cure rate of 97% is achieved in patients undergoing surgery, one large study revealed an increased risk of premature death, with better survival for patients who underwent parathyroidectomy at an early stage of disease.[39] Additional mortality due mainly to cardiovascular disease was also reported for mild and non-progressive forms of disease. The death rate attributable to 1°HPT in the USA in 1986, however, was only 57 for the entire population, with an additional 157 deaths attributable to hypercalcaemic complications.[40]

Normocalcaemic hyperparathyroidism

Normocalcaemic hyperparathyroidism is defined as completely normal total serum calcium concentrations in the presence of symptoms or complications of 1°HPT. Factors known to decrease calcium concentrations (such as decreased serum albumin concentration, vitamin D deficiency, severe pancreatitis, increased phosphate intake and hypomagnesaemia) should be eliminated during diagnostic investigations.

Most patients are identified because of presentation with a renal calculus, and most have hypercalciuria.[41] They present a diagnostic challenge to differentiate from idiopathic hypercalciuria (assumed to be due to increased intestinal absorption, and diminished tubular resorption, of calcium resulting in a renal leak or a primary urinary phosphate leak). A failure to distinguish these two possibilities may lead to either inappropriate neck exploration in patients with idiopathic hypercalciuria or an overlooked diagnosis in those with 1°HPT.

Hypercalcaemic crisis

Hypercalcaemia is a common metabolic emergency, occurring in 0.5% of hospitalised patients. The severity of clinical manifestations often correlates with the degree of hypercalcaemia. Neuromuscular, renal and gastrointestinal manifestations are influenced by the time course of developing hypercalcaemia and any intercurrent medical conditions.

Hypercalcaemia associated with malignancy is the most common cause. Generally, the higher the concentration of plasma calcium, the more likely that malignancy is the underlying cause. Acute 1°HPT is more common in patients with longstanding hypercalcaemia, very large parathyroid adenomas, radiographic evidence of osteitis fibrosa cystica (50%) and a history of nephrolithiasis (60%).[42] Sarcoidosis, milk-alkali syndrome and adrenal insufficiency are rare causes of hypercalcaemic crisis. For a biochemical diagnosis it is important to use calcium values corrected for concentration of albumin (reduced in patients with anorexic and catabolic states associated with neoplasia) or ionised calcium.

Marked dehydration owing to anorexia, nausea or vomiting leads to more severe hypercalcaemia. Weakness and lethargy lead to immobilisation, which accentuates bone resorption. Confusion and frequent and major cognitive impairment and coma are possible. If untreated, the condition proceeds to oliguric renal failure, cardiac arrhythmia and death.

Familial HPT is described in Chapter 4.

Differential diagnosis of hypercalcaemia

The main differential diagnosis of hypercalcaemia is summarised in **Table 1.1**. Other causes previously considered are rare in today's practice: milk-alkali syndrome (H_2-blockers and proton-pump inhibitors make the excessive use of alkaline compounds unnecessary), immobilisation associated with fractures, acute renal failure and other endocrine diseases (thyrotoxicosis, phaeochromocytoma, adrenal crisis). More than 80% of patients with persistent hypercalcaemia have either 1°HPT or malignancy.

Malignancy	Multiple myeloma
	Skeletal metastasis from breast, lung or other cancers
	Skeletal carcinomatosis
Iatrogenic	Treatment with thiazide diuretics
	Excess intake of vitamin D and/or calcium
	Treatment with lithium
Familial diseases	
Familial hypocalciuric hypercalcaemia	Must be checked by 24-hour urinary calcium excretion
Metaphyseal chondrodysplasia Jansen	Constitutive activity of parathyroid hormone/parathyroid hormone-related protein receptor (rare)
Granulomatous diseases	Sarcoidosis
	Tuberculosis
Endocrine diseases	Thyrotoxicosis
	Phaeochromocytoma
	Adrenal crisis
Renal failure	

Table 1.1 *Other causes of hypercalcaemia*

Breast and lung cancer account for 60% of hypercalcaemia of malignancy; renal cell cancer for 10–15%, head and neck carcinomas for 10% and haematological malignancies for 10%. Many neoplastic tissues express high concentrations of PTH-related peptide (PTH-RP), a hormone with possible paracrine/autocrine functions in multiple adult and fetal tissues. Although its coding genes and chemical structure differ from those of PTH, the two peptides act on similar/identical receptors (reviewed in reference 43).

The history should uncover a positive family history of hypercalcaemia (the possibility of familial hypocalciuric hypercalcaemia) or other endocrine tumours (the possibility of MEN syndromes).

Familial hypocalciuric hypercalcaemia (FHH) is an autosomal dominant disorder associating hypercalcaemia, low urinary calcium excretion and few symptoms. Serum PTH concentrations are usually within the normal range but are considered inappropriately increased considering the calcium concentration. Several mutations in the *CaR* gene have been demonstrated to decrease its affinity for Ca^{2+}. Patients heterozygous for such *CaR* mutations present with FHH, whereas homozygous patients have neonatal severe HPT.

Investigative techniques

Laboratory tests

Plasma and serum electrolytes

High total calcium/ionised calcium concentrations. Determination of total calcium concentrations continues to be used as a screening tool because it is widely available, inexpensive and has a low experimental error. Because most protein-bound calcium is in the form of calcium albuminate, corrected values for plasma albumin concentrations offer more reliability. When an abnormality of calcium metabolism is suspected, however, the investigation of choice is the direct measurement of the ionised fraction.[44] An increased plasma concentration of ionised calcium should raise the suspicion of 1°HPT in patients with minimal, intermittent or no increase of the total calcium concentration. The diagnosis is then supported by non-suppressed intact PTH (iPTH) concentrations

Hypophosphataemia and phosphaturia

Hyperchloraemia and increased chloride to phosphate ratio

Hypercalciuria (>10 mmol d^{-1}) is present in 75% of hypercalcaemic patients. Excess calcium spillage supports the diagnosis of 1°HPT but, more importantly, loss of less than 2 mmol of calcium per day must alert the clinician to the diagnosis of familial hypercalcaemic hypocalciuria. This condition may mimic 1°HPT, with normal/high concentrations of PTH inappropriate in the face of hypercalcaemia. Repeated measurements of urinary calcium concentration, enquiry into family history and measurement of serum calcium concentration in first-degree siblings (being an autosomal dominant disorder) will confirm the correct diagnosis and save the patient an unnecessary neck exploration.

PTH concentration

An increased serum iPTH concentration is essential for diagnosis. New assays using two antibodies identify only iPTH and overcome the previous pitfalls generated by measuring the biologically inactive C-terminal fragments of PTH. More recently, rapid iPTH immunoradiometric and immunochemiluminometric assays have been developed. These can be used intraoperatively to confirm removal of all overactive parathyroid tissue, and because the half-life of circulating iPTH is 3–4 minutes, a decline by 50% or more at 5–10 minutes after excision of an enlarged gland provides evidence of a complete procedure.[45] A similar method has been proposed for lateralisation of parathyroid adenomas by PTH estimation in left versus right internal jugular veins at the beginning of surgery.[46]

Serum alkaline phosphatase concentration

An increased serum alkaline phosphatase concentration is not usually seen since bone involvement is currently decreasing in severity and frequency.

cAMP and hydroxyproline

Increased urinary excretion of nephrogenous cAMP (marker of PTH action on renal tubules) and hydroxyproline (marker of bone breakdown) are useful but not essential for diagnosis. Intraoperative measurement of nephrogenous cAMP can be used to prove the adequacy of exploration, because its short half-life (2–4 minutes) allows detection of an early decline after removal of hyperfunctional parathyroid tissue.

Dynamic studies

An EDTA infusion test consists of infusion of disodium EDTA or an intramuscular injection of salmon calcitonin as a hypocalcaemic stimulation test for the differential diagnosis of hypercalcaemia. In 1°HPT, EDTA always, and calcitonin usually, induces an increase in PTH concentrations. No such increase is demonstrated in patients with other causes of hypercalcaemia.

  A calcium infusion test can be used to demonstrate the reduced suppressibility of PTH concentrations (the set-point abnormality). Patients with 1°HPT do not have a major PTH response, whereas in normal individuals an iPTH concentration is suppressed below 70% of baseline at 60 minutes after a 1000 mg calcium load. Simultaneous abnormal suppression of nephrogenous cAMP with oral calcium loading has also been used as a diagnostic test.

MEN syndromes

As 1°HPT is the commonest component of the MEN syndromes, it might be assumed that patients presenting with 1°HPT represent a population at increased risk for either of the two syndromes, but serum gastrin, prolactin and calcitonin concentrations are needless determinations in patients without any clinical indication of MEN syndromes.[47]

Radiological studies

Parathyroid imaging is not needed before initial surgery. Failure to localise does not refute the biochemically confirmed diagnosis. Equally, a unilateral positive image does not obviate the need for bilateral neck exploration. All the imaging techniques available have insufficient sensitivity and specificity, and none is adequate alone.

  Ultrasonography is easily available but ineffective in localising small adenomas (weighing less than 500 mg). It produces satisfactory results in localising adenomas weighing more than 1 g, but these adenomas should not present a problem to an experienced endocrine surgeon. Intraoperative ultrasonography with a

10 MHz probe is useful in locating intrathyroidal adenomas and during surgical re-exploration of the neck.

Thallium–technetium subtraction scanning relies on the fact that thallium (TI-chloride) is trapped in both thyroid and parathyroid tissue, whereas technetium (^{99m}Tc-pertechnetate) is trapped only in thyroid tissue (**Fig. 1.2**). It seems that the uptake of thallium by parathyroids relates to mitotic activity (DNA profile) rather than gland weight.[48] A sensitivity of up to 85% and a specificity of about 90% have been reported.

Technetium–sestamibi scanning is becoming the initial investigation of choice[49] if localisation studies are required. Sestamibi accumulates in the mitochondria of parathyroid cells in a manner similar to that described for thallium, but its emission spectrum enhances the sensitivity for both smaller and deeper lesions. In addition, sestamibi permits imaging by single photon emission computed tomography (SPECT), with a tridimensional data display and markedly improved spatial resolution.

Magnetic resonance imaging (MRI) is best suited for locating ectopic glands because the signal intensity of parathyroid adenomas is similar to that of thyroid gland and fat, and MRI will therefore miss adenomas in close vicinity to the thyroid gland. Comparison of the short tau inversion recovery (STIR) sequence images (which differentiate from fat tissue) with concomitant T1 images (which have better image detail) provides improved anatomical localisation.[50] In some centres MRI is the most accurate non-invasive localisation study, especially when gadolinium enhancement is used. Computed tomography (CT) can also be used to localise ectopic and mediastinal glands but is limited by artefacts if metallic clips have been used in previous surgery.

Positron emission tomography with [^{11}C]methionine or glucose analogues is still experimental.[51]

The advantage and cost-effectiveness of preoperative localisation and unilateral neck exploration in 1°HPT are controversial issues. Some say preoperative localisation of a solitary parathyroid adenoma (eventually coupled with confirmation of excision of all hyperfunctional tissue by quick PTH assay) may optimise operative time with unilateral neck exploration.[52,53] Others report unacceptably high failure rates for unilateral neck exploration guided by preoperative localising studies compared with a bilateral neck exploration by an experienced endocrine surgeon.[54] No localisation test can accurately identify multigland disease, which occurs in up to 20% of patients.

Tests for localisation after initial operative failure

Localisation procedures should be carried out before re-exploration. The less invasive test described above should be used first, and several other additional options are available.

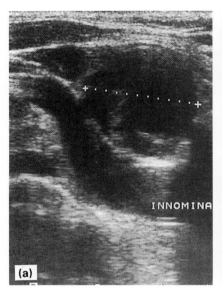
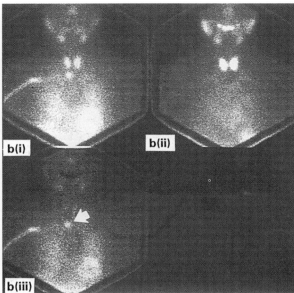

Figure 1.2
*Parathyroid imaging.
(a) Ultrasound image of a
parathyroid adenoma in close
vicinity with the innominate
artery. (b) Technetium–thalium
subtraction scan: (i) thallium
uptake by both thyroid and
parathyroid; (ii) technetium
uptake by the thyroid; (iii) the
subtracted image, demonstrating
an area of increased uptake on
the left side of the neck,
corresponding to left lower
parathyroid (c) Magnetic
resonance image of the same
adenoma in T2 (i) and short tau
inversion recovery sequence (ii).
(Courtesy of Dr J Kaballa,
Department of Radiology, Bristol
Royal Infirmary, Bristol, UK.)*

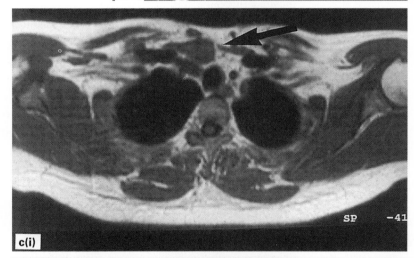
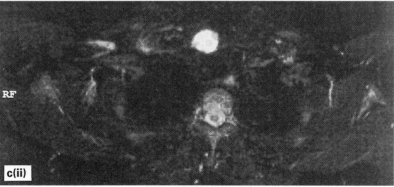

1. Venous sampling for PTH concentrations may demonstrate important gradients between neck and peripheral blood. The test may help in both the diagnosis of a mediastinal parathyroid as the cause of 1°HPT and the 'mapping' of the neck before a second exploration.

2. Measuring PTH concentration by immunoradiometric assay in percutaneous needle aspirates of cervical masses might confirm parathyroid adenomas,[55] but the small size and profound position of most parathyroid tumours make this method difficult to apply.

3. Methylene blue is rarely used. The dye is selectively taken up by parathyroid adenomas and helps in their localisation during dissection, but many surgeons achieve excellent results without its use.

4. Limited arteriography is possible but rarely used in current practice.

5. Combined use of ^{99m}Tc-sestamibi and a hand-held gamma-detecting probe may prove feasible for intraoperative localisation of abnormal parathyroid tissue, but the technique is still experimental.

Bone lesions

The earliest changes are seen on radiographs of the hands, where subperiosteal erosions can be detected in the phalanges (especially the radial aspect of the middle phalanges) and terminal tufts. The skull demonstrates a mottled appearance with lucent cystic areas ('pepperpot skull' in its most florid form; **Fig. 1.3**), and any bone may demonstrate cystic lesions due to osteoclastomas or brown tumours. These lesions may lead to pathological fractures. Subtle bone changes are rarely detected on skeletal surveys and there is little justification for this investigation unless there are specific symptoms.

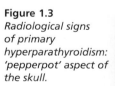

Figure 1.3
Radiological signs of primary hyperparathyroidism: 'pepperpot' aspect of the skull.

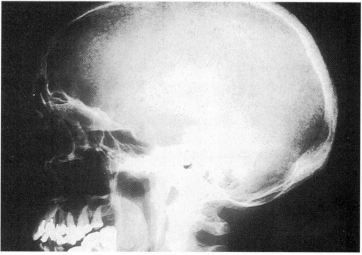

Abnormal bone density can be demonstrated by bone densitometry, X-ray spectrophotometry or single-photon absorptiometry. The densitometric site at which evidence of PTH-mediated bone resorption is greatest is the cortical distal third of the radius. Bone mass can be evaluated by single-photon absorptiometry and dual-photon absorptiometry, quantitative CT and dual-energy X-ray absorptiometry (DEXA scan). In many patients there is an initial rapid loss in bone mass followed by a period of stable disease, with little progression at the time of diagnosis of 1°HPT.

Pathological basis for primary hyperparathyroidism

Adenomas are found in approximately 80% of patients. Chief cells, oxyphil cells and water clear cells are present in differing proportions in parathyroid adenomas. An acinar pattern can be observed in some tumours. The presence of a rim of compressed normal tissue supports the diagnosis of an adenoma. Their weight ranges from 70 mg to 20 g.

Double adenomas are probably a distinct entity. Patients with persistent or recurrent 1°HPT caused by missed/not recognised double adenomas are older, nephrolithiasis is less common, and muscle weakness, neuropsychiatric disorders, constipation and weight loss are more severe than in patients with persistent or recurrent 1°HPT caused by hyperplasia.[56]

Diffuse hyperplasia can be found in as many as 15–20% of patients. It can occur alone or in association with certain familial endocrinopathies. The first intimation of hyperplasia might be the uncovering of multigland disease in a patient presenting in a conventional way. Intraoperative assessment is not always easy, even with the help of frozen sections and a skilled pathologist. Four gland enlargement is unusual in the hyperplasia of sporadic 1°HPT, and the marked heterogeneity in gland size may result in failure to recognise multigland disease.[57] Even the histological diagnosis may be difficult in such patients.

Carcinomas occur in about 1% of all patients, with an equal incidence in women and men at a mean age of 55 years. Data have been reported from the first prospectively accrued series of 286 patients with parathyroid carcinomas treated in the USA between 1985 and 1995.[58] There were no clinical or biochemical markers to allow the preoperative recognition of patients with carcinoma. Furthermore, even in centres with experienced endocrine surgeons, up to 86% of cases were not appreciated initially by the surgeons, and carcinoma was often confirmed only when the patient subsequently developed local recurrence or metastases. Tumours were rather large (median size 3.3 cm) and lymph node metastasis was identified in 16 of the 105 patients when lymph node status was evaluated at the time of the initial operation.[58]

The accurate histological diagnosis of malignancy is difficult. Vascular and capsular invasion, the presence of fibrous bands, trabecular or rosette-like cellular architecture or mitotic figures have all been used to help distinguish carcinoma from adenoma, but the specificity of these criteria is low. Chief cells predominate in carcinomas, but oxyphil and transitional oxyphil cells may also be found. The architecture varies from a more solid to a trabecular pattern, but there are no great differences between adenoma and carcinoma.[59] Flow cytometry analysis of DNA content in parathyroid lesions does little to enhance the distinction between benign and malignant lesions. In patients with clinically or pathologically demonstrated parathyroid cancer, however, flow cytometry may differentiate the likely indolent disease (diploid tumours) from tumours more likely to behave aggressively (aneuploid).[60] Mitotic activity constitutes a prognostic risk factor but is of limited diagnostic importance. In half the carcinomas, the frequency of mitoses does not exceed values recorded in benign parathyroid lesions.[61]

Parathyroid carcinomas usually continue to function, and troublesome hypercalcaemia adds considerably to the patient's suffering. Occasionally the carcinomas are non-secretory, although they have consistent light and electron microscopic features, and PTH immunoreactivity is demonstrable.

Ectopic PTH secretion is extremely rare, and examples of patients with small-cell lung cancer and ovarian carcinoma have been reported,[63] where DNA rearrangement and amplification in the regulatory region of one PTH gene allele have been demonstrated.[63]

Neonatal HPT is a genetically transmitted autosomal dominant disease characterised by life-threatening marked hypercalcaemia and intense parathyroid hyperplasia and hypercellularity. The disease is due to a mutation in the calcium receptor gene, which induces hyperplasia of the chief cells leading to severe hypercalcaemia. This is fatal if not recognised and treated early. Patients seem to be homozygous for *CaR* mutations, which determine familial benign hypocalciuric hypercalcaemia in heterozygotes (reviewed in reference 64). Near-total parathyroidectomy controls the disease.

HPT in familial syndromes is presented in Chapter 4.

Management options

Treatment should be adapted to the severity of 1°HPT (**Table 1.2**).

Medical treatment

All patients diagnosed with 1°HPT should be advised to avoid prolonged bed rest or dehydration and to ask medical advice if persistent vomiting or diarrhoea develop (since it can trigger a hypercalcaemic crisis). A moderate dietary calcium

Mild hypercalcaemia (2.6–2.9 mmol l⁻¹)	Moderate hypercalcaemia (2.9–3.3 mmol l⁻¹)	Severe hypercalcaemia (>3.4 mmol l⁻¹)
50% symptomatic patients—surgery	Surgical treatment	Emergency treatment (see Table 1.3)

50% asymptomatic patients
  Mobilise
  Keep well hydrated
  Provide diet with moderate calcium
  Oestrogens to menopausal women
  Clodronate orally
		Surgical treatment on equilibrated patient

Table 1.2 *Therapeutic options adapted to the severity of primary hyperparathyroidism*[56]

intake is advisable because low intake further stimulates the parathyroids and high intake accentuates hypercalcaemia. However, a high calcium intake (up to 60 mmol d⁻¹ *vs.* the currently recommended 20 mmol d⁻¹) over a 3-year period is reported to reverse the degree of age-dependent HPT in postmenopausal women.[65]

No satisfactory medical therapy exists for the treatment of 1°HPT.[66]

Calcitonin and bisphosphonates do not give good long-term control. The efficacy of the somatostatin analogue **octreotide** in the management of 1°HPT is low. It produces a significant decrease in urinary calcium concentration, but reductions in serum calcium and PTH concentration are not significant,[67] and parathyroid tissue is usually negative for somatostatin–receptor expression.[68] Hormone replacement therapy in postmenopausal women may offer the advantage of oestrogenic effects on the bone.

CaR agonists The cloning of the CaR has triggered efforts to develop drugs that could increase the affinity of CaR for [Ca²⁺]ext and thereby potentially correct the biochemical abnormalities in 1°HPT. One such compound is NPS R-568, an allosteric modulator of the CaR that potentiates the effects of cation agonists on CaR.[69] Pharmacological activation of CaR *in vivo* with NPS R-568 inhibits PTH secretion. In clinical studies, NPS R-568 inhibited PTH secretion in healthy postmenopausal women.

A randomised, placebo-controlled, double-blinded trial concluded that single and increasing doses of NPS R-568 (20–160 mg) inhibit PTH secretion by up to 70% for up to 4–8 hours in postmenopausal women with mild 1°HPT.[70]

Clinical trials to establish the therapeutic potential of this CaR agonist are in progress. Treatment of a woman with hypercalcaemia secondary to parathyroid carcinoma with NPS R-568 over 2 years produced no adverse clinical effects, and the drug seemed effective in the long-term control of hypercalcaemia.[71]

PTH-autoantibodies A recent report of a single patient with parathyroid carcinoma treated with autoantibodies against human PTH offers an intriguing prospect.[73]

Emergency treatment of hypercalcaemic crisis

It often takes 4–6 litres to restore the volume status in the first 24 hours of a hypercalcaemic crisis, and this increases calcium excretion by 100–300 mg d^{-1} but rarely normalises serum calcium concentration if used alone.

Forced saline diuresis Loop antidiuretics depress the proximal tubular reabsorptive mechanisms for calcium and increase urinary calcium excretion by 800–1000 mg d^{-1}. Frusemide, ethacrynic acid or bumetamide are used but should not be initiated until volume repletion has been achieved. The risks of forced diuresis include cardiac decompensation (need central venous pressure monitoring), hypophosphataemia, hypokalaemia and hypomagnesaemia.

Antiresorptive agents Bisphosphonates have become one of the mainstays of therapy for severe hypercalcaemia. All active bisphosphonates reduce bone turnover, inhibit the recruitment of osteoclasts to the bone surface, inhibit osteoclast activity and shorten osteoclast lifespan.[73] The most potent bisphosphonate is pamidronate, which is widely used in the treatment of acute hypercalcaemia. Details about each of the three main agents are presented in **Table 1.3**. For moderate hypercalcaemia, oral formulations are available (clodronate). The resulting decrease in bone turnover could potentially reduce the severity and magnitude of the 'hungry bone syndrome' post-parathyroidectomy.[74] The calcium-lowering effect is, however, incomplete and ill sustained owing to the unopposed effect of PTH on renal tubular reabsorption of calcium. Bisphosphonates could be used for assessing the beneficial effects of parathyroidectomy on renal function and thus could help identify patients who would benefit from surgery.

Gallium nitrate is an antiresorptive drug, which did not prove as clinically efficient as hoped.

Calcitonin This is a non-toxic therapy with a rapid onset of action (within minutes) but limited usefulness because of its short-lived effects. Its main indication remains for the first 24–48 hours of treatment of acute severe hypercalcaemia, in conjunction with more potent but slower acting therapies (as bisphosphonates).

Glucocorticoids These may be useful in treating patients with other causes of hypercalcaemia, i.e. myeloma/lymphoma, granulomatous diseases (it decreases vitamin D production by activated macrophages in granulomas) and vitamin D intoxication.

Dialysis This is reserved for patients with renal failure. Peritoneal dialysis removes 500–2000 mg of calcium in 24 hours, whereas haemodialysis clears 250 mg h^{-1}.

Treatment	Dose	Onset of action	Duration of action	Advantages	Disadvantages
Saline	4–6 l	Hours	During infusion	Rehydration	Cardiac overload, electrolyte disturbances (potassium, magnesium, phosphates)
Loop diuretics	Frusemide 40 mg i.v. every 1–2 hours	Hours	During infusion	Enhanced renal calcium excretion	Cardiac overload, electrolyte disturbances (potassium, magnesium, phosphates)
Calcitonin	2–8 U kg^{-1} i.v., s.c. or i.m.	Hours	2–3 days	Rapid onset of action	Only modest reduction of plasma calcium concentrations, for only few days
Etidronate	25 mg kg^{-1} (single i.v. dose) or 7.5 mg kg^{-1} over few days	24–48 hours	5–7 days	33–80% of patients are normocalcaemic by 7 days	Hyperphosphataemia
Pamidronate	30–90 mg (single i.v. or infusion over 24 hours)	24–48 hours	10–14 days	Potency: 70–100% of patients become normocalcaemic Immediate onset Prolonged duration of action	Adverse effects (1 of 3 patients) Limited/transient fever (20%), myalgias, hypophosphataemia, hypomagnesaemia
Clodronate	4–6 mg kg^{-1} in 2–4 hours			Well tolerated	Potential nephrotoxicity
Galium nitrate		48–72 hours	10–14 days	High potency	Contraindicated if renal impairment
Mithramycin	15–25 µg kg^{-1} over 4 hours	6–12 hours	Not sustained		Local/soft tissue irritation if extravasation occurs Increases in hepatic transaminases Nephrotoxicity, thrombocytopenia

Table 1.3 *Treatment of acute hypercalcaemia*

Intravenous phosphate therapy This is dramatically effective but has serious potential hazards, such as precipitation of calcium phosphate in the skeleton, kidney, soft tissues and heart. With the availability of potent and hazard-free drugs, phosphates are rarely used in current practice.

Mitomycin This was one of the first-line drugs used especially for hypercalcaemia of malignancy despite its potentially disturbing side effects (**Table 1.3**). It is little used since the availability of bisphosphonates.

Treatment of asymptomatic HPT

The debate about the optimum treatment of asymptomatic 1°HPT continues.

Because most patients with 1°HPT have few or no symptoms, the need for parathyroidectomy to treat all patients has been questioned. A recent study followed the clinical course and complications in 121 patients (101 (83%) of whom were asymptomatic) for up to 10 years. During the study, 61 patients underwent parathyroidectomy and 60 were followed without surgery. Parathyroidectomy in patients with or without symptoms led to normalisation of serum calcium concentrations and an increase in lumbar spine and femoral neck bone mineral density. The 52 asymptomatic patients who did not undergo surgery had no change in serum calcium concentration, urinary calcium excretion or bone mineral density. However, 14 of these 52 patients had progression of disease, defined as the development of at least one new indication for parathyroidectomy. All 20 patients with symptoms had kidney stones. None of the 12 who underwent parathyroidectomy had recurrent kidney stones, whereas 6 of the 8 patients who did not undergo surgery did have a recurrence. Most asymptomatic patients who did not undergo surgery did not have progression of disease, but approximately one quarter of them did.[75]

Some advocate parathyroidectomy for all patients with symptomless mild 1°HPT because:

1.   Subtle physical and psychological changes are only appreciated on restoration of biochemical normality;
2.   There is risk of developing renal failure in the long term;
3.   There is a risk of bone loss—especially important in elderly females;
4.   Hypercalcaemia may contribute to confusion in elderly people;
5.   There is a risk of hypercalcaemic crisis in elderly people, especially if an intercurrent illness produces dehydration;
6.   The incidence and mortality from cardiovascular disease may be increased;
7.   The cost of definitive diagnosis and surgical treatment would be exceeded by the cost of 6 years' medical follow-up.

The workload of adopting such a policy would be considerable, and it should be kept in mind that the preoperative risk factor profile is altered. Impairments in cardiovascular, respiratory and renal function and abnormal glucose control are found often in these patients, and they seem more likely to have a history of congestive heart disease, thromboembolic diseases, stroke and diabetes mellitus. The literature on the role of surgical treatment in elderly patients with asymptomatic or middly symptomatic 1°HPT has recently been reviewed.[76]

Surgical treatment of 1°HPT

Once the biochemical diagnosis of 1°HPT is confirmed there is no need to proceed to localisation procedures, and neck exploration can be undertaken forthwith.

A consensus conference by the National Institutes of Health in 1990 recommended surgery for patients with major adverse effects of 1°HPT, for patients with complicating coexistent illnesses, for younger patients and for those in whom long-term follow-up could not be assured.[77] However, a recent cross-sectional survey of over 100 members of the American Association of Endocrine Surgeons showed that criteria for surgery diverge from these guidelines and that high-volume surgeons (>50 cases per year) had significantly lower thresholds for surgery with respect to abnormalities in biochemical parameters.[78]

More recently, the demonstrated prevalence of non-classic symptoms and their reversibility, the evidence of 'asymptomatic' but harmful effects and the accumulating evidence for reduction of increased long-term mortality risk after surgery substantially strengthen the argument for recommending parathyroidectomy to any patient with a secure diagnosis of 1°HPT.[79] Furthermore, improvement of glucose control in diabetic patients suggests that such patients with 1°HPT should have surgery.[80]

Over 50 years ago, Albright and Reifenstein wrote 'there is no time like the first operation to uncover a small adenoma.'[81] The identification of all glands is important, as the search for a specific missing gland can then proceed logically based on anatomical and embryological knowledge. Excellent monographs exist that describe the technical details of neck exploration, and those by Gunn[82] and Wells et al.[83] are recommended.

The strap muscles are separated in the midline and elevated from the underlying thyroid. They need never be divided; there may be a need to divide the middle thyroid vein or the inferior thyroid veins, but this should be avoided if possible. Preservation of the veins may be important if the exploration is unsuccessful and selective venous sampling is subsequently required.

The thyroid lobe is gently retracted toward the midline to allow examination of those areas where the glands are most likely to be found—just above the inferior artery and around the lower thyroid pole. The recurrent nerve must be protected; undue dissection or palpation near or directly on the nerve may interfere with its function. The nerve is sometimes closely applied to an abnormal parathyroid, and it must be carefully dissected free. Diathermy should not be used in the vicinity of the nerve.

The glands are often enclosed within a fat pad beneath fascia and this has to be opened before the gland 'pops out.' This is particularly the case for glands within the thyrothymic ligament or thymus.

The vessels supplying a normal gland can be seen coursing into its substance, and care must be taken not to devascularise these structures unwittingly. If a biopsy sample is taken it should be a sliver from the distal pole of the gland away from the feeding vessels. A silver clip placed across the distal third of a gland both marks the gland and allows a bloodless biopsy.

All four glands should be visualised before a policy of resection and biopsy is decided. Too aggressive a biopsy policy leads to an unacceptably high incidence of hypoparathyroidism. By concentrating on the likely sites of the parathyroids, a competent surgeon can successfully identify and remove abnormal tissue in 95% of patients. The presence of four normal glands probably means a wrong diagnosis as a fifth ectopic and abnormal gland is rare. The exploration must be carried superiorly above the upper thyroid pole and behind the pharynx and oesophagus. A full exploration and excision of the thymic upper poles should be performed, opening the carotid sheath and examining the lower thyroid poles. Intrathyroidal adenomas may be detected by intraoperative ultrasonography. In any event a careful description with a map should be kept with the location of all glands, with a notation whether biopsy was proven or not and the presence of identifying landmarks, e.g. non-absorbable sutures or clips, which might mark retained glands or biopsy sites.

Drains need not be placed. Most surgeons reapproximate the strap muscles and platysma and close the skin with clips or staples. No dressing is required.

If a parathyroid adenoma is not found in any of the 'usual' positions, a step-by-step systematic search is needed. Useful tips for such a dissection have recently been formulated as rules that should be followed in succession if the previous one fails to help identifying the abnormal parathyroid gland:[84]

1. The majority of parathyroid glands are located within a 1–2 cm circle around the intersection of the inferior thyroid artery and the recurrent laryngeal nerve;
2. Rule of symmetry: it can be assumed that the glands on one side are located similarly to the ones on the other side;
3. The upper gland can be displaced posteriorly and caudally to lie beside the oesophagus, just in front of the vertebral column;
4. The lower gland can be either below the lower pole of the thyroid in the thyrothymic ligament or thymus itself or in the carotid sheath;
5. According to embryology, the lower parathyroid gland may be high up in the neck, above the upper thyroid pole and medial to the carotid sheath, as high as the submandibular gland;
6. Only <1% are truly intrathyroid glands.

Successful parathyroidectomy in an ambulatory setting seems to be feasible and acceptable for at least half of the patients (42 of 85) studied in one centre.[85] Furthermore, despite using ^{99m}Tc-sestamibi scintigraphy and intraoperative measurements of iPTH concentration for all the patients, a decrease to 40% of overall hospitalisation costs can be obtained by using this approach.[85] Whether this experience could be extended or attempted in other centres is yet to be elucidated.

In recent years, two alternative approaches to parathyroid surgery have been reported but are yet to demonstrate their advantage over the 'traditional' technique. Endoscopic procedures with or without carbon dioxide insufflation have been reported to be feasible.[86] In addition, a new bilateral oblique approach has been described, avoiding infrahyoid dissection and enabling exploration of unusual locations of parathyroid glands (e.g. retro-oesophageal space, jugulo-carotid sheath, thymus), without additional morbidity in 600 patients.[87]

Parathyroid adenomas Unilateral parathyroidectomy without exploration of the contralateral side is claimed to eliminate the risk of persisting hypocalcaemia but may not uncover double adenomas or hyperplasia (may be 10% of any population of patients with 1°HPT). Methods proposed to ensure complete excision of sources of the excess PTH include urinary cAMP and intraoperative PTH concentrations.[88] PTH concentrations are reduced to half baseline values within 10–15 minutes after successful parathyroidectomy whereas calcium concentrations are reduced to the normal range within 24–36 hours. Hypocalcaemic symptoms and the need for supplements in the early postoperative period are not predicted by determination of an early plasma calcium concentration.[89]

Sporadic multigland hyperplasia Excision of the enlarged glands, leaving 'normal-sized' glands intact, is adopted by some surgeons,[90] whereas others recommend 3 and $3\frac{1}{2}$ glands excision.[91] Recent data in favour of conservative surgery (i.e. resecting the grossly enlarged glands without biopsying the macroscopically normal glands) come from a series of 1204 patients with 1°HPT, 250 of whom presented with multigland enlargement in seemingly sporadic cases.[92] When followed-up for an average of 90 months, 90% were normocalcaemic, 5% hypocalcaemic and 5% hypercalcaemic, suggesting that conservative surgery is an acceptable treatment for such patients.[92]

MEN syndromes Treatment of HPT in patients with MEN syndromes is described in Chapter 4.

Parathyroid carcinoma If parathyroid carcinoma is recognised preoperatively (perhaps by suggestive features on a CT scan or palpable lymphadenopathy) *en bloc* resection offers the best results, with central compartment dissection when there is evidence of regional node metastases. Combination with ipsilateral thyroidectomy is also recommended by some.[58] The role of adjuvant radiotherapy remains unclear.

The overall survival for 134 patients followed-up prospectively was reported to be 85% at 5 years and 49% at 10 years, with no relationship between survival and tumour size or lymph node status.[58] These values are similar to those reported in a retrospective review of 95 cases.[93]

Measurements of serum calcium and PTH concentrations are postoperative markers of tumour recurrence. Recurrence in the neck or lungs can often be treated surgically with *en bloc* radical dissection, mediastinal lymph node clearance and limited pulmonary resections. Palliation is obtained by reducing hypercalcaemia with mithramycin or disodium clodronate.

Multiple resections for local recurrence or metastases in patients with recurrent or distant disease seem to prolong survival and palliate the symptoms of hypercalcaemia.[94]

The outlook is variable and, as with many endocrine tumours, some patients survive for many years with indolent metastatic disease.

Overall results of parathyroidectomy

The increased set-point seen in 1°HPT is normalised on the first postoperative day, and baseline serum PTH concentrations are within the normal range 24–48 hours after excision of the adenoma. The suppression of PTH concentrations during an oral calcium load is already normalised on the second postoperative day. A given decrease in extracellular calcium concentration is counteracted by a progressively larger increase in serum concentrations of iPTH after parathyroid surgery; the reason for this increase in the 'secretory reserve' is not well understood.[95]

More than 95% of first-time patients and 83% of those requiring reoperations were reported to have been cured of 1°HPT 6 months postoperatively. The self-reported outcomes differ significantly between surgeons performing less than 15 parathyroidectomies per year and those operating on more than 50 patients per year[78]: complication rates after primary operation were 1.89 *vs.* 0.91%, respectively, and after reoperations were 3.77 *vs.* 1.49, respectively, whereas in-hospital mortality was 1% *vs.* 0.04%, respectively.

Persistent hyperparathyroidism is the commonest cause of postoperative hypercalcaemia, which is defined as continued hypercalcaemia in the immediate postoperative period or occurring within 1 year of surgery.

Recurrent hyperparathyroidism can be strictly defined as hypercalcaemia occurring after the following criteria have been met.[96]

1. Identification and biopsy proof of all four parathyroids at the initial operation;
2. Complete removal of all abnormal tissue;
3. A normocalcaemic phase of 1 year or longer;

4. Abnormal tissue uncovered at re-exploration at a site of a previously normal gland.

These extremely rigorous criteria are not usually fulfilled in today's surgical practice, when it is unusual to biopsy all glands.

Recurrent disease as defined above might account for 1% of patients with persistent hypercalcaemia. If persistent disease is suspected, the diagnosis must be checked and confirmed. If HPT is confirmed, the next steps require careful thought. There is no virtue in attempting to localise the abnormal tissue if the patient's general condition would not withstand re-exploration and its associated morbidity. If a decision is made to offer re-exploration, then most surgeons would use localisation procedures preoperatively. This would be carried out while consulting previous operation notes, operative maps and histology reports as these often indicate the likely site of abnormality. If, for example, all glands had been identified and biopsied as normal except the left lower parathyroid, then techniques that looked specifically in this area would be used to detect intrathyroid masses or mediastinal adenomas.

Reoperative surgery After unsuccessful surgery, the diagnosis of 1°HPT must be reconfirmed and the severity of the condition assessed because, even when successful, reoperation is associated with some increased morbidity. Operative and pathology reports are reviewed to assess the adequacy or extent of the previous operation. Localisation studies have a major influence on planning subsequent reoperation.

Current areas of research

Although major insights into the management and pathophysiology of 1°HPT have been gained since Mandl performed the first parathyroidectomy in 1924, 1°HPT remains an area with many unsolved questions. Genetic alterations and molecular pathways involved in parathyroid gland physiology and pathology and the relationship between abnormal parathyroid cell growth and hormone secretion in 1°HPT are not yet integrated into a simple model. Furthermore, understanding why and how high cytoplasmic calcium concentration inhibits secretion from parathyroid cells whereas it stimulates secretion from all other endocrine cells continues to challenge numerous research groups. The recent development of CaR agonists promises to offer effective pharmacological control of PTH secretion and to expand significantly the medical therapy for 1°HPT. The appropriate aggressiveness of treatment for patients with mild symptomatic disease is still not agreed. There is continued controversy concerning the advantages of unilateral exploration versus bilateral neck dissection in patients with positive imaging of one parathyroid adenoma.

Secondary hyperparathyroidism

Secondary HPT (2°HPT) is the condition in which PTH is secreted to compensate for a chronic imbalance of calcium and/or phosphate concentration. There is presumably no initial abnormality inherent within the parathyroid glands. Possible causes of 2°HPT are presented in **Table 1.4**.

Some of the conditions listed are rare and this section concentrates on renal 2°HPT. Nearly all patients with chronic renal failure develop some degree of 2°HPT, with a wide variation in the extent of disease. The prevalence of 2°HPT has been assessed at 67% with a bone biopsy technique,[97] but improved and early medical treatment means that less then 5% of these patients require parathyroidectomy.[98]

Mechanisms of 2°HPT

In most patients on long-term haemodialysis an increase in parathyroid size is noted, progressing from diffuse to nodular hyperplasia and possible adenoma formation. A deficit of calcitriol synthesis is an important factor for inducing 2°HPT and is aggravated by a reduced expression of vitamin D receptors. With advanced chronic renal failure, hyperphosphataemia is an additional important factor in worsening 2°HPT. A low calcium intake and the use of dialysate containing low calcium concentrations may place the patients at a higher risk for developing 2°HPT.

These metabolic abnormalities are amplified by the decreased expression of the calcium-sensing receptor (CaR) in the parathyroid cells in the presence of uraemia. In a rat model of renal failure, CaR mRNA and CaR protein expression were reduced only in uraemic rats fed with a high phosphate diet, and CaR down-regulation was primarily in areas of active proliferation.[99] As in 1°HPT,

Chronic renal failure

Rickets
    Vitamin D deficiency
    Vitamin D resistance syndromes
    Renal tubular phosphate-wasting disorders

Osteomalacia
Malabsorption
Pseudohypoparathyroidism
Complication of high-dose phosphate therapy in patients with X-linked hypophosphataemia

Table 1.4 *Possible causes of secondary hyperparathyroidism*

no point mutations in the coding sequence of the *CaR* gene have been detected in renal 2°HPT.[100]

Although the process starts as a four gland response to a metabolic drive, worsening 2°HPT involves monoclonal recruitment of cell subpopulations. Morphologically, this is demonstrated by replacement of diffuse hyperplasia by nodular areas. Compared with cells obtained from diffuse hyperplasia, cells in areas of nodular hyperplasia have a higher proliferation rate,[101], higher set-point for Ca^{2+}-controlled PTH secretion,[102] lower density of CaR and calcitriol receptor and higher expression of parathyroid adenoma 1 (*PRAD1*) cyclin D_1 and retinoblastoma (RB) gene products.[103]

In vivo dynamic tests of parathyroid gland function suggest that calcium-regulated PTH secretion does not differ with the degree of 2°HPT. Set-point values in patients with 2°HPT do not correspond to basal serum PTH concentrations, maximum serum PTH concentrations in response to hypocalcaemia or minimum serum PTH concentrations during hypercalcaemia. Some propose that variations in parathyroid gland size are the major contributor to excessive PTH secretion in patients with chronic renal failure and not a functional abnormality.[104]

Increased plasma concentrations of PTH have an extensive metabolic influence. The effects on bone are discussed in a later section. Detrimental effects on remnant nephrons and a suppressive effect on tubular proteinase activities have been described in an experimental model.[105]

Presentation

The frequency and severity of symptoms of 2°HPT are highly variable.

Bone disease

Patients with chronic renal failure present with osteitis fibrosa cystica (OFC) or less frequently with osteomalacia, which may eventually lead to skeletal deformities or fractures. OFC occurs to some degree in up to 5% of patients. Physical findings may include a funnel chest deformity and sternal bowing owing to rib deformities, height reduction from kyphosis and vertebral crush fractures. Bone pain occurs primarily in the thoracolumbar spine and lower extremity and it is exacerbated by weight bearing, sudden movements and pressure. Progressive bone demineralisation leads to thinning and weakening of the bones, with lytic lesions involving the skull ('pepperpot' radiographic aspect; see **Fig 1.3**) or subperiosteal resorptions.

Pathogenic factors for bone lesions associated with 2°HPT are deficiency of vitamin D and/or its receptors, skeletal resistance to the calcaemic effects of PTH (**Fig. 1.4**), aluminium toxicity, osteoporosis linked to ageing and the recently described dialysis-associated amyloidosis of the β2-microglobulin type.[106] In

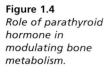

Figure 1.4
Role of parathyroid hormone in modulating bone metabolism.

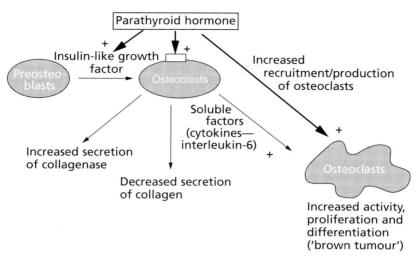

contrast, low serum PTH concentrations accompany the dynamic bone disease, the pathogenesis of which as part of renal osteodystrophy is poorly understood. PTH binds to its receptors on the osteoblasts. PTH, together with tumour necrosis factor (TNF-α) and interleukin-1 (IL-1), activate the remodelling cycle through actions on the layer of osteoblasts covering bone surfaces. PTH stimulates osteoblastic proliferation at a discrete undetermined point in osteoblast ontogeny, in part by stimulating the production of insulin–like growth factor (IGF–1). Activated osteoblasts release soluble factors (as IL-6, IL–11, granulocyte-macrophage colony-stimulating factor), which induce the proliferation and differentiation of osteoclast precursors and activate the function of osteoclasts.

Aluminium-associated osteomalacia is a serious complication of advanced renal disease and should be differentiated from the effects of 2°HPT. In an experimental model of azotaemic rats, aluminium seemed to alter the relationship between concentrations of serum PTH and calcium. Sources of aluminium include the water used for haemodialysis and the gastrointestinal absorption of aluminium from some phosphate binders. Serum aluminium levels and bone biopsy may be necessary to confirm this diagnosis.

Soft tissue calcification

Soft tissue calcification is a common manifestation of 2°HPT, affecting 27% of patients with renal failure at the outset of dialysis and 58% of those who have been dependent on dialysis for more than 5 years.[107] Calcification may involve soft tissues, blood vessels, kidneys (nephrocalcinosis), lungs, heart and skin. Calcification in soft tissues may compress adjacent structures, causing pain, organ dysfunction and cosmetic deformities.

Although debatable, a likely mechanism for metastatic calcification is the increased serum calcium-phosphate product, and values greater than 4.5–5 are considered an indication for parathyroidectomy.

Calciphylaxis

Calciphylaxis is a rare condition associated with haemodialysis or transplantation, high PTH values and an increased serum calcium-phosphate product. Patients present with severe calf pain and tenderness due to extensive non-ulcerating large, hard and tender subcutaneous plaques in the calves. These painful, violaceous, mottled cutaneous lesions progress to skin and subcutaneous necrosis, deep non-healing ulcers and gangrene. The lesions are reticular in pattern and may be large (up to 20 cm). Involvement of the distal fingers and toes is characteristic; lesions less commonly involve the forearms, arms, trunk, buttocks, thighs and legs. This severe complication can threaten digits and limbs and even a patient's life. Calcium deposition can be confirmed radiologically and by bone scanning. Before urgent parathyroidectomy is performed, medical treatment with phosphate binders might be useful. The condition is no longer rare and is not confined to patients on haemodialysis; it has been described in predialysis renal failure.[108]

Pruritus

Pruritus is a disabling symptom that affects 15–90% of patients with chronic renal failure treated by dialysis. 2°HPT is considered to be a possible cause of uraemic pruritus.[109] Parathyroidectomy seems to reduce pruritus both in short-term and long-term follow-up.[110]

Other symptoms

Muscle weakness, proximal myopathy and easy fatigability are often disclosed by careful history. Peptic ulcer disease (20%) and neuropathy (1%) can be associated with 2°HPT.

The severity of 2°HPT seems to accentuate the resistance to erythropoietin (in addition to iron deficiency, aluminium toxicity and marrow dysfunction), and most patients need a higher dose to achieve an adequate haematocrit.[111]

'Cardiotoxicity' of PTH

In a five-year longitudinal echocardiographic study including 52 patients dependent on haemodialysis, one of the best clinical predictors for the presence of left ventricular hypertrophy was an increased PTH concentration. This direct effect is mediated by specific receptors for PTH in the cardiomyocytes and by a permissive role on activation of interstitial cells in the heart. Increased cytosolic calcium concentration in the cardiomyocytes contributes to reduced myocardial performance, and an increased value for the calcium-phosphate product leads to myocardial and valve calcification.[112]

Investigative techniques

Hyperphosphataemia with normocalcaemia/hypercalcaemia is demonstrated in all patients.

Increased concentrations of intact PTH (iPTH) are decisive for diagnosis and this excludes diagnostic confusion created by measuring C-terminal fragments of PTH (as in previous assays), which accumulates owing to decreased renal clearance. Because uraemia induces a bone resistance to the effects of PTH, the target range of optimal plasma concentration of iPTH for these patients is not necessarily the absolute range recommended for healthy non-uraemic patients. Some centres therefore consider optimal concentrations for patients on haemodialysis to be 2–3 times the upper limit of normal and 2–5 times the upper limit of normal when they are on continuous ambulatory peritoneal dialysis.

Increased alkaline phosphatase concentrations confirm bone disease.

Serum concentrations of vitamin D can be measured to confirm adequate substitution.

Serum aluminium concentrations are monitored to exclude aluminium toxicity as a cause of bone disease.

Histopathological findings The typical histopathological findings are asymmetrical enlargement, nodularity and increased numbers of oxyphil cells. Diffuse and nodular hyperplasia can coexist within the same gland. The macroscopic difference in involvement of each gland (i.e. size and degree of nodularity) is striking. Because of the chronicity of the process, a prolonged period of biochemical surveillance allows the disease to be seen in evolution.

Radiological investigations

Preoperative parathyroid scanning in 2°HPT is not necessary[113] as none of the methods available are sensitive enough to detect small glands that could be missed by a systematic surgical exploration.[114]

Subperiosteal bone resorption is seen in up to 86% of these patients, especially in the phalanges, pelvis, distal clavicles, ribs, femur, mandible and skull. Classically, the earliest lesion seen on radiography is an irregularity of the radial aspect of the second digit of the middle phalanx. Increased alkaline phosphatase concentrations correlate well with the severity of bone disease. In a patient maintained on dialysis with appropriate medical treatment, progressive radiographic findings of bone disease should serve as an indication for operation.

Management options

Medical treatment

Goals The aims of medical treatment are to maintain calcium and phosphate concentrations close to normal levels, to suppress PTH secretion and to ameliorate the bone disease. The methods available are diet, calcium supplementation, phosphate binders, routine vitamin D and bisphosphonates.

Dietary phosphate restriction (<1000 mg per 24 hours) is complemented with phosphate-binding agents in a dose adapted to the meal's content of phosphate. Calcium acetate and calcium carbonate are preferred to aluminium hydroxide (to reduce the risk of aluminium toxicity).

A daily calcium intake of at least 1500 mg is necessary and can be assured by using oral supplementation. If the patient is still hypocalcaemic, calcium may be added to the dialysis bath to achieve normocalcaemia.

Calcium-α-ketoglutarate Long-term treatment with calcium-α-ketoglutarate (4.5 g day^{-1}) is reported to normalise 2°HPT by simultaneously binding phosphate and correcting the serum calcium:phosphate ratio without vitamin D treatment.[115]

Routine vitamin D supplementation is now started before a patient commences dialysis, and plasma concentrations should be monitored to ensure adequate dosage.[116] High peak plasma concentrations are more efficient at suppressing PTH secretion, and once weekly intravenous bolus administration seems to be a safe and cost effective protocol.[117,118] Good results have also been reported with oral therapy. The risks of vitamin D treatment include the development of hypercalcaemia and persistent hyperphosphataemia.

Aluminium toxicity has been treated successfully with desferoxamine.

Pruritus is ameliorated by charcoal haemoperfusion in conjunction with standard haemodialysis.

Bisphosphonates The use of bisphosphonates in the treatment of 2°HPT is still experimental. Details about their properties are presented in Table 1.3.

PTH removal during continuous ambulatory peritoneal dialysis is greater than with haemodialysis but has the disadvantage that protein losses are greater and vitamin D and its binding protein are lost in the peritoneal dialysate.

NPS R-568 In an experimental model of 2°HPT, chronic administration of the CaR agonist NPS R–568 inhibits PTH synthesis and secretion and decreases parathyroid cell volume.

Surgical treatment for 2°HPT

Parathyroidectomy is indicated in patients with severely advanced renal 2°HPT that is refractory to medical treatment (5–10% of patients on long-term dialysis).

Symptoms	Improvement after parathyroidectomy (%)	Comments
Bone pain	85	Alkaline phosphatase concentrations generally correlate with the extent of bone resorption
Joint pain	80	
Pruritus	85	
Malaise	73	
[Ca] × [P] >70 (in mg dl^{-1}) C-terminal parathyroid hormone fragments >3000 μEq l^{-1}		Associated with resolution of symptoms after parathyroidectomy[98]

Table 1.5 *Improvement of symptoms after parathyroidectomy*

Indications for operation are based in part on the knowledge of which symptoms and signs are likely to improve after parathyroidectomy (**Table 1.5**) and from an assessment of the rate of progression of biochemical abnormalities. When parathyroid hyperplasia progresses to nodular hyperplasia, parathyroidectomy should be required, but there are still no definite clinical/biochemical tests to demonstrate this stage of the disease.

When offering a surgical option, patients should be informed of the potential risks (recurrent HPT, injury to the recurrent laryngeal nerves).

Perioperative care

Patients should undergo dialysis within one day of operation and then 48 hours postoperatively or as needed. The risk of bleeding should be kept in mind as heparin is used during haemodialysis and platelets are dysfunctional in severely uraemic patients. Preoperative vitamin D treatment should continue because it decreases the chance of postoperative hypocalcaemia.

Marked hypocalcaemia may occur after parathyroidectomy, due to the hungry bone syndrome, hypomagnesaemia and hypofunction of parathyroid remnants or grafts. Oral supplementation (up to 6 g of elemental calcium daily) suffices for mild symptoms, whereas more severe hypocalcaemia is treated with intravenous calcium and magnesium.

Surgical strategies

After standard transverse neck incision, all four glands are located and resected tissue confirmed by frozen section. Transcervical thymectomy (by dissection along the thyrothymic ligament) should be routine, aiming to remove supranumerary glands or embryonic rests. If all four glands are not found in the 'classical' locations, the retro-oesophageal space, superior thyroid pedicles and areas along the carotid sheath should be explored. If, despite a rigorous search, all four glands are not identified, the operation should be concluded. Median sternotomy is not performed as part of the initial operation. The pathology report, postoperative concentrations of PTH and calcium and the clinical response should influence further decisions about localisation studies (see previous section) in anticipation of re-exploration.

Subtotal parathyroidectomy involves resection of three glands, leaving approximately 50 mg of viable tissue *in situ*. If permanent dialysis is anticipated, the remnant should be small (owing to long-term hypertrophy of the remnant) whereas it should be larger if renal transplant is likely (to avoid subsequent hypoparathyroidism). The disadvantage of this approach is that a second cervical exploration would be needed if persistent or recurrent HPT occurs.

Total parathyroidectomy plus autotransplantation was introduced around 1975 by Wells,[83] and in some centres it is still the preferred procedure. The gland, which macroscopically looks most normal and on frozen section shows predominantly diffuse hyperplasia (and not nodular hyperplasia), is selected for autografting. The gland is sliced into 3 mm × 1 mm × 1 mm pieces, which are placed in a bath of ice-cold saline. The forearm flexor mass is exposed through a longitudinal incision below the antecubital fossa, and about 15 such parathyroid fragments are placed—each in its own muscle pocket. Each pocket is closed by reapproximating the fascia with a non-absorbable suture (to prevent graft extrusion, mark the site of implantation and aid re-exploration if necessary). Some fragments can be cryopreserved.

Primary graft failure is extremely rare. Graft function can be evaluated by measuring PTH concentrations in the ipsilateral antecubital vein and comparing this with the contralateral non-grafted forearm. A gradient between grafted versus non-grafted arm proves graft viability and function; lack of gradient suggests either failure of the graft (when PTH concentrations are low) or persistent HPT due to missed gland in the neck. Grafting of cryopreserved cells is successful in only 60% of patients.

Total parathyroidectomy alone may now be preferred, and in a small series recently reported it seems to be a safe and effective option, with all patients having symptomatic and biochemical improvement. If followed-up for several years, most patients are found to have detectable concentrations of PTH,[119] suggesting that total parathyroidectomy was not 'complete' and residual parathyroid cells or parathyroid cell rests become activated under the continued biochemical stimulus of chronic renal failure.

Results

The clinical effect of parathyroidectomy is striking, but skeletal deformity, vessel calcification and severe reduction of bone content are irreversible.

Both subtotal parathyroidectomy and total parathyroidectomy plus autotransplantation have been preferred before in the hope of avoiding the need for long-term calcium supplementation, and equivalent results have been cited with both procedures. A randomised trial concluded that total parathyroidectomy is superior to subtotal parathyroidectomy in terms of recurrence rate (no recurrence *vs.* 4/20) and symptom amelioration scores (pruritus, 100% *vs.* 45%; weakness, 3% *vs.* 20%).[120]

A wide range of recurrence rates has been reported for both procedures (10–70%). In an analysis of 73 patients with chronic renal failure, recurrent HPT was diagnosed in 4 of 39 patients who underwent total parathyroidectomy with autograft and 2 out of 34 patients who underwent subtotal parathyroidectomy, indicating that there is little to choose between the two techniques.[107] In a series of 782 patients, the function of autografted parathyroid tissue was satisfactory and no retransplantation of cryopreserved parathyroid tissue was necessary but graft-dependent recurrent HPT occurred in 20%.[121]

Persistent HPT is diagnosed if hypercalcaemia recurs within 6 months after initial surgery. The most common reasons for recurrent hypercalcaemia include unrecognised asymmetrical hyperplasia of all four glands, too large a remnant left behind, unrecognised hyperfunctioning supranumerary glands and hyperfunction of the autotransplanted parathyroid tissue. Reoperation in such patients can be successful, a recurrence rate of only 10.5% being reported for a large series of 152 such patients.[122]

A rare cause is **parathyromatosis**, where multiple rests of hyperfunctioning parathyroid tissue are scattered throughout the fibrofatty tissue of the lower neck and superior mediastinum. Various authors speculate that abnormally placed parathyroid tissue is either inadvertent autoimplantation of tissue from the handling of abnormal glands during previous operations or hyperfunction of tissue left behind during ontogenesis.[123]

Permanent hypocalcaemia can ensue after reoperations for persistent or recurrent hyperparathyroidism. If cryopreserved material is available, it may subsequently be used to restore normocalcaemia, sometimes long after surgery.

Tertiary hyperparathyroidism

Tertiary HPT is the condition in which reactive parathyroid hyperplasia results in autonomous hypersecretion, which continues despite correction of the underlying renal disease. On the basis of calcium concentrations, it is estimated to occur in 25–50% of patients, but PTH concentrations and bone biopsies suggest a prevalence of up to 70%. These early postrenal transplant findings improve with time, such that 60% of these patients become normocalcaemic within 12 months and only few require operation.

Transplant patients usually present with less severe disease, have better normalisation of biochemical parameters after parathyroidectomy and rarely develop recurrent HPT compared with those on haemodialysis.

References

 1. Heath H, Hodgson SF, Kennedy MA. Primary hyperparathyroidism—incidence, morbidity and potential economic impact in a community. N Engl J Med 1980; 302: 189–93.

2. Arnold A, Staunton CE, Kim HG et al. Monoclonality and abnormal PTH genes in parathyroid adenomas. N Engl J Med 1988; 318: 658–62.

3. Friedman E, Bale AE, Marx SJ et al. Genetic abnormalities in parathyroid adenomas. J Clin Endocrinol Metab 1990; 71: 293–7.

4. Arnold A, Brown MF, Urena P et al. Monoclonality of parathyroid tumours in chronic renal failure and in primary parathyroid hyperplasia. J Clin Invest 1995; 95: 2047–53.

 5. Thakker RV, Bouloux P, Wooding C et al. Association of parathyroid tumours in MEN type I with loss of alleles on chromosome 11. N Engl J Med 1989; 321: 218–24.

6. Friedman E, Sakaguci K et al. Clonality of parathyroid tumours in familial MEN type 1. N Engl J Med 1989; 321: 213–8.

7. Vasef MA, Brynes RK, Sturm M et al. Expression of cyclin D1 in parathyroid carcinomas, adenomas, and hyperplasias: a paraffin immunohistochemical study. Mod Pathol 1999; 12: 412–6.

8. Bates S, Peters G. Cyclin D1 as a cellular proto-oncogene. Semin Cancer Biol 1995; 6: 73–82.

9. Rosenberg CL, Kim HG, Shows TB et al. Rearrangement and overexpression of D11S287E, a candidate oncogene on chromosome 11q13 in benign parathyroid tumours. Oncogene 1991; 6: 449–53.

10. Motokura T, Bloom T, Kim HG et al. A novel cyclin encoded by a bc11-linked candidate oncogene. Nature 1991; 350: 512–5.

11. Cryns VL, Thor A, Xu HJ et al. Loss of the retinoblastoma tumour-suppressor gene in parathyroid carcinoma. N Engl J Med 1994; 330: 757–61.

12. Weinberg RA. The retinoblastoma protein and cell cycle control. Cell 1995; 81: 323–30.

13. Cryns VL, Yi SM, Tahara H et al. Frequent loss of chromosome arm 1p DNA in parathyroid adenomas. Genes Chrom Cancer 1995; 13: 9–17.

14. Tahara H, Smith AP, Gas RD et al. Genomic localization of novel candidate tumour suppressor gene loci in human parathyroid adenomas. Cancer Res 1996; 56: 599–605.

15. Hakim JP, Levine MA. Absence of p53 point mutations in parathyroid adenoma and carcinoma. J Clin Endocrinol Metab 1994; 78: 103–6.

16. Cryns VL, Rubio MP, Thor AD et al. p53 abnormalities in human parathyroid carcinoma. J Clin Endocrinol Metab 1994; 78: 1320–4.

17. Heppner C, Kester MB, Agarwal SK et al. Somatic mutation of the MEN1 gene in parathyroid tumours. Nat Genet 1997; 16: 375–8.

 18. Carling T, Correa P, Hessman O et al. Parathyroid MEN1 gene mutations in relation to clinical characteristics of nonfamilial primary hyperparathyroidism. J Clin Endocrinol Metab 1998; 83: 2960–3.

19. Farnebo F, Teh BT, Kytola S et al. Alterations of the MEN1 gene in sporadic parathyroid tumors. J Clin Endocrinol Metab 1998; 83: 2627–30.

20. Willeke F, Hauer MP, Buchcik R et al. Multiple endocrine neoplasia type 2-associated RET proto-oncogene mutations do not contribute to the pathogenesis of sporadic parathyroid tumors. Surgery 1998; 124: 484–90.

21. Schneider AB, Gierlowski TC, ShoreFreedman F et al. Dose-response relationships for radiation-induced hyperparathyroidism. J Clin Endocrinol Metab 1995; 80: 254–7.

 22. Brown EM, Gamba G, Riccardi E et al. Cloning and characterisation of an extracellular Ca^{2+}-sensing receptor from bovine parathyroid. Nature 1993; 366: 575–80.

23. Pollak MR, Brown EM, Chou YHW. Mutations in the human calcium-sensing receptor gene cause familial hypocalciuric hypercalcaemia and neonatal severe hyperparathyroidism. Cell 1993; 75: 1297–303.

 24. Hosokawa Y, Pollak MR, Brown EM et al. The extracellular calcium-sensing receptor gene in human parathyroid tumours. J Clin Endocrinol Metab 1995; 80: 3107–10.

25. Cetani F, Pinchera A, Pardi E et al. No evidence for mutations in the calcium-sensing receptor gene in

sporadic parathyroid adenomas. J Bone Miner Res 1999; 14: 878–82.

26. Thomson DB, Samowitz WS, Odelberg S et al. Genetic abnormalities in sporadic parathyroid adenomas: loss of heterozygosity for chromosome 3q markers flanking the calcium receptor locus. J Clin Endocrinol Metab 1995; 80: 3377–80.

27. Kifor O, Moore FD, Wang JP et al. Reduced immunostaining for the extracellular Ca^{2+} sensing receptor in primary and uremic secondary hyperparathyroidism. J Clin Endocrinol Metab 1996; 81: 1598–606.

28. Kaneko C, Mizunashi K, Tanaka M et al. Relationship between Ca-dependent change of serum PTH and extracellular Ca^{2+}-sensing receptor expression in parathyroid adenoma. Calcif Tissue Int 1999; 64: 271–2.

29. Saito A, Pietromonaco S, Kwor–Chieh Loo A et al. Complete cloning and sequencing of rat gp330/'megalin,' a distinct member of the low density lipoprotein receptor gene family. Proc Natl Acad Sci USA 1994; 91: 9725–9.

30. Juhlin C, Klareskog L, Nygren P et al. Hyperparathyroidism is associated with reduced expression of a parathyroid calcium receptor mechanism defined by monoclonal antiparathyroid antibodies. Endocrinology 1988; 122: 2999–3001.

31. Brown EM, Segre GV, Goldring SR. Serpentine receptors for parathyroid hormone, calcitonin and calcium ions. Baillière's Clin Endocrinol Metab 1996; 123–61.

32. Harms HM, Schlinke E, Neubauer O. Pulse amplitude and frequency modulation of parathyroid hormone in primary hyperparathyroidism. J Clin Endocrinol Metab 1994; 78: 53–7.

33. Carling I, Kindmark A, Hellman P et al. Vitamin D receptor genotypes in primary hyperparathyroidism. Nature Med 1995; 1: 1309–11.

34. Chan AK, Duh QY, Katz MH et al. Clinical manifestations of primary hyperparathyroidism before and after parathyroidectomy. Ann Surg 1995; 222: 402–14.

35. Elvius M, Lagrelius A, Nygren A et al. Seventeen year follow–up study of bone mass in patients with mild asymptomatic hyperparathyroidism some of whom were operated on. Eur J Surg Acta Chir 1995; 161: 863–9.

36. Benishin CG, Lewanczuk RZ, Shan J et al. Purification and structural characterization of parathyroid hypertensive factor. J Cardiovasc Pharmacol 1994; 23(S2): 9–13S.

37. Lewanczuk RZ, Benishin CG, Shan J et al. Clinical aspects of parathyroid hypertensive factor. J Cardiovasc Pharmacol 1994; 2(S2): 23–6S.

38. Piovesan A, Molineri N, Casasso F et al. Left ventricular hypertrophy in primary hyperparathyroidism. Effects of successful parathyroidectomy. Clin Endocrinol (Oxford) 1999; 50: 321–8.

39. Hedback G, Oden A, Tissel LA. Parathyroid adenoma weight and the risk of death after treatment for primary hyperparathyroidism. Surgery 1995; 117: 134–9.

40. National Center for Health Statistics: vital statistics of the United States, 1986, Vol 2, Part A, Mortality. Washington, DC: US Government Printing Office, DHHS Publ No (BHS) 1986; 88–1122.

41. Monchik JM. Presidential address: normocalcemic hyperparathyroidism. Surgery 1995; 118: 917–23.

42. Fitzpatrick LA, Bilezikian JP. Acute primary hyperparathyroidism. Am J Med 1987; 82: 275–82.

43. Strewler GJ. The physiology of parathyroid hormone-related protein. N Engl J Med 2000; 342: 177–85.

44. White TF, Farndon JR, Conceicao SC et al. Serum calcium status in health and disease: a comparison of measured and derived parameters. Clin Chim Acta 1986; 157: 199–214.

45. Irvin GL, Dembrow VD, Prudohomme DL. Operative monitoring of parathyroid gland hyperfunction. Am J Surg 1991; 162: 299–302.

46. Taylor J, Fraser W, Banaszkiewicz P et al. Lateralization of parathyroid adenomas by intraoperative parathyroid hormone estimation. Br J Surg 1995; 82: 1428–9.

47. Farndon JR, Geraghty JM, Dilley WG et al. Serum gastrin, calcitonin, and prolactin as markers of multiple endocrine neoplasia syndromes in patients with primary hyperparathyroidism. World J Surg 1987; 11: 253–7.

48. Carlson GL, Farndon JR, Shenton BK et al. Thallous chloride uptake and DNA profile in parathyroid adenomas. Br J Surg 1990; 77: 1302–4.

49. Mitchell BK, Kinder BK, Cornelius E et al. Primary hyperparathyroidism: preoperative localisation using technetium-sestamibi scanning. J Clin Endocrinol Metab 1995; 80: 7–10.

50. Wright AR, Goddard PR, Nicholson S et al. Fat-suppression magnetic resonance imaging in the preoperative localisation of parathyroid adenomas. Clin Radiol 1992; 46: 324–8.

51. Hellman P, Ahlstrom H, Bergstrom M. Positron emission tomography with ^{11}C-methionine in hyperparathyroidism. Surgery 1994; 116: 974–81.

52. Wei JP, Burke GJ. Analysis of savings in operative time for primary hyperparathyroidism using localization with technetium 99m sestamibi scan. Am J Surg 1995; 170: 488–91.

53. Irvin GL, Prudhomme DL, Deriso C *et al.* A new approach to parathyroidectomy. Ann Surg 1994; 219: 574–81.

54. Zmora O, Schachter PP, Heyman Z *et al.* Correct preoperative localization: does it permit a change in operative strategy in primary hyperparathyroidism? Surgery 1995; 118: 932–5.

55. Sacks BA, Pallotta JA, Cole A *et al.* Diagnosis of parathyroid adenomas: efficacy of measuring parathormone levels in needle aspirates of cervical masses. Am J Roentgenol 1994; 163: 1223–6.

56. Tezelman S, Shen W, Siperstein AE *et al.* Persistent or recurrent hyperparathyroidism in patients with double adenomas. Surgery 1995; 118: 1115–24.

57. Berger AC, Libutti SK, Bartlett DL *et al.* Heterogeneous gland size in sporadic multiple gland parathyroid hyperplasia. J Am Coll Surg 1999; 188(4): 382–9.

 58. Hundahl SA, Fleming ID, Fremgen AM *et al.* Two hundred eighty-six cases of parathyroid carcinoma treated in the U.S. between 1985–1995: a National Cancer Data Base Report. The American College of Surgeons Commission on Cancer and the American Cancer Society. Cancer 1999; 86: 538–44.

59. LiVolsi VA, Hamilton R. Intraoperative assessment of parathyroid gland pathology. A common view from the surgeon and the pathologist. Am J Clin Pathol 1994; 102: 365–73.

60. August DA, Flynn SD, Jones MA *et al.* Parathyroid carcinoma: the relationship of nuclear DNA content to clinical outcome. Surgery 1993; 113: 290–6.

61. Bondeson L, Sandelin K, Grimelius L. Histopathological variables and DNA cytometry in parathyroid carcinoma. Am J Surg Pathol 1993; 17: 820–9.

62. Yoshimoto K, Yamasaki R, Sakai H. Ectopic production of parathyroid hormone by small cell lung cancer in a patient with hypercalcaemia. J Clin Endocrinol Metab 1989; 68: 976–81.

63. Nussbaum SR, Gaz RL, Arnold A. Hypercalcaemia and ectopic secretion of parathyroid hormone by an ovarian carcinoma with rearrangement of the gene for parathyroid hormone. N Engl J Med 1990; 323: 1324–8.

64. Pearce SHS, Brown EM. Calcium-sensing receptor mutations: insights into a structurally and functionally novel receptor. J Clin Endocrinol Metab 1996; 81: 1309–11.

65. McKane WR, Khosla S, Egan KS *et al.* Role of calcium intake in modulating age-related increases in parathyroid function and bone resorption. J Clin Endocrinol Metab 1996; 81: 1699–703.

 66. Bilezikian JP. Management of hypercalcaemia. J Clin Endocrinol Metab 1993; 77: 1445–9.

67. Lucarotti ME, Hamilton JA, Farndon JR. Somatostatin and primary hyperparathyroidism. Br J Surg 1994; 81: 1141–3.

68. Hasse C, Zielke A, Bruns C *et al.* Influence of somatostatin to biochemical parameters in patients with primary hyperparathyroidism. Exp Clin Endocrinol Diab 1995; 103: 391–7.

69. Hammerland LG, Garrett JE, Hung BCP *et al.* Allosteric activation of the Ca²⁺ receptor expressed in Xenopus laevis oocytes by NPS-467 R NPS-568. Mol Pharmacol 1998; 53: 1083–8.

 70. Silverberg SJ, Bone III HG, Marriott TB *et al.* Short-term inhibition of parathyroid hormone secretion by a calcium-receptor agonist in patients with primary hyperparathyroidism. N Engl J Med 1997; 337: 1506–10.

71. Collins MT, Skarulis MC, Bilezikian JP *et al.* Treatment of hypercalcaemia secondary to parathyroid carcinoma with a novel calcimimetic agent. J Clin Endocrinol Metab 1998; 83: 1083–8.

72. Bradwell AR, Harvey TC. Control of hypercalcaemia of parathyroid carcinoma by immunisation. Lancet 1999; 353: 370–3.

73. Rodan GA, Fleisch HA. Bisphosphonates: mechanisms of action. J Clin Invest 1996; 97: 2692–6.

74. Hamdy NAT, McCloskey EV, Kanili JA. Role of bisphosphonates in the medical management of hyperparathyroidism. Acta Chir Aust 1994; 26(S112): 6–7.

75. Silverberg SJ, Shane E, Jacobs TP *et al.* A 10-year prospective study of primary hyperparathyroidism with or without parathyroid surgery. N Engl J Med 1999; 341: 1249–55.

76. Roche NA, Young AE. Role of surgery in mild primary hyperparathyroidism in the elderly. Br J Surg 2000; 87:1640–49.

77 Potts JT. Proceedings of the NIH consensus development conference on diagnosis and management of asymptomatic primary hyperparathyroidism. J Bone Miner Res 1990; 6(S2): 9–13.

78. Sosa JA, Powe NR, Levine MA *et al.* Profile of a clinical practice: thresholds for surgery and surgical outcomes for patients with primary hyperparathyroidism: a national survey of endocrine surgeons. J Clin Endocrinol Metab 1998; 83: 2658–65.

79. Silverberg SJ, Bilezikian JP, Bone HG *et al.* Therapeutic controversies in primary hyperparathyroidism. J Clin Endocrinol Metab 1999; 84: 2275–85.

80. Richards ML, Thompson NW. Diabetes mellitus with hyperparathyroidism: another indication for parathyroidectomy? Surgery 1999; 126: 1160–6.

81. Albright F, Reifenstein EC. The parathyroid glands and metabolic bone disease. Baltimore: Williams & Wilkins, 1948.

82. Gunn A. Parathyroid exploration. London: Wolfe, 1988.

83. Wells SA, Leight GS, Ross AJ. Primary hyperparathyroidism. Chicago: Year Book Medical Publishers, 1980.

84. Rothmund M. A parathyroid adenoma cannot be found during neck exploration of a patient with presumed primary hyperparathyroidism. Br J Surg 1999; 86: 725–6.

85. Irvin GL, Fishman LM, Molinari AS et al. Ambulatory parathyroidectomy for primary hyperparathyroidism. Arch Surg 1996; 131: 1074–8.

86. Miccoli P, Bendinelli C, Vignali E et al. Endoscopic parathyroidectomy: report of an initial experience. Surgery 1998; 124: 1077–80.

87. Chaffanjon PCJ, Brichon PY, Sarrazin R. Bilateral oblique approach to parathyroid glands. Ann Surg 2000; 231: 25–30.

88. Tommasi M, Brocchi A, Benucci A et al. Intraoperative fall in plasma levels of intact parathyroid hormone in patients undergoing parathyroid adenomectomy. Int J Biol Markers 1995; 10: 206–10.

89. Wong NACS, Wong WK, Farndon JR. Early postoperative calcium concentrations as a predictor of need for calcium supplementation after parathyroidectomy. Br J Surg 1996; 83: 532–4.

90. Thompson NW, Sandelin K. Primary hyperparathyroidism caused by multiple gland disease (hyperplasia) long-term results in familial and sporadic cases. Acta Chir Aust 1994; 26(S112): 44–7.

91. Grant CS, Weaver A. Treatment of primary parathyroid hyperplasia: representative experience at Mayo Clinic. Acta Chir Aust 1994; 26(S112): 41–4.

92. Proye C, Carnaille B, Quievreux JL et al. Late outcome of 304 consecutive patients with multiple gland enlargement in primary hyperparathyroidism treated by conservative surgery. World J Surg 1998; 22: 526–9.

93. Sandelin K, Auer G, Bondeson L et al. Prognostic factors in parathyroid cancer: a review of 95 cases. World J Surg 1992; 16: 724–31.

94. Vetto JT, Brennan MF, Woodruf J et al. Parathyroid carcinoma: diagnosis and clinical history. Surgery 1993; 114: 882–92.

95. Bergenfelz A, Valdermarsson S, Ahren B. Functional recovery of the parathyroid glands after surgery for primary hyperparathyroidism. Surgery 1994; 116: 827–36.

96. Muller H. True recurrence of hyperparathyroidism: proposed criteria for recurrence. Br J Surg 1975; 62: 556–9.

97. Llach F, Felsenfeld A, Coleman M et al. Renal osteodistrophy in 131 unselected hemodialysis patients. Kidney Int 1984; 25: 187.

98. Demeure M, McGee D, Wilkes W et al. Results of surgical treatment for hyperparathyroidism associated with renal disease. Am J Surg 1990; 160: 337–40.

99. Brown AJ, Ritter CS, Finch JL, Slatopolsky EA. Decreased calcium-sensing receptor expression in hyperplastic parathyroid glands of uremic rats: role of dietary phosphate. Kidney Int 1999; 55: 1284–92.

100. Degenhardt S, Toell A, Weidemann W et al. Point mutations of the human parathyroid calcium receptor gene are not responsible for non-suppressible renal hyperparathyroidism. Kidney Int 1998; 53: 556–61.

101. Loda M, Lipman J, Cukor B et al. Nodular foci in parathyroid adenomas and hyperplasia: an immunohistochemical analysis of proliferative activity. Hum Pathol 1994; 25: 1050–6.

102. Tominaga Y, Sato K, Tanaka Y et al. Histopathology and pathophysiology of secondary hyperparathyroidism due to chronic renal failure. Clin Nephrol 1995; 44(SI): 42–7S.

103. Tominaga Y, Tsuzuki T, Uchida K et al. Expression of PRAD1/cyclin D1, retinoblastoma gene products, and Ki67 in parathyroid hyperplasia caused by chronic renal failure versus primary adenoma. Kidney Int 1999; 55: 1375–83.

104. Goodman WG, Belin T, Gales B et al. Calcium-regulated parathyroid hormone release in patients with mild or advanced secondary hyperparathyroidism. Kidney Int 1995; 48: 1553–8.

105. Schaefer L, Malchow M, Schaefer RM et al. Effects of parathyroid hormone on renal tubular proteinases. Miner Electrolyte Metab 1996; 22: 182–6.

106. Hruska KA, Teitelbaum SL. Renal osteodistrophy. N Engl J Med 1995; 333: 166–74.

107. Nichols P, Owen JP, Ellis HA et al. Parathyroidectomy in chronic renal failure: a nine-year follow-up study. Q J Med 1990; 77: 1175–93.

108. Fine A, Fleming S, Leslie W. Calciphylaxis presenting with calf pain and plaques in four continuous ambulatory peritoneal dialysis patients and in one predialysis patient. Am J Kidney Dis 1995; 25: 498–502.

109. Cho YL, Liu HN, Huang TP et al. Uremic pruritus: role of parathyroid hormone and substance P. J Am Acad Dermatol 1997; 36: 538–41.

110. Cho FF, Ho JC, Huang SC et al. A study of pruritus after parathyroidectomy for secondary

hyperparathyroidism. J Am Coll Surg 2000; 190: 65–70.

111. Rao DS, Shih MS, Mohini R. Effect of serum parathyroid hormone and bone marrow fibrosis on the response to erythropoietin in uremia. N Engl J Med 1993; 328: 171–5.

112. Timio M. Cardiotoxicity of parathyroid hormone in chronic renal failure. Ital J Miner Electrolyte Metab 1995; 9: 119–24.

113. Pattou F, Huglo D, Proye C. Radionuclide scanning in parathyroid disease. Br J Surg 1998; 85: 1605–16.

114. Wheeler MH. Preoperative scanning in secondary hyperparathyroidism. Lancet 2000; 353: 2174.

115. Zimmermann E, Wassmer S, Steudle V. Long-term treatment with calcium-alphaketoglutarate corrects secondary hyperparathyroidism. Miner Electrolyte Metab 1996; 22: 196–9.

116. Llach F, Hervas J, Cerezo S. The importance of dosing intravenous calcitriol in dialysis patients with severe hyperparathyroidism. Am J Kidney Dis 1995; 26: 845–51.

117. Stim JA, Lowe J, Arruda JAL *et al*. Once weekly intravenous calcitriol suppresses hyperparathyroidism in hemodialysis patients. ASAIO J 1995; 41: 693–8M.

118. AlaHouhala M, Holmberg C, Ronnholm K *et al*. Alphacalcidol oral pulses normalize uremic hyperparathyroidism prior to dialysis. Pediatr Nephrol 1995; 9: 737–41.

119. Nicholson ML, Feehally J. Br J Surg 1995; 82: 1427.

120. Rothmund M, Wagner P, Schark C. Subtotal parathyroidectomy vs. total parathyroidectomy and autotransplantation in secondary hyperparathyroidism—a randomised trial. World J Surg 1991; 15: 745–50.

121. Tominaga Y. Surgical management of secondary hyperparathyroidism in uremia. Am J Med Sci 1999; 317: 390–7.

122. Henry J-FR, Denizot A, Audiffret J *et al*. Results of reoperations for persistent or recurrent secondary hyperparathyroidism. World J Surg 1990; 14: 303–7.

123. Kollmorgen CF, Aust MR, Ferreiro JA *et al*. Parathyromatosis—a rare yet important cause of persistent or recurrent hyperparathyroidism. Surgery 1994; 116: 111–5.

2 The thyroid gland

Gregory P. Sadler
Malcolm H. Wheeler

Embryology

The median thyroid diverticulum in the floor of the pharynx gives rise to the thyroid gland. It grows downwards between the ventral ends of the first and second pharyngeal arches, the stalk of the diverticulum elongating to become the thyroglossal duct. This duct, later obliterated, extends from the foramen caecum at the base of the tongue to the isthmus, its distal part remaining as the pyramidal lobe of the thyroid. The ultimobranchial bodies, arising from the fourth pharyngeal pouch on each side, become applied to the lateral portion of each thyroid lobe and contribute the parafollicular or C-cells. These cells of neural crest origin become secondarily involved with the thyroid, produce calcitonin and may later assume clinical importance as the cells giving rise to medullary thyroid carcinoma.

Investigation of the thyroid

Thyroid hormones

Measurement of thyroid hormone concentrations in the serum allows precise assessment of thyroid status to confirm the clinical diagnosis or clarify a difficult diagnostic problem. The thyroid hormones thyroxine (T4) and triiodothyronine (T3) are stored in thyroid colloid bound to thyroglobulin. The immediate control of synthesis and release of these hormones is achieved by thyroid stimulating hormone (TSH), released from the anterior pituitary. By a negative feedback mechanism, TSH secretion is regulated by the concentration of thyroid hormones in blood. Thyrotrophin releasing hormone (TRH) from the hypothalamus also influences TSH secretion. The thyroid hormones in the circulation are bound to thyroxine-binding globulin (TBG), thyroxine-binding pre-albumin (TBPA) and albumin. The principal metabolic effects of the thyroid hormones are due to unbound free T4 and T3 (0.03–0.04% and 0.2–0.5% of the total circulating hormones, respectively). Because almost all T4 and T3 is protein bound, measurement of total hormone concentrations is influenced by conditions that change the serum con-centrations of thyroxine-binding proteins. For example, increased concentrations are found in pregnancy and in women taking oral contraceptives, and low concentrations occur in the nephrotic syndrome. Drugs such as salicylates and some antibiotics compete for protein binding. Radioimmunoassays for free T4 and T3 are now readily available and give a precise assessment of thyroid function. T3 is the more active physiological hormone, with 80% being produced in the periphery by mono deiodination of T4. Measurement of T3 is particularly important in T3 toxicosis when there is a clinical picture of thyrotoxicosis with normal serum T4 concentrations.

TSH concentration can also be measured precisely by a sensitive immuno-chemiluminometric assay (normal range 0–5 mU l^{-1}). Increased TSH concentrations are found in primary hypothyroidism, e.g. autoimmune thyroiditis, after treatment of thyrotoxicosis by surgery or radioiodine. Suppressed TSH concentrations occur in hyperthyroidism.

Thyroid antibodies

Thyroglobulin

Antibodies to thyroglobulin, the major constituent of colloid and precursor of thyroid hormones, are found in most people with Graves' disease and virtually 100% of those with Hashimoto's thyroiditis.[1] Thyroglobulin measurement is used either in place of, or as an adjunct to, radioiodine scanning to detect residual or recurrent tumour in patients who have undergone total thyroidectomy for differentiated thyroid malignancy and who are receiving replacement T4.[2]

Thyroid peroxidase

Antibodies to thyroid peroxidase (TPO), previously know as thyroid microsomal antigen, are found in most patients with Graves' disease or Hashimoto's thyroiditis.[3] Raised titres are also detected in patients with postpartum thyroiditis and non–organ specific autoimmune diseases such as rheumatoid arthritis.

TSH receptor autoantibodies

Most TSH receptor autoantibodies (TRAbs) have a stimulatory action, but in some instances antibodies bind to the receptor and block activity. Measurement of TRAbs is especially valuable in the diagnosis of Graves' disease, being detected in approximately 90% of patients.[4] Neonatal hyperthyroidism may result from transplacental passage of TRAbs.

Calcitonin

Increased serum concentrations of calcitonin (from the parafollicular or C-cells) are found in patients with medullary thyroid carcinoma (MTC).[5] Measurement of basal or stimulated calcitonin concentrations is employed to assess the completeness of surgical resection of MTC and is valuable in the follow-up and detection of metastases after thyroidectomy. Screening for the detection of familial MTC, usually as part of the multiple endocrine neoplasia type-2A (MEN-2A) or -2B (MEN-2B) syndrome, has until recently depended on measurement of stimulated calcitonin concentrations. Identification of germ-line mutations in the RET proto-oncogene on chromosome 10 is now replacing biochemical screening in these disorders[6] (see Chapter 4).

Carcinoembryonic antigen

Measurement of carcinoembryonic antigen (CEA) is a useful adjunct to calcitonin assay in the follow-up of patients with MTC.

Thyroid isotope scanning

Traditionally, the thyroid gland has been scanned either with radioactive ^{123}I or technetium pertechnetate (^{99m}Tc), classifying nodules into those that are non-functioning 'cold' (**Fig. 2.1**), normally functioning 'warm' and hyperfunctioning 'hot.' Although the finding of a hot nodule is usually consistent with benign pathology, more than 80% of nodules are cold and only 20% of these will be malignant. Iodine scanning is therefore not helpful in the diagnosis of malignancy and has only a limited role in the investigation of euthyroid patients with a solitary nodule. Discrepant imaging is well documented, with hot ^{99m}Tc images being cold on ^{123}I scanning.[7] It has therefore been suggested that all ^{99m}Tc hot scans should be re-evaluated with ^{123}I. Isotope scanning has most utility in the investigation of a solitary autonomous toxic nodule (**Fig. 2.2**) or toxic multinodular goitre (**Fig. 2.3**). Iodine scanning is helpful in the evaluation of patients

Figure 2.1
I^{123} scan of 'cold' thyroid nodule.

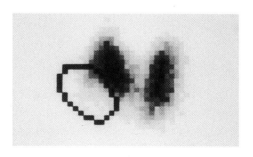

Figure 2.2
*Toxic autonomous
thyroid nodule.*

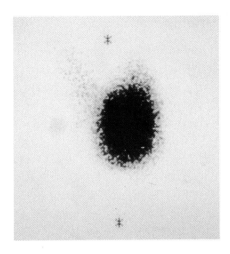

Figure 2.3
*I^{123} scan of toxic
multinodular goitre.*

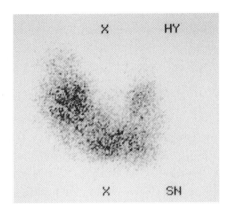

Figure 2.4
*I^{123} scan of ectopic
submental thyroid.*

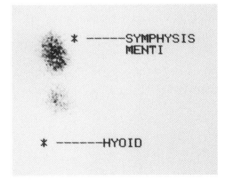

with metastatic thyroid tumours and in the localisation of ectopic thyroid tissue (**Fig. 2.4**). Other isotopes are occasionally used, especially in the evaluation of patients with MTC and include pentavalent dimercapto succinic acid[8] (DMSA), thallium[9] and metaiodobenzyl guanidine (MIBG).[10]

Radioiodine uptake

Radioactive ^{123}I is taken into the thyroid gland in an identical manner to inorganic iodine. Measurement of the uptake of an administered dose after 4 and 48 hours is useful in the assessment of patients with thyrotoxicosis. Increased uptake is seen in most forms of the disorder, with the notable exceptions of thyrotoxicosis due to subacute thyroiditis and after excessive T4 intake.

Ultrasonography

This technique is operator dependent but capable of identifying impalpable nodules as small as 0.3 mm in diameter. Ultrasonography also discriminates cystic lesions from solid lesions but is not reliable in distinguishing benign disease from malignant disease. Cystic nodules constitute 15–25%[11] of all thyroid nodules and when 4 cm or more in diameter may have a malignancy rate of approximately 20% (**Fig. 2.5**).[12]

Figure 2.5
Ultrasound scan of mixed thyroid nodule with cystic and solid component.

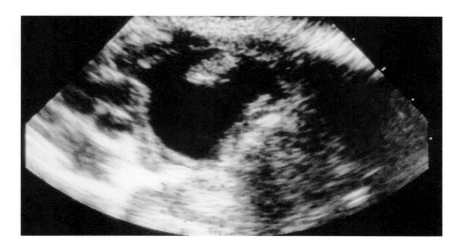

Computed tomography and magnetic resonance imaging

Computed tomography (CT) and magnetic resonance imaging (MRI) play an increasingly important part in thyroid disease, particularly in the evaluation of retrosternal goitres and glands producing major pressure effects and distortion of adjacent structures (**Fig. 2.6**).

Needle biopsy

Needle biopsy is a most valuable complement to clinical examination, particularly in the assessment of thyroid nodular disease. There are two quite distinct

Figure 2.6
CT scan showing extensive intrathoracic goitre posterior to the trachea.

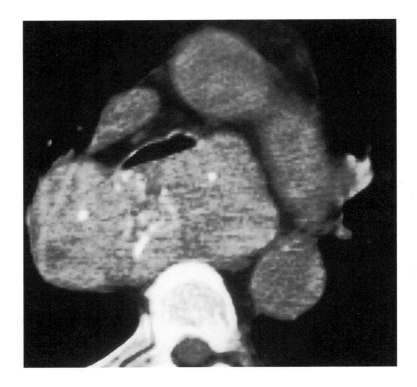

types of needle biopsy; the cutting biopsy needle and fine needle aspiration cytology.

Cutting needle biopsy

Cutting needle biopsy produces a core of tissue suitable for histological examination and has high diagnostic accuracy but has the disadvantages of being a painful procedure with poor compliance. Potential complications include haematoma, tracheal puncture and recurrent laryngeal nerve damage. Lesions less than 3 cm in size may not be amenable to this technique. The risk of seeding malignancy along the needle tract has been greatly exaggerated.[13]

Fine needle aspiration cytology

Fine needle aspiration cytology (FNAC, ABC) employs a fine gauge (21 or 23) needle to obtain a thyroid sample suitable for cytological assessment. First used in Scandinavia in the early 1950s,[14] it is now universally accepted as being a highly accurate, cost effective method with low morbidity and good patient compliance. In experienced hands the high diagnostic accuracy is such that the method can diagnose:

● Colloid nodules
● Thyroiditis

- Papillary carcinoma
- Medullary carcinoma
- Anaplastic carcinoma
- Lymphoma

Its major limitation is its inability to distinguish benign from malignant follicular neoplasms,[15] this distinction being dependent on the histological criteria of capsular and vascular invasion.

Four possible results are available from FNAC:

- Malignant
- Benign
- Suspicious
- Inadequate

The first two categories are well defined, and indeed Lowhagen *et al.*[15] reported no false positive results with respect to malignancy and a false negative rate of 2.2%, which later decreased to 0.[15] Grant *et al.*[16] found a false negative rate of only 0.7% in 439 patients studied and concluded that FNAC was a safe, reliable and accurate means of discriminating between benign and malignant lesions.

Suspicious lesions are mostly the follicular tumours, and because of the inability of the technique to provide histological details all such lesions should be resected. An inadequate sample rate of 15% is not uncommon but such a result should not be regarded as being benign but is an indication for repeat aspiration.

Goitre

The term goitre, derived from the Latin guttur, meaning throat, is used as a non-specific term to indicate diffuse enlargement of the thyroid gland. A classification of goitre is shown in **Table 2.1**.

Simple goitre

Simple goitre is the result of TSH stimulation, usually secondary to inadequate concentrations of circulating thyroid hormones. In these circumstances, TSH stimulation causes diffuse hyperplasia and an increase in hormone output. Iodine deficiency is a key factor in simple endemic goitre, associated with a low iodine content of water and food.[17] There are 5 to 10 mg of iodine in the thyroid pool, with a turnover rate of 1% daily. The minimum daily dietary requirements of iodine are therefore small, about 50 to 100 µg. Endemic goitrous areas are

Simple goitre (endemic or sporadic)	Diffuse hyperplastic goitre Nodular goitre
Toxic goitre	Diffuse (Graves' disease) Toxic multinodular goitre Toxic solitary nodule
Neoplastic goitre	Benign Malignant
Thyroiditis	Subacute (granulomatous)—de Quervain's Autoimmune (Hashimoto's) Riedel's Acute suppurative
Miscellaneous	Chronic bacterial infection (e.g. tuberculosis or syphilis) Actinomycosis Amyloidosis Dyshormonogenesis

Table 2.1 Classification of goitre

mountainous regions such as the Alps, Andes and Himalayas. In Britain, recognised regions include the Chilterns, Cotswolds, Derbyshire and South Wales.

Iodine deficiency in its most extreme form is associated with cretinism, congenital hypothyroidism and various degrees of mental impairment. Usually an endemic goitre commences as a soft diffuse enlargement appearing in childhood, which can evolve into a colloid goitre at a later stage when TSH stimulation has diminished. Times of physiological stress, such as puberty and pregnancy, result in increased demands for T4 and are accompanied by TSH stimulation of the thyroid and diffuse hyperplasia. The natural history of thyroid stimulation by TSH is such that there are fluctuating levels of stimulation, but eventually active and inactive lobules coexist. At this stage nodules form, and throughout the thyroid there are changes of hyperplasia, cystic degeneration, hemorrhage, colloid-filled follicles, fibrosis and later calcification. Simple goitre occurring in a non-endemic area is usually described as sporadic, but the nodules of endemic goitre appear earlier. All types of simple goitre occur more often in women.

Environmental factors such as the dietary goitrogen thiocyanate in cassava or vegetables of the brassica family may cause thyroid enlargement.[18] The interaction of environmental goitrogens and iodine deficiency may explain some of the differences in the prevalence of endemic goitre seen with similar degrees of iodine deficiency. Other environmental agents, including calcium and drugs such as the antithyroid agent carbimazole, are capable of acting at various sites within the thyroid gland, and by interfering with the process of hormone synthesis lead to hyperplasia with goitre formation.

Paradoxically, excess iodine intake can inhibit proteolysis and release of thyroid hormones leading to goitre and hypothyroidism.[18]

Deficiency of one or more of the enzymes in the thyroid responsible for T4 synthesis may be the cause of sporadic goitre. These deficiencies, either complete or partial, are usually genetic and are well illustrated by the dyshormonogenic Pendred's syndrome in which thyroid enlargement progresses to nodular goitre. These is associated deafness. Severe forms of dyshormonogenesis result in hypothyroidism and cretinism in the infant. Treatment consists of T4 and thyroidectomy if the goitre produces pressure symptoms or cosmetic concerns.

Prevention and treatment

Prevention of the development of simple endemic goitre can be achieved by the addition of iodine to the diet as, for example, in table salt. At a prenodular stage a hyperplastic goitre can be made to regress in size by giving T4 0.1–0.15 mg daily, often over several years. Thyroidectomy may be indicated for cosmetic reasons or because of pressure effects if the gland does not regress.

Thyroid nodules

Thyroid nodules are common, being a feature of many different thyroid diseases. In a nongoitrous area, the prevalence of palpable thyroid nodules in a population aged 30 to 59 years was 4.2%.[19] At adult autopsy the prevalence of thyroid nodules, many less than 1 cm in diameter and impalpable, is much greater, perhaps even as high as 50%.[20] Although the majority of thyroid nodules are benign and include colloid lesions, follicular adenomas, nodular thyroiditis and degenerative cysts, the essential clinical problem, particularly when the lesion is solitary, remains the distinction between benign and malignant diseases.

Clinical assessment

Most thyroid nodules are asymptomatic but the acute development of a painful swelling in the thyroid is usually due to haemorrhage into a pre-existing colloid nodule. This is an important condition to recognise as spontaneous resolution, sometimes aided by aspiration, occurs in a few weeks without intervention.

Rapid growth of an existing nodule, with discomfort radiating into the face or jaw, may be due to malignancy, but often a malignant nodule may be slow growing and be present for many years before a diagnosis is made. Thyroid nodules, like most thyroid conditions, occur more often in women, but it is thought that a solitary nodule in a man carries a greater risk of malignancy. In elderly people a rapidly growing firm painful lesion is likely to be an anaplastic carcinoma. Young people are particularly at risk for malignancy and, for example, a solitary nodule is likely to be malignant in 50% of children under 14 years of age.[21,22] A family history of thyroid or other endocrine disease may be relevant to the diagnosis of MTC in MEN-2A, MEN-2B and non-MEN familial syndromes (see Chapter 4).

Several key environmental and geographic factors require consideration. The incidence of follicular cancer is increased in endemic goitrous areas,[23] for example, whereas iodine-rich regions such as Iceland have an increased incidence of papillary cancer.[24] The Chernobyl nuclear reactor accident demonstrated the tumour-inducing effects of irradiation. Although the association between thyroid carcinoma and a history of head and neck irradiation in children was first recorded in 1950,[25] the true magnitude of the problem was only identified by DeGroot and Paloyan in the Chicago area in 1973.[26] Irradiation also increases the incidence of benign thyroid nodules, but the reported risk of malignancy in a palpable nodule found in a previously irradiated thyroid ranges from 20 to 50%. High dose external irradiation to the neck for conditions such as Hodgkin's lymphoma may also increase the risk of thyroid malignancy.[27] The latent period for developing post-irradiation tumours ranges from 6 to 35 years. Therapeutic radioiodine used in the treatment of Graves' disease and the administration of diagnostic isotopes are not associated with any increased risk of malignancy.

A preliminary clinical examination of the patient is directed towards assessment of thyroid status, although most patients with a solitary thyroid nodule will be euthyroid. A nodule in a hyperthyroid patient is highly unlikely to be malignant. Previously much emphasis was placed on the distinction between a clinically solitary nodule and a multinodular gland in the mistaken belief that multinodular goitres were unlikely to contain a malignancy. When a dominant lesion is present within a multinodular gland, the malignancy rate may be virtually identical to that of the true solitary nodule.

A hard fixed nodule is likely to be malignant, but it is not uncommon for papillary lesions to be cystic and follicular lesions to be soft as a result of haemorrhage. A very hard lesion may be an entirely benign calcified colloid nodule. Lymphadenopathy either in the central paratracheal groups or in the lateral deep cervical region is a common finding in papillary and medullary carcinomas.

Although voice change and hoarseness may be non-specific findings, a proven recurrent laryngeal nerve palsy on the side of a palpable thyroid nodule is likely to indicate malignant infiltration. Rarely, direct pressure from a benign lesion can also produce vocal cord paralysis. Although the presence of pressure symptoms and clinical identification of tracheal deviation or retrosternal extension does not aid the distinction of malignant from benign lesion, these features nevertheless will be major considerations in the selection of patients for surgery.

Following this careful clinical assessment, the clinician will have formed an opinion as to the likelihood of malignancy. Further supportive and diagnostic tests are now appropriate. The thyroid status will be confirmed by measurement of T4 and TSH, and a radiograph of the neck and chest will delineate a retrosternal goitre or airway distortion. Most calcified thyroid nodules are benign, but some papillary and medullary neoplasms have a characteristic fine stippled or punctate calcification. Measurement of calcitonin concentration is not routinely performed, although some recent studies have suggested that this determination can facilitate the identification of a patient with an unsuspected medullary carcinoma (J.F. Henry, personal communication). Hypercalcitonaemia is not absolutely specific for medullary tumours, in that increased concentrations may be seen in patients with carcinoma of the breast, pancreas or lung or in those with carcinoid tumours, phaeochromocytoma and bony metastases.

Positive thyroid antibody titres are non-specific, being raised in patients with thyroiditis and sometimes malignancy.

Thyroglobulin measurement, although valuable in the follow-up of patients with malignant tumours, has no value in their initial diagnosis.

Diagnostic investigation

Needle biopsy and FNAC

This highly accurate and cost-effective technique is the method of choice for achieving a precise diagnosis in most patients with thyroid nodular disease. A recent refinement of the method using an immunocytochemical technique for the detection of TPO may be a useful adjunct to FNAC in the preoperative diagnosis of follicular malignancy.[28] Delbridge et al.[29] have shown that proton magnetic resonance spectroscopy (PMRS) analysis of FNAC specimens helps to make the distinction between benign and malignant lesions and thereby reduces unnecessary surgery for patients with benign follicular neoplasms.

Ultrasonography

Ultrasonography has limited diagnostic value in the assessment of thyroid nodules but allows a clear delineation of multinodularity. An apparently solitary nodule may be shown on ultrasonography to be surrounded by small impalpable nodules.

Isotope scanning

Unless the patient has thyrotoxicosis scintigraphy of the thyroid either with ^{123}I or technetium pertechnetate (^{99m}Tc) has little value in the investigation of the patient with a thyroid nodule.

Treatment

Thyroid hormone administration

There is little evidence that the administration of T4 is capable of reducing the size of benign nodules. The possibility of reducing the size of an incorrectly diagnosed malignant nodule by T4 is clearly a potential pitfall.

Summary of indications for surgery

Selection of patients for surgery is based primarily on clinical features aided by preoperative FNAC yielding either a diagnostic or suspicious appearance of malignancy. Another large group of patients will require surgery because of pressure and mechanical symptoms, including dyspnoea, choking and dysphagia. A scheme of management of patients with solitary thyroid nodular disease is shown in **Figure 2.7**. Clinical features such as characteristics of nodule, lymphadenopathy, recurrent laryngeal nerve palsy, family history and history of irradiation may override cytological findings in the decision for surgery.

Surgery for thyroid nodules

The minimum surgical procedure for adequate treatment of the solitary thyroid nodule is a unilateral *total* lobectomy with removal of the isthmus and pyramidal lobe. This is a safe operation with minimal risk of damaging either the parathyroids or the recurrent laryngeal nerve. A full histological examination of the nodule is permitted with no risk of tumour spillage in the operative field. This surgical procedure completely obviates the need to reoperate and remove a posterior thyroid lobe remnant if the definitive histology should be returned as malignant or if there should be any benign nodule recurrence at a later date. These are most important benefits compared with the outmoded procedure of unilateral *subtotal* lobectomy.

Frozen section histology can be employed to confirm the preoperative diagnosis and aid decision making, particularly with respect to benign pathology where lobectomy alone will be sufficient.

Thyroid cysts

Confirmation of the diagnosis of a thyroid cyst is usually made by fine needle aspiration and this simple technique can be both diagnostic and therapeutic (**Fig. 2.8**). A full cytological assessment usually requires sampling thyroid tissue adjacent to the cyst to avoid missing a carcinoma in the cyst wall. If a cyst refills it is appropriate to reaspirate but after two or three such manoeuvres surgery is likely to be indicated. A large cyst (greater than 4 cm in diameter), a significantly blood-stained aspirate, cytological findings of neoplasia or a history of irradiation are all indications for surgery.

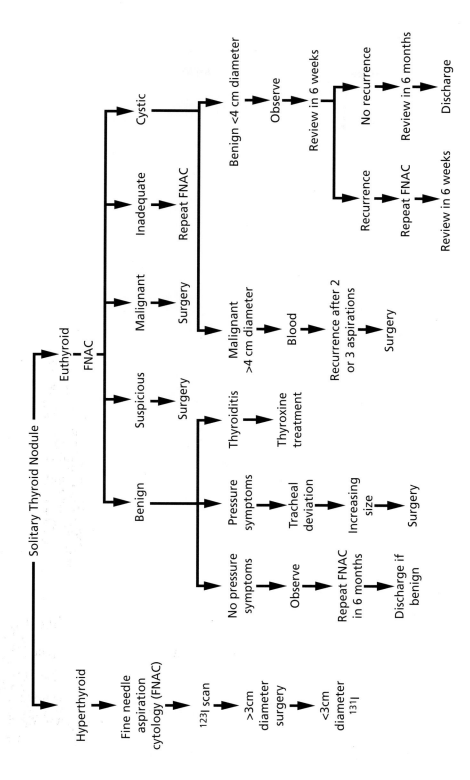

Figure 2.7
Scheme of management for solitary thyroid nodule.

Figure 2.8
Aspiration of cystic thyroid nodule demonstrating therapeutic as well as diagnostic value of fine needle aspiration.

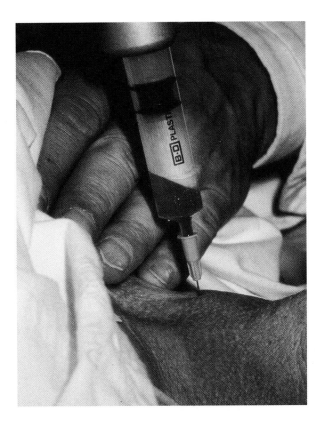

Multinodular disease

The usual indications for surgery are cosmetic or pressure effects, a dominant nodule perhaps increasing in size or showing cytological features that raise the possibility of malignancy, thyrotoxicosis or retrosternal extension (**Fig. 2.9**). The surgical procedure will be tailored to the situation found at surgery, and although a bilateral subtotal thyroidectomy is often appropriate, if there is asymmetrical nodularity with one lobe significantly larger than the other, a unilateral total lobectomy with a subtotal procedure on the opposite side may be indicated.

There is increasing support for the more radical approach of performing a total thyroidectomy when the multinodularity is both bilateral and extensive, often with no normal thyroid tissue to be left as a remnant.[30]

Retrosternal goitre

Almost all retrosternal goitres arise from growth of the lower half of the thyroid lobes, extending down into a substernal position. The degree of descent of the gland is variable, but when palpable in the neck it is usually classified as substernal whereas a gland entirely within the chest is intrathoracic. In some instances a retrosternal goitre may be asymptomatic and found as a coincidental observation

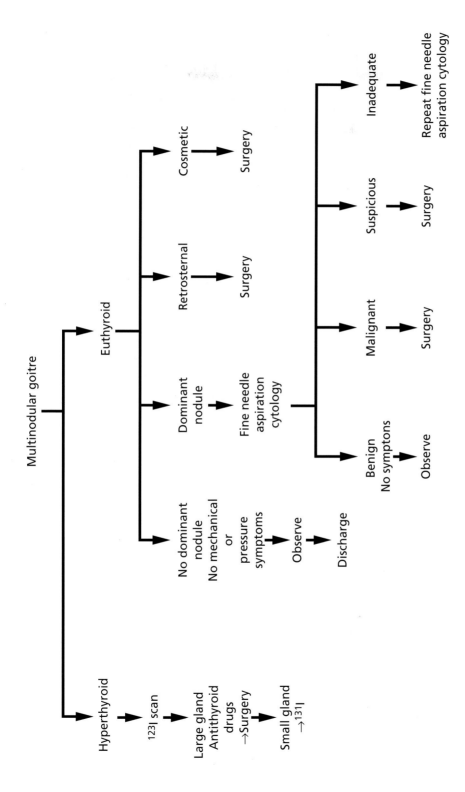

Figure 2.9
Scheme of management for multinodular goitre.

Figure 2.10
Chest radiograph of large retrosternal goitre producing tracheal deviation and extending posterior to the trachea into the right thoracic cavity.

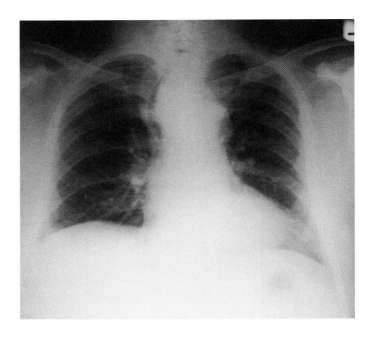

on a chest radiograph (**Fig. 2.10**). Many patients are symptomatic with problems of airway compression, 'asthma,' dysphagia, hoarseness of the voice and even thyrotoxicosis. Recurrent laryngeal nerve palsy may occur rarely as a direct effect of pressure from a benign lesion. More dramatic pressure effects can lead to superior vena cava compression syndrome (**Fig. 2.11**). The incidence of malignancy in retrosternal glands is probably no different to that of other nodular goitres, but of course a gland behind the sternum is not amenable to palpation or FNAC for diagnosis.

Confirmation of the diagnosis can be made by a combination of plain radiographs and either CT (**Fig. 2.12**) or MRI. The last two investigations will give precise information concerning airway compromise. Respiratory function tests with flow loop studies are also helpful in patient assessment.

The diagnosis of a retrosternal goitre is usually an indication for surgery both to obtain a precise histological diagnosis and to remove the significant risk of progressive airway obstruction resulting from growth of the gland or from haemorrhage into a benign colloid lesion.

Thyroid cancer

Thyroid cancer is rare (3.7–4.7 per 100 000 population)[31] accounting for fewer than 1%[32] of all malignancies and 0.5% of all cancer deaths.[33] Thyroid cancer constitutes an extremely heterogeneous group of tumours, with a wide spectrum

Figure 2.11
Venogram of a patient with retrosternal goitre producing obstruction of the superior vena cava.

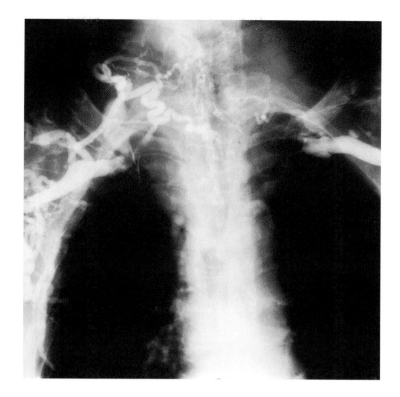

Figure 2.12
CT scan of multinodular goitre producing extreme tracheal narrowing.

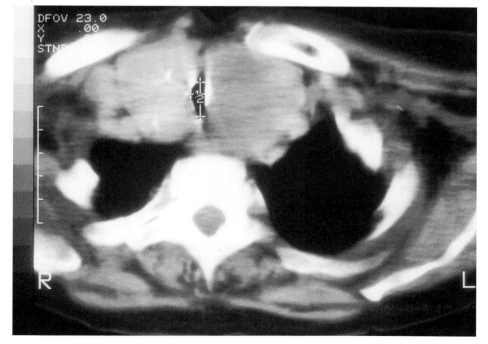

of biological behaviour. In most instances if treated appropriately there is a high survival rate. Disappointingly, because of the lack of long-term follow-up studies or large randomised trials comparing various procedures, the optimal management for many of these tumours remains controversial.

The role of molecular genetic changes

Thyroid cancer results from complex alterations and disorders of the genetic content of a single cell, which is subsequently inherited by its daughter cells. Several genetic aberrations have been well studied and shown to be implicated in thyroid tumorigenesis.

Oncogenes when activated stimulate tumour growth.[34] Important members of this gene family which play a part in thyroid tumour development include the *Ras* genes,[35] growth factors, such as epidermal growth factor (EGF)[36] (and its receptor EGFr), insulin-like growth factor 1 (IGFI), fibroblast growth factor (FGF), TSH, *Gsα* gene and the RET proto-oncogene (see section on familial MTC).

Tumour suppressor genes, especially *p53*,[37] exert an influence on thyroid cell growth by inhibiting tumorigenesis. Mutations in *p53* can lead to its inactivation, which may be important in thyroid tumour initiation and progression especially leading to anaplastic change.

Papillary carcinoma

This is the commonest thyroid tumour and occurs with an increased incidence in iodine-rich areas and usually affects children and young adults. Previous neck irradiation, particularly in young people, may predispose to thyroid cancer, and approximately 85% of such irradiation-induced tumours are papillary.[26] A rare familial form of the disease has also been described.[38]

Pathology

This tumour has a propensity for lymphatic spread both within the thyroid and to the paratracheal and cervical lymph nodes, is usually a hard whitish lesion infiltrating the thyroid gland and presents as a thyroid nodule. The lesion is frequently multifocal (30–87.5%)[39] and rarely encapsulated. Blood-borne spread is usually a late feature.

These tumours can be divided into three main types based on their size and extent.

Minimal

These lesions are less than 1 cm in diameter and usually not clinically obvious. They are also called papillary microcarcinoma. They readily metastasise to regional lymph nodes and are a common finding at autopsy, being detected in 6–13% of thyroid glands of patients dying from causes other than thyroid disease. Many of these clinically inapparent tumours present with cervical lymphadenopathy—the so-called lateral aberrant thyroid. Although rarely associated with metastatic disease, deaths have been reported. The Mayo Clinic group described four deaths in 396 patients with tumours 1.5 cm or less in diameter,[40] and Noguchi *et al.* documented two deaths in 867 patients.[41]

Intrathyroidal

These lesions are larger than minimal tumours, have a less favourable prognosis, are situated totally within the thyroid and do not invade adjacent structures.

Extrathyroidal

This is a locally advanced condition extending through the thyroid capsule, often involving adjacent structures such as the trachea, oesophagus and recurrent laryngeal nerve. The prognosis of this disease type is the least favourable.

Histology

The typical lesion has a mixture of papillary projections and follicular structures. The cuboidal cells with pale abundant cytoplasm have intranuclear cytoplasmic inclusions, nuclear overlapping and grooves (Orphan Annie cells). Psammoma bodies occur and are associated with a high incidence of lymphatic spread. The presence of involved lymph nodes, however, does not seem to adversely affect the prognosis. Follicular, encapsulated, diffuse sclerosing and tall cell varieties of papillary carcinoma have been described.

Clinical presentation

The commonest presentation of papillary carcinoma is a thyroid nodule often associated with enlarged cervical lymph nodes, especially in children. Cystic change in metastases is not unusual and the differential diagnosis may include a branchial cyst. Involvement of adjacent structures by a locally invasive tumour may cause hoarseness of the voice owing to recurrent laryngeal nerve palsy, airway symptoms because of tracheal involvement and dysphagia as a result of oesophageal invasion. Less than 1% of patients at the time of initial presentation will show features of distant metastases. The highest frequency of metastases at initial presentation is seen in children, but up to 20% of patients overall ultimately develop distant spread.[42]

Diagnosis

Diagnosis is based on a combination of careful clinical assessment and FNAC.

Follicular carcinoma

This tumour, less common than papillary carcinoma, has a higher incidence in iodine-deficient areas owing to chronic TSH stimulation. It can also be caused by previous irradiation. The disease has a female to male ratio of 3:1, affects an older age group (mean age 50 years) than papillary carcinoma and rarely occurs in familial form (**Fig. 2.13**).[43]

Pathology

Follicular carcinoma is invariably encapsulated, solitary, frequently exhibits vascular invasion and spreads via the blood stream. In contrast with papillary tumours, lymphatic spread is usually a late phenomenon, seen with advanced tumours. Follicular carcinoma is classified into two types according to histopathological features.

Figure 2.13
Patient with longstanding multinodular goitre and coexisting follicular thyroid carcinoma.

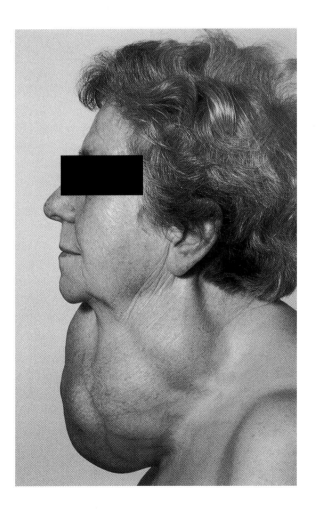

Minimally invasive

This tumour is seen on histology to demonstrate only slight capsular or vascular invasion in contrast with frankly invasive tumours.

Frankly invasive

This more aggressive tumour, the diagnosis of which depends on histological confirmation of capsular and angioinvasive features, may demonstrate at surgery gross venous extension, particularly into the middle thyroid and internal jugular veins. Although most well differentiated tumours have a well formed follicular structure, the oxyphilic Hurthle cell lesion is composed mostly of cells with eosinophilic granular cytoplasm, large clear nuclei and trabecular architecture. Some consider this variety to be a particularly aggressive form of follicular carcinoma, with a greater propensity for multifocality and lymph node metastases.[44] Furthermore, therapeutic options in Hurthle cell tumours are limited by the inability of the lesion to concentrate radioactive iodine. They do, however, synthesise thyroglobulin.

Clinical features

Follicular thyroid cancer presents as a discrete solitary thyroid nodule increasing in size. Although many tumours are firm they can be soft because of haemorrhage within the lesion. Metastatic disease may already be present at the time of diagnosis, with bone and lung involvement.

Diagnosis

Unlike papillary thyroid carcinoma, follicular carcinoma cannot be diagnosed precisely by FNAC. The cytology report will describe a follicular tumour, usually showing a microfollicular pattern, and only 20% of these will subsequently be identified as follicular carcinoma.

Treatment of differentiated thyroid cancer

There is general agreement that thyroidectomy is the treatment of choice, but the precise extent of the procedure (excisional biopsy to total thyroidectomy) remains controversial.[45] The treatment objectives are to irradicate the primary tumour, reduce the incidence of distant or local recurrence, facilitate treatment of metastases, cure the maximum number of patients and achieve all of these objectives with minimal morbidity.

Patients with papillary carcinoma can be separated into high and low risk groups in terms of risk for recurrence and long-term survival on the basis of patient age at diagnosis; younger subjects (patients under 45 years) usually having a more favourable outlook. Several more sophisticated prognostic scoring systems have been introduced to identify patients with high risk tumours and aid comparison between different surgical therapies. The AGES scoring system from the Mayo Clinic considers: *A*ge of patients, histological *G*rade and *E*xtent and *S*ize of tumour.[46] Most patients being assessed by the scoring system fit into the low risk group, with an excellent long-term prognosis. Other scoring systems include AMES (*A*ge, *M*etastasis and *E*xtent and *S*ize) and MACIS (*M*etastasis, *A*ge, *C*ompleteness of resection, *I*nvasion and *S*ize).

Total thyroidectomy has been advocated because of its ability to treat multifocal tumour, decrease local recurrence, decrease distant recurrence, reduce the risk of anaplastic change in remaining remnants, facilitate treatment with ^{131}I and permit postoperative measurements of thyroglobulin concentration for monitoring the patient's subsequent progress. Papillary carcinoma is usually multifocal and this would not be effectively treated by unilateral or even near total thyroidectomy. It is likely, however, that many small foci of microscopic tumour remaining after less than total thyroidectomy stay dormant and do not necessarily progress and achieve clinical importance. Nevertheless, local tumour recurrence is an extremely serious event, carrying a high risk of death. Retrospective studies of patients undergoing thyroidectomy have demonstrated a reduced local recurrence rate with total thyroidectomy compared with a subtotal resection.[47] With respect to mortality risk, it has been shown that high risk patients have a lower mortality rate at 25 years when treated by bilateral resection than by ipsilateral lobectomy.[46] The life-threatening complication of anaplastic transformation in an inadequately resected papillary carcinoma can be avoided by initial total thyroid clearance.

Most patients with differentiated thyroid cancer will have presented with a unilateral thyroid nodule and should be treated by the minimum surgical procedure of total lobectomy on the side of the lesion, isthmusectomy and removal of the pyramidal lobe. If papillary carcinoma is confirmed, usually by a combination of the preoperative FNAC and intraoperative frozen section, a total thyroidectomy is the most appropriate surgical treatment for intrathyroidal and extrathyroidal tumours. Thyroidectomy must always include clearance of pretracheal and paratracheal lymph nodes. The thymus should not be disturbed to avoid devascularising the inferior parathyroids often situated within the superior thymic horns. Lymph nodes in the lateral carotid chain group are biopsied and, if they give a positive result on frozen section histology, should be cleared by a modified neck dissection, leaving the internal jugular vein and sternomastoid muscle intact. There is no evidence to support the use of the more extensive and mutilating classic block dissection. More extensive extrathyroidal papillary carcinomas, however, may require radical excision of adjacent structures, even including part of the trachea with construction of a temporary tracheostomy.

Recently the concept of sentinel node assessment has been applied to the operative management of patients with differentiated thyroid cancer, although the precise role of this technique has yet to be defined.

A unilateral total lobectomy and isthmusectomy is adequate for minimal (<1 cm) lesions and the rare encapsulated papillary cancers that generally have an excellent prognosis. The recurrent laryngeal nerve must be identified throughout its course in these procedures so that damage may be avoided. Rarely is it necessary to sacrifice the nerve to achieve tumour clearance. The incidence of permanent postoperative hypoparathyroidism should be no more than 3%, care being taken to identify the parathyroid glands and leave their blood supply intact.

Follicular tumours diagnosed on FNAC are treated by total lobectomy, isthmusectomy and removal of the pyramidal lobe. Frozen section is usually unhelpful, failing to demonstrate capsular or vascular invasion, because of sampling difficulties. If the definitive histology is returned as a minimal lesion, then a unilateral procedure is all that is required. A lesion shown to be frankly invasive requires a total thyroidectomy, either performed within a few days of the initial lobectomy or after a period of 3–4 months. Lymph node dissection is not routinely performed for follicular tumours. A decision to proceed to a total thyroidectomy can often be made at the time of surgery on the basis of the macroscopic appearances of the lesion, especially when the tumour size is in excess of 4 cm.

Hurthle cell lesions, considered by some to have a bad prognosis, should be treated by total thyroidectomy and central neck node dissection.[44]

Postoperative treatment

T4

Any patient who has undergone total thyroidectomy requires replacement treatment with T4, and in those with papillary carcinoma there is a compelling argument for prescribing T4 to suppress TSH concentrations, which may well influence the biological behaviour of the tumour.

Thyroglobulin

Measurement of thyroglobulin concentration is a sensitive indicator of residual or recurrent differentiated thyroid cancer after total thyroidectomy and when the patient is on full replacement/suppressive T4 dosage.[2] This measurement is now performed routinely at each postoperative clinic attendance and has markedly reduced the need for routine serial radioactive iodine scanning.

Measurement of thyroglobulin concentration may be difficult when there are circulating autoantibodies to thyroglobulin (TgAb). In these circumstances there is the potential to underestimate the risk or likelihood of metastatic malignancy.[48]

Radioactive iodine

Radioactive iodine is a most useful means of detecting metastatic disease when total thyroidectomy has been performed, but approximately 20% of papillary carcinomas in patients older than 50 years of age cannot concentrate ^{131}I.[47] Most follicular carcinomas, with the exception of the Hurthle cell variety, can be imaged by radioiodine. If total thyroidectomy has been performed for differentiated cancer, patients are initially given T3 20 μg t.d.s. and sent home to await an ^{131}I scan approximately 6 weeks later. T3 is discontinued 2 weeks before the scan to allow an increase in TSH concentration before administering 2–5 mCi of ^{131}I. If there are no metastases or residual remnants of thyroid, the uptake at 24 hours should be less than 1%. When there is significant uptake in the thyroid bed, this can be ablated with radioiodine and any metastatic disease subsequently treated with a therapeutic dose of 150–200 mCi^{131}I. Patients are then given T4 (0.15–0.2 mg daily) and scanned repeated at 6-monthly intervals, and repeated therapeutic doses of ^{131}I are given as necessary until all residual uptake is ablated. The maximum cumulative dose of ^{131}I should be no greater than 800–1000 mCi. Patients whose metastases are visible only on radioiodine scanning despite negative results on chest radiography or tomography have an excellent prognosis.[49] Once the patient is stable and disease free, subsequent follow-up is achieved by a combination of clinical examination and measurement of serum thyroglobulin concentration.

Anaplastic carcinoma

This tumour has a peak incidence between 60 and 70 years of age, occurs slightly more often in women and has a higher incidence in endemic goitrous areas. The tumour rapidly infiltrates local structures and metastasises via the blood stream and lymphatics. The frequent finding of foci of papillary or follicular carcinoma in anaplastic tumours gives rise to the view that this disease originates in an unrecognised or untreated differentiated tumour.[50] The clinical findings are typically those of an elderly woman, often with a long history of goitre that suddenly starts to grow rapidly. Involvement of adjacent structures results in hoarseness, dysphonia, dysphagia and a compromised airway.

Although the clinical findings are virtually diagnostic, confirmation can be obtained by FNAC, the aspirate showing bizarre giant, multinucleated and pleomorphic tumour cells. Resection of the thyroid is rarely possible because of the local extent of disease. Incision biopsy for diagnostic purposes should be avoided for fear of initiating uncontrollable local spread of the disease. If surgery is possible, it should relieve an obstructed airway by excision of the isthmus. Radiotherapy and doxorubicin are the main modalities of treatment, but invariably the tumour rapidly progresses usually leading to death of the patient within 6 months.

Malignant lymphoma

Thyroid lymphoma, usually of the non-Hodgkin's B-cell type, can develop as part of a generalised lymphomatous process involving other viscera, but the disease is usually confined as a primary tumour to the thyroid. The majority of such lymphomas arise in a background of longstanding autoimmune Hashimoto's thyroiditis.[51] It must be emphasised that only a very small number of patients with this relatively common disorder ultimately go on to develop lymphoma.

These tumours infiltrate throughout lymphatics and blood vessels, spreading directly into adjacent tissue and involving cervical nodes.

As in the case of anaplastic carcinoma, this is primarily a disease of elderly women, a typical patient presenting with a painless firm thyroid mass, rapidly increasing in size. There may be a history of goitre or autoimmune disease, and some patients will be frankly hypothyroid or already receiving T4. This tumour grows to involve adjacent cervical structures, and lymphadenopathy is invariably present. The diagnosis can be confirmed by FNAC although full characterisation of the lymphoma may require the histological assessment of a core biopsy. Radiotherapy and chemotherapy are the main treatment modalities. Chemotherapy is of most value for extrathyroidal and disseminated disease. Surgery may be necessary to free the trachea when there is impending obstruction. Although 5-year survival of 85% has been reported,[52] the overall prognosis of the disease is significantly influenced by the histopathological grade of the lesion and the presence of locally extensive or disseminated disease.

Squamous cell carcinoma

This is a rare tumour, distinct from the squamous metaplasia often seen in papillary carcinomas. It is an aggressive disease with a clinical course similar to that of anaplastic carcinoma. Most squamous cell tumours are unresectable.

Metastatic carcinoma of the thyroid

The thyroid gland can be the site of metastatic spread from tumours such as breast and kidney. Careful clinical assessment may suggest the correct diagnosis but confirmation is usually obtained by FNAC. In some instances resection of the thyroid gland is indicated if the primary disease is otherwise well controlled.

Medullary carcinoma

This is a tumour arising from the C-cells and derived from neural ectoderm. It accounts for approximately 8% of malignant thyroid tumours. In 1959 Hazard[53] described the tumour as a solid, non-follicular carcinoma with coexisting amyloid. In 1966 Williams[54] while further defining the histology of the tumour,

Figure 2.14
Tongue of patient with multiple endocrine neoplasia type-2B syndrome showing ganglioneuromata.

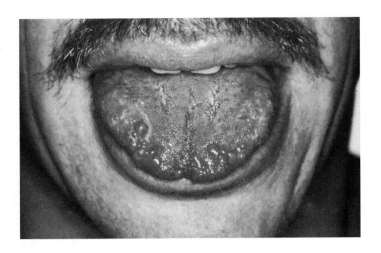

proposed that the disease arose from the parafollicular or C-cells, later shown to secrete calcitonin, a peptide capable of lowering the blood calcium concentration and amenable to measurement by radioimmunoassay.[55] MTC is a sporadic tumour in 80% of patients and familial in 20%. The familial syndromes, which are inherited in an autosomal dominant manner with almost complete penetrance but variable expressivity, consist of the MEN-2A and MEN-2B syndromes (**Fig. 2.14**) and the rarer non-MEN familial form (see Chapter 4).

Pathology

MTC is a solid tumour usually occurring in the upper two thirds of the thyroid and is often multicentric and bilateral when occurring in the familial form. The typical histological picture is one of infiltrating neoplastic cells invading the thyroid, forming glandular and solid areas with amyloid stroma. The tumour grows locally but readily spreads by lymphatics to regional nodes and via the blood stream to distant sites such as liver, lungs and bones (**Fig. 2.15**). The tumour synthesises and secretes calcitonin, which proves to be a most valuable biochemical and histochemical marker for MTC, CEA and calcitonin gene-relate peptide (CGRP) are also produced by C-cells, but they have little clinical value as tumour markers.

Clinical features

As with most thyroid tumours, the disease typically presents as a mass in the neck, often with enlarged cervical and mediastinal lymph nodes. Involvement of adjacent organs and the recurrent laryngeal nerve may cause respiratory or swallowing difficulties and voice changes. Sporadic disease has a peak incidence at 40–50 years of age whereas inherited, familial disease is usually seen at a younger age. Diarrhoea is often a prominent clinical feature, but the ability of this tumour to secrete a range of hormones and peptides, including calcitonin, prostaglandins,

Figure 2.15
Thoracic vertebral metastases from medullary thyroid cancer.

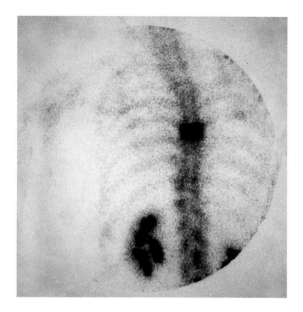

5-hydroxytryptamine and adrenocorticotrophic hormone can give rise to a range of clinical syndromes, which may include Cushing's syndrome.

Although the familial varieties of the disease can present in an identical manner to sporadic disease, biochemical and, more recently, genetic screening allow detection of the condition at a preclinical stage before there is histological or macroscopic evidence of the disease.

Diagnosis

Clinical assessment and the taking of a careful family history are fundamental to establishing a precise diagnosis. Confirmation is obtained by FNAC and measurement of serum calcitonin concentration when there is a high index of suspicion. At this stage although the diagnosis of MTC is secure it may still not be possible to distinguish the sporadic from familial variety. Because of the close association of phaeochromocytoma and MTC in the MEN familial forms, measurement of urinary vanillylmandelic acid and metanephrine concentrations is mandatory in all patients with MTC before progressing to any invasive procedure such as surgery. A thyroidectomy performed on a patient with an undiagnosed, untreated phaeochromocytoma is likely to have disastrous physiological and clinical consequences.

Treatment

Total thyroidectomy is the appropriate procedure to adequately treat multicentric and bilateral disease. The central and paratracheal lymph nodes are cleared from the level of the thyroid cartilage to the upper mediastinum, including thymectomy as necessary. The lateral nodes in the carotid sheath are sampled and, if involved with tumour, a modified radical node dissection is performed, preserving the internal jugular vein, sternomastoid muscle and spinal accessory nerve. Even when the primary tumour is extensive, the recurrent laryngeal nerve can usually be preserved. Because of the multifocal nature of hereditary tumours, a bilateral lymph node clearance is advised.

Prognosis

The presence or absence of distant metastases and lymph node positivity are major factors in determining the ultimate prognosis. Excellent 10-year survival figures of approximately 90% have recently been reported,[56] but when lymph node metastasis is present this survival rate is reduced to 45%. Sporadic disease and MEN-2B tumours are associated with the worst prognosis. A better outlook is seen in patients with non-MEN familial and MEN-2A syndromes.

Follow-up

After surgery, regular clinical and biochemical follow-up is carried out with measurement of calcitonin and CEA concentrations. When increased concentrations of these agents persist after thyroidectomy or develop subsequently this may signify presistent and recurrent disease. Ultrasonography, CT, MRI and scanning with MIBG, octreotide or DMSA can be utilised to detect this disease (**Fig. 2.16**). For occult disease, selective venous catheterisation and sampling for calcitonin

Figure 2.16
CT scan demonstrating laryngeal metastatic deposit from medullary thyroid carcinoma. Patient treated by hemilaryngectomy.

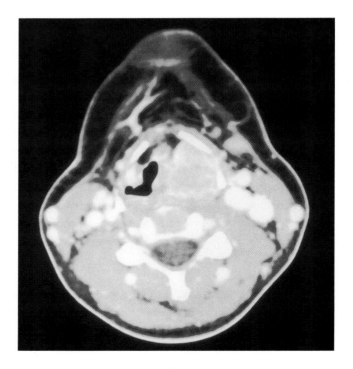

concentration have been used.[57] Laparoscopic assessment of the liver may detect small metastases not visible by conventional scanning. A proportion of these patients can be helped by reoperative surgery, but the benefits of radical reoperative surgery remain controversial. External irradiation can occasionally produce some benefit, but chemotherapy with doxorubicin is both toxic and disappointing.

Hyperthyroidism

Hyperthyroidism has a prevalence in the UK of approximately 27 per 1000 women and 2.3 per 1000 men.[58] Although Graves' disease is the most common cause of hyperthyroidism, there is an extensive list of other causes which require consideration (**Table 2.2**).

Graves' disease (diffuse toxic goitre) is an immunological disorder in which thyroid-stimulating antibodies (TsAbs) of the IgG type bind to the TSH receptor and stimulate the thyroid cell to produce and secrete an excess of thyroid hormones. Human leucocyte antigen (HLA) studies demonstrate that patients positive for HLA B8 and HLA DR3 have an increased susceptibility to the disease. The thyroid gland hypertrophies, producing diffuse enlargement, although nodular varieties of the condition are recognised. An important subgroup is that of internodular hyperplasia in a background of multinodular goitre. Histologically there is acinar hyperplasia, high columnar epithelium, increased vascularity and often lymphoid infiltration.

Clinical features

Most of the symptoms and signs of thyrotoxicosis (**Table 2.3**) result from excess thyroid hormones stimulating metabolism, heat production and oxygen

Common	Diffuse toxic goitre (Graves' disease)
	Toxic multinodular goitre (Plummer's disease)
	Toxic solitary nodule
	Toxic multinodular goitre with internodular hyperplasia
	Nodular goitre with hyperthyroidism due to exogenous iodine
	Exogenous thyroid hormone excess (factitious)
	Thyroiditis (subacute and autoimmune)—transient
Rare	Diffuse thyroid autonomy
	Metastatic thyroid carcinoma[60]
	Struma ovarii
	Pituitary tumour secreting thyroid stimulating hormone
	Choriocarcinoma and hydatidiform mole
	Neonatal thyrotoxicosis
	Postpartum hyperthyroidism
	After ^{131}I therapy

Table 2.2 *Causes of thyrotoxicosis*

Palpitations, tachycardia, cardiac arrhythmias, cardiac failure
Sweating
Tremor
Hyperkinetic movements
Nervousness
Myopathy
Tiredness and lethargy
Weight loss (occasional weight gain due to increased appetite)
Heat intolerance
Diarrhoea
Vomiting
Irritability
Emotional disturbance
Behavioural abnormalities
Ophthalmic signs
Irregular menstruation and amenorrhoea
Pretibial myxoedema
Thyroid acropathy
Vitiligo
Alopecia

Table 2.3 *Clinical features of thyrotoxicosis (see Fig. 2.17)*

consumption. Cardiac features are caused by β-adrenergic sympathetic activity. Although Graves' disease can occur at any age, it is especially common in young women between 20 and 40 years of age (Fig. 2.17). The onset may be gradual or abrupt, with an extremely variable subsequent course often characterised by exacerbations and remissions. Clinical features due to hypermetabolism tend to predominate, although in elderly people the cardiovascular and neurological features usually dominate. Hyperthyroidism may be severe and even fatal. In children the condition often causes growth abnormalities.

The immunological changes in Graves' disease are complex and undoubtedly cause many of the ophthalmic symptoms and signs.

Ophthalmopathy has two major components:

- *Non-infiltrative ophthalmopathy*, resulting from increased sympathetic activity leading to upper lid retraction, a stare and infrequent blinking;
- *Infiltrative ophthalmopathy*, causing oedema of the orbital contents, lids and periorbital tissues, cellular infiltration and deposition of mucopolysaccharide material within the orbit. Although the ophthalmopathy is usually bilateral, it may affect only one eye. Diplopia, particularly on upward outward gaze, results from weakening and paralysis of the external ocular muscles. The cornea is vulnerable to damage, and in extreme cases ulceration may occur. Papilloedema, retinal haemorrhage and optic nerve damage (malignant exophthalmos) can progress to blindness (Fig. 2.18).

Figure 2.17
I^{131} scan in a patient with Graves' disease with ophthalmopathy and small diffuse goitre.

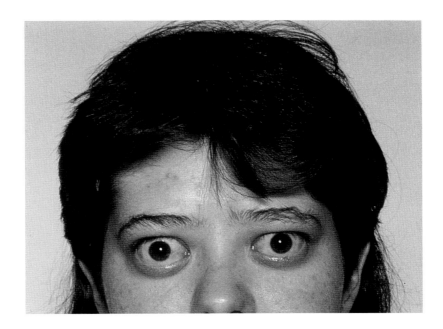

Figure 2.18
CT scan of orbit in Graves' ophthalmopathy demonstrating marked infiltration of the extraocular muscles.

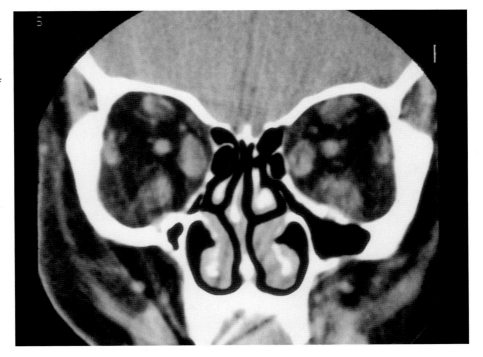

Investigation

Measurement of free T4, T3 and TSH concentrations will confirm the diagnosis (in T3 toxicosis, T4 concentrations will be normal whereas concentrations of T3 will be increased and TSH suppressed). A radioactive iodine or technetium scan is not essential in the diagnosis of Graves' disease, although is necessary in the assessment of toxic solitary and multinodular goitre to determine the site of nodular overactivity. Radioactive iodine uptake studies are particularly appropriate when a diagnosis of thyroiditis or factitious hyperthyroidism is being considered.

In Graves' disease there are three treatment options that can be used either alone or in combination to restore the euthyroid state:

- Antithyroid drugs
- Radioactive iodine
- Surgery

Each of these treatments has an important role, but for each patient all factors, medical, personal and social are carefully considered to produce a treatment plan individualised for each patient.

Medical treatment

Antithyroid drugs (propylthiouracil, carbimazole and methimazole)

These drugs interfere with the incorporation of iodine into tyrosine residues and prevent the intrathyroglobulin coupling of iodotyrosines into iodothyronines. Carbimazole may also have some immunosuppressive action on TsAb production. Medical treatment with thionamides has two principal roles:

1. Treatment of patients with a new diagnosis of Graves' disease in the hope of inducing a permanent remission;
2. To render the toxic patient euthyroid in preparation for surgery.

Although most patients can be rendered euthyroid with antithyroid drugs there is a less than optimum remission rate after an 'adequate' course of medication. A relapse rate of approximately 43% is seen in the first year after stopping drugs, and approximately 20% of the remaining patients relapse in each of the subsequent 5 years.[60] Antithyroid drugs are therefore only a satisfactory long-term solution to the problems of hyperthyroidism for less than 50% of patients. Carbimazole is prescribed in a dose of 10–15 mg 8 hourly reducing to 5 mg 8 hourly once the euthyroid state has been achieved. Iatrogenic hypothyroidism may be prevented by the administration of a small dose of T4 in a so-called blocking/replacement regimen. Patients must be followed-up carefully, with regular clinical assessment and measurement of thyroid function tests. All patients should be warned concerning side effects, particularly those relating to effects on the bone marrow resulting in leucopenia, agranulocytosis and aplastic anaemia. Instructions are given to discontinue carbimazole and seek medical advice immediately should buccal ulceration or a sore throat develop. Other side effects include rashes, pruritus, arthritis and nausea.

Propylthiouracil is more widely used in the USA than elsewhere and can be used effectively if *mild* side effects have occurred with carbimazole. The other major indication for administration of antithyroid drugs is to render the patient euthyroid once a decision has been made to proceed with surgery.

β-Adrenergic blockers

Many of the manifestations of hyperthyroidism, particularly those relating to the cardiovascular system, can be ameliorated by the administration of β-blockers, such as propranolol. This agent also reduces peripheral conversion of T4 to T3. β-Blockers are usually used in combination with one of the thionamides, particularly in patients who are severely toxic and in those being prepared for surgery. The usual dose of propranolol is 20–40 mg 8 hourly. New long-acting β-blockers can be administered once daily. β-Blockers are absolutely contraindicated in patients with asthma. When used as preoperative preparation, propranolol must not be omitted on the morning of surgery and must be continued for at least 5 days postoperatively because of the 8-day half-life of circulating T4.

Radioactive iodine

^{131}I can be used to control thyrotoxicosis by destruction of overactive thyroid tissue. There would seem to be no adverse effects of ^{131}I treatment with respect to leukaemia, thyroid carcinoma, fetal damage or genetic mutation, and in the USA the therapy is even given to children. ^{131}I (555 MBq) is administered as an ablative dose and the patient covered with carbimazole 10 mg t.d.s. started 3 days after the administration and continued for approximately 1 month to counter the effects of thyroid hormone release which might precipitate a thyroid crisis. Although some patients require additional doses of ^{131}I as a result of an inadequate initial response, most patients will be cured of toxicity. An ablative dose (555 MBq) renders more than 60% of patients hypothyroid in 1 year.[61] Regular long-term surveillance is required and T4 replacement given as necessary. Thyroid eye disease may worsen after radioactive iodine treatment. Steroids should be given to reduce this risk.

Surgery

Thyroidectomy in patients with Graves' disease is safe and rapidly renders the patient euthyroid. The principal indications for surgery are:

- Relapse after an adequate course of antithyroid drugs
- Severe thyrotoxicosis with a large goitre

- Difficulty in controlling toxicity with antithyroid drugs (including poor compliance)
- High T4 concentrations (>70 pmol l^{-1})

Surgery would be offered to most patients under 40 years of age fulfilling the above criteria.

Operative strategy

Details of thyroidectomy are covered in the section dealing specifically with surgical technique, but essentially the procedure is one of bilateral subtotal thyroidectomy, leaving a 3–4 g posterior remnant of thyroid tissue on each side of the trachea. When there is a very small goitre (less than 20 g), much smaller remnants should be left.

Special circumstances in Graves' disease

Children

Treatment should be started with antithyroid drugs and continued for no more than 12–18 months. When treatment is discontinued, relapse may follow in up to 50% of patients. These children are usually candidates for surgery, and the resection must be more radical than in adults because remnant growth and recurrent hyperthyroidism are more likely.

Pregnancy

Hyperthyroidism occurring in pregnancy[62] poses a difficult management problem. Radioactive iodine is absolutely contraindicated. Antithyroid drugs are used, propylthiouracil being the drug of choice as it crosses the placenta less readily than carbimazole. Once control of thyrotoxicosis has been achieved, the dose of antithyroid drugs should be reduced as far as possible and the thyroid status of the mother carefully measured. A blocking/replacement regimen must not be used as T4 does not cross the placenta in sufficient amounts to avoid fetal hypothyroidism. In a patient still requiring high doses of antithyroid drugs or in whom hyperthyroidism is difficult to control, surgery may be safely performed in the second trimester.

Recurrent hyperthyroidism after surgery

Further surgery is not indicated as it is likely to be unsuccessful and carries a significant risk of damage to recurrent laryngeal nerves and parathyroid glands. Over the age of 40, ^{131}I is the treatment of choice, whereas under 40 years of age, antithyroid drugs are prescribed in the hope of achieving lasting remission.

Neonatal hyperthyroidism

TsAbs crossing the placenta may stimulate the fetal thyroid, to produce transient hyperthyroidism.[63] Active supportive treatment with antithyroid drugs is necessary and the whole process is usually self-limiting within a period of 1–2 months.

Ophthalmic Graves' disease

The effect of surgery on this condition is somewhat unpredictable, although in the past total thyroidectomy has been advocated in an attempt to arrest the progress of the eye disease. Patients must be warned that effective treatment of the thyrotoxicosis is not a guarantee that ophthalmopathy will regress. Mild symptoms can be treated by the administration of methyl cellulose eye drops, but more severe disease may require steroids, lateral tarsorrhaphy or even orbital decompression.

Toxic multinodular goitre

Antithyroid drugs are of no value as a long-term treatment because toxicity is due to autonomy and will recur once any medication is discontinued. ^{131}I can be used for small goitres, but usually a subtotal thyroidectomy is most appropriate after achievement of the euthyroid state with antithyroid drugs.

Toxic solitary nodule

This condition, caused by a single autonomous thyroid nodule, can be treated by either a unilateral thyroid lobectomy or ^{131}I.

Follow-up

Because of the risk of developing postoperative hypothyroidism, patients who have undergone any form of treatment for hyperthyroidism must be followed-up on a long-term basis, with regular clinical and biochemical assessment.

Thyroiditis

The thyroid gland may be subject to inflammatory change in a variety of conditions, which may be focal or diffuse and often associated with thyroid dysfunction.

Subacute thyroiditis

This condition, often called granulomatous or de Quervain's thyroiditis, is probably of viral origin. It is characterised by painful swelling of one or both thyroid lobes, with associated malaise and fever. Often there is a preceding history of sore throat or viral infection a week or two before the onset of thyroid symptoms. Approximately one third of patients are asymptomatic apart from enlargement of the thyroid gland, but 10–15% have a more acute illness with symptoms and signs of hyperthyroidism resulting from the outpouring of thyroid hormones into the circulation from the damaged inflamed thyroid. Thyroid hormone concentrations are increased, but in contrast to Graves' disease there is low uptake of radioactive iodine on scintigraphy. The erythrocyte sedimentation rate is invariably raised. The disease process of subacute thyroiditis is usually self-limiting, with resolution of local symptoms and thyroid dysfunction. A few patients, however, pass through a mild hypothyroid phase. Local symptoms can be controlled with aspirin but, if severe and prolonged, a course of steroids can be helpful. The transient hyperthyroidism does not require treatment with antithyroid drugs.

Autoimmune thyroiditis

Focal thyroiditis is often seen in association with other thyroid disease, particularly Graves' hyperthyroidism, and is a common finding in autopsy studies. A condition of lymphomatous thyroiditis was described by Hashimoto and occurs as a diffuse process throughout the gland, which usually enlarges to several times normal size. Although classically the gland enlargement is diffuse, there may be nodularity and lobulation making the distinction from simple multinodular goitre or even malignant disease difficult. Histologically there is infiltration of the thyroid by lymphocytes and plasma cells, frequently secondary lymphoid nodules and adjacent stromal fibrosis. The condition is due to an immunological disorder characterised by thyroid antibodies (antithyroglobulin and antimicrosomal (TPO)) in the serum. A positive family history of other autoimmune disease such as pernicious anaemia, gastritis, vitiligo, diabetes mellitus, Addison's disease, autoimmune liver disease and thyrotoxicosis is often obtained.[64] As a result of destructive changes within the infiltrated thyroid, hypothyroidism usually ensues and when present requires treatment with T4. This medication suppresses TSH and leads to shrinkage of the thyroid gland with relief of any local symptoms. Pressure symptoms and involvement of adjacent structures are rare and surgery is usually not required. Occasionally a satisfactory reduction in the size of the goitre can be achieved by the administration of steroids. The risk of developing lymphoma of the thyroid, although small, is increased several times in the presence of Hashimoto's thyroiditis.[51] When a gland which is involved with autoimmune disease is seen to enlarge rapidly or develop a firm asymmetrical nodular area, exclusion of lymphoma by FNAC or core biopsy is required.

Riedel's thyroiditis

This condition, sometimes called invasive fibrous thyroiditis, is characterised by a dense fibrous inflammatory infiltrate throughout the gland, sometimes extending through the capsule to involve adjacent structures. The condition is rare but is important because the clinical picture mimics thyroid malignancy. Sclerosing cholangitis and retroperitoneal, mediastinal and retro-orbital fibrosis may coexist.

Needle biopsy is likely to be uninformative, and often an open incision biopsy is required to establish a precise diagnosis. Surgical resection of the isthmus will be required to free a compromised airway. Steroid medication has been tried without much success, and recently there have been reports of benefit from tamoxifen.[65]

Acute suppurative thyroiditis

The thyroid gland can be affected by a variety of bacterial or fungal agents, producing clinical features of an acute painfully inflamed organ. Confirmation of diagnosis and bacteriology is obtained by needle aspiration and appropriate antibiotics administered. The condition is rare in Western practice.

Postpartum thyroiditis

Postpartum thyroiditis[66] is now recognised much more often and is characterised by an early thyrotoxic phase usually with mild symptoms and transient dysfunction.[67] There is a later hypothyroid phase, sometimes requiring treatment with T4, long-term hypothyroidism occurring in up to 25% of patients.

Developmental abnormalities of the thyroid

Thyroglossal cyst

This condition results from persistence of part of the thyroglossal duct and is usually found as a midline cyst (occasionally more laterally) just below the hyoid bone or above the thyroid cartilage. Less commonly the cyst is found at a higher level above the hyoid bone. The essential diagnostic feature is that of upward movement on swallowing, and because of the attachment of the thyroglossal tract to the foramen caecum, the cyst rises on protrusion of the tongue. These cysts are prone to infection and therefore should be excised. The most appropriate and successful operation is the Sistrunk's procedure, with excision of the central portion of the hyoid bone. Malignancy, usually of a papillary type, can occur within the thyroglossal cyst as a primary phenomenon.[68]

Thyroglossal fistula

This results from infection or inadequate removal of a thyroglossal cyst, the opening being found at a lower level in the neck than the original cyst. Complete excision of the fistula is achieved by careful tracing of the tract superiorly to the foramen caecum and excision of the central portion of the hyoid bone.

Lingual thyroid

When the thyroid gland fails to descend it may be found in the back of the tongue close to the foramen caecum. If large it can result in respiratory or swallowing difficulties and haemorrhage. Diagnosis is confirmed by radioactive iodine scanning, and treatment with T4 should result in shrinkage. Radioactive iodine is an alternative therapeutic measure and excision is rarely necessary.

Ectopic thyroid

Arrested descent of the thyroid results in the gland being found at any point along the line of the thyroglossal tract, and in these circumstances this may be the only thyroid tissue present. If excision is carried out, full replacement T4 dosage is required.

Hypothyroidism

Hypothyrodism is a hypometabolic state resulting from insufficient thyroid hormone or a resistance of the tissues to T4. Causes can be classified as congenital, to which the term cretinism is usually applied, and acquired (adult type). Retardation of growth and mental development are the serious features of hypothyroidism in the infant. The child fails to thrive, is constipated and displays the classic physical signs of a puffy face, large tongue and protuberant abdomen. In adults the extreme presentation is that of myxoedema, characterised by weight gain, facial puffiness and pallor, dry skin, hair loss, hoarseness of the voice, declining intellect and, in extreme cases, psychiatric disturbance and even coma.

The causes of hypothyroidism are given in **Table 2.4**.

The diagnosis of hypothyroidism is confirmed by measurement of free T4 and T3 concentrations (which will be low in primary hypothyroidism whereas TSH concentrations will be high). Treatment is by T4, starting cautiously in

Primary hypothyroidism
    Thyroid agenesis
    Disorders of thyroid hormone synthesis
    Iodine deficiency
    Dyshormonogenesis
    Antithyroid drugs
    Thyroid gland damage
    Hashimoto's thyroiditis
    Surgical resection of the thyroid
    Radioactive iodine ablation
    Post subacute thyroiditis

Secondary hypothyroidism (pituitary)
    Pituitary tumour
    Autoimmune hypophysitis

Tertiary hypothyroidism (hypothalamic)
    Hypothalamic tumour
    Generalised or peripheral thyroid hormone resistance

Table 2.4 *Causes of hypothyroidism*

myxoedematous and elderly patients (who may already be suffering from heart disease) with a low dose (0.025 mg) increasing gradually over a period of 2–3 months to a full replacement level.

Thyroidectomy

The term 'thyroidectomy' embraces a variety of surgical procedures but the precise procedure should be tailored to the existing pathology (**Table 2.5**).

Unilateral total thyroid lobectomy

After obtaining informed consent from the patient, the preoperative preparation should include examination of the vocal cords by indirect laryngoscopy to exclude an unsuspected, pre-existing unilateral nerve palsy, this being particularly important if the patient has undergone previous thyroid surgery.

General anaesthesia, with endotracheal intubation and muscle relaxation, is used and the patient is placed supine on an operating table tilted 15 degrees upwards at the head end to reduce venous engorgement. Neck extension and access to the thyroid are facilitated by placing a sand bag pillow in the inter-scapular region. The head must be well supported and care taken, particularly in elderly patients, not to over-extend the neck.

A curved skin incision is placed 3–4 cm above the sternal notch, extending laterally to the sternomastoid muscles. The incision is deepened through the platysma, and upper and lower skin flaps are then raised by a combination of sharp and blunt dissection in the plane anterior to the anterior jugular vessels. The upper flap is freed to the level of the thyroid notch and the lower flap to the suprasternal notch. These skin flaps are held apart with two wishbone self-retaining retractors and a midline incision made through the fascia over the thyroid. It is the

Procedures	Indications
Unilateral total lobectomy, including pyramidal lobe and isthmus	Solitary nodules Unilateral multinodular disease
Bilateral subtotal thyroidectomy (unilateral lobectomy and contralateral resection)	Diffuse toxic goitre of Graves' disease Bilateral non-toxic and toxic multinodular goitre Hashimoto's thyroiditis
Total thyroidectomy	Most cases of papillary, follicular and medullary carcinoma
Excision of isthmus	May be only procedure possible in anaplastic carcinoma or lymphoma to free airway Riedels thyroiditis

Table 2.5 *Thyroid surgery*

length of this vertical incision that determines access to the thyroid. The strap muscles will be separated, dissected from the thyroid and retracted laterally. These muscles are not routinely divided. If greater exposure is required to gain safe access to a large or vascular goitre, the strap muscles may be divided.

The thyroid lobe is dislocated and delivered forward by the insertion of the index finger between the thyroid lobe and strap muscles. The middle thyroid veins, if apparent at this stage, should be ligated and divided. Any adhesions lateral to the thyroid lobe are divided by a combination of sharp and blunt dissection and the thyroid lobe retracted further medially, usually with a gauze swab between the operator's thumb and the gland. Tissue forceps must not be placed on the thyroid when performing surgery for a solitary nodule, in case the lesion should prove to be malignant and cell spillage occur.

Full mobilisation of the thyroid lobe is then achieved by ligation and division of the superior thyroid vessels at the upper pole. To gain access to these vessels it is often helpful to pass a finger upwards in the plane behind the vessels, breaking down adhesions, and then with gentle downward traction on the thyroid the vessels come clearly into view. The space medial to the superior thyroid artery is carefully opened with a pledget or artery forceps to expose the external branch of the superior laryngeal nerve (ESLN), which is usually easily identified on the inferior pharyngeal constrictor before entering the cricothyroid muscle. A non-toothed forcep is then passed under the vascular pedicle to lift the vessels forward. The branches of the superior thyroid artery and vein must be individually tied close to the thyroid gland to avoid damage to the ESLN. In approximately 20% of patients, this nerve may pass between the branches of the vessels and is in great danger if mass ligation is carried out (**Fig. 2.19**). In a further 20% of patients the nerve runs its distal course through the inferior pharyngeal constrictor muscle, is not visible at surgery and is at no risk of damage.

The recurrent laryngeal nerve (RLN) should now be identified before continuing with dissection of the thyroid lobe. The nerve may run close to the tracheo-oesophageal groove but there is enormous variability of its position, course and relationship to key anatomical structures in the neck. If damage is to be avoided, an accurate knowledge of the normal anatomy and these variations is of paramount importance. Palpation of the RLN as a cord-like structure against the trachea is often a useful initial guide to the nerve's location. The nerve can then be exposed by gentle dissection of the overlying fascial layers with a small artery clip. The nerve often has a small blood vessel running on its surface. Vulnerability is somewhat greater on the right than on the left because of the obliquity of the nerve's course in the lower third of the wound. The nerve usually lies deep to the inferior thyroid artery but can be rendered vulnerable by anterior fixation in a fork formed by the glandular branches of this artery (**Fig. 2.20**). Precise definition of the nerve/artery relationship is most important. A potential

Figure 2.19
The external superior laryngeal nerve (ESLN) passing medial to the superior thyroid artery before entering the cricothyroid muscle. The ESLN is in a vulnerable position when passing between branches of superior thyroid artery (see inset).

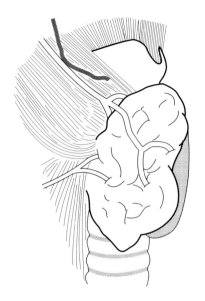
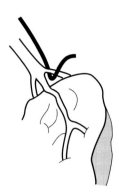

Figure 2.20
Recurrent laryngeal nerve held in a vulnerable anterior position by fork of inferior thyroid artery branches.

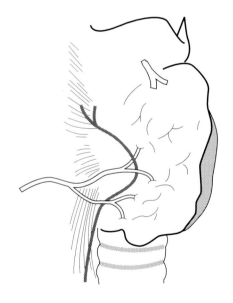

pitfall for the unwary exists when the RLN passes superficial to the inferior thyroid artery, appears to pulsate and may therefore be mistaken for a vessel and ligated.

The RLN can be displaced from its usual position by nodules, particularly in the posterior part of the thyroid lobe and occasionally is displaced anteriorly, close to the lower pole of the thyroid into a dangerous position where it may be ligated and divided with the inferior thyroid veins. Clearly these veins must not be clipped until the nerve has been identified in its lower third. During unilateral lobectomy, the small arterial branches to the thyroid must all be individually clipped and tied close to the gland, staying on the thyroid capsule. The main inferior thyroid artery trunk is not ligated.

The nerve is perhaps in most danger close to its point of entry into the larynx as it passes through Berry's ligament, often adopting a curving, looping course before entering the larynx. To identify the nerve in this region the suspensory fascia must be carefully divided. This manoeuvre is most safely accomplished by staying close to the thyroid and picking up superficial layers one at a time with fine haemostats, being absolutely certain that at each stage only fascia and small arterial branches are included. The nerve is soon seen at a deeper level, glistening, with its fine accompanying arterial blood vessel aiding identification. The inferior cornu of the thyroid cartilage is a most dependable land mark for the point of entry of the RLN into the larynx.

In approximately 1% of patients the nerve on the right is non-recurrent, arising from the vagus and passing medially close to the inferior thyroid artery before turning to ascend and enter the larynx (**Fig. 2.21**). Ligation of the main trunk of the inferior thyroid artery in these circumstances could result in permanent damage to the nerve. It is well recognised that the RLN can divide into several branches before entering the larynx and therefore clear identification of all divisions is necessary for their preservation.

Figure 2.21
Non-recurrent laryngeal nerve passing in close proximity to the inferior thyroid artery before ascending to the larynx.

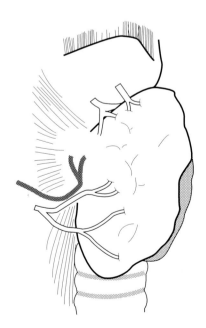

The parathyroid glands must now be identified. When they are in their usual positions, the inferior gland can be located close to the lower pole of the thyroid anterior to the RLN. The superior gland is usually seen just above the inferior thyroid artery, in more than 90% of patients being within a 1 cm radius of the junction of the inferior thyroid artery and the RLN. The dissection of the thyroid should continue close to the capsule of the gland, with ligation and division of the individual branches of the inferior thyroid artery, preserving those branches that supply the parathyroid glands. It is possible to tease the parathyroid glands away from the thyroid with their blood supply intact, leaving them free but perfectly viable. It must be remembered that enlargement of the thyroid can carry the parathyroid glands far forward onto the anterolateral surface of the thyroid when they may be devascularised or inadvertently excised. In these circumstances they should be diced into 1 mm cubes and autotransplanted into several pockets in the sternomastoid muscle.

It is important to keep diathermy usage to a minimum as heat conduction may damage the RLN, the blood supply to the parathyroids or the delicate joints within the larynx.

The thyroid lobe is now almost completely free and is dissected further medially by dividing the vascular fascia binding it to the trachea and larynx. The division of Berry's ligament is completed, taking care to re-identify the RLN. Small vessels close to the nerve at this point require careful clipping and ligation otherwise troublesome bleeding may obscure the nerve's entry point to the larynx. Indeed, safe thyroidectomy is utterly dependent on careful haemostasis as it is only by this discipline that the RLN and parthyroid glands can be identified and left undamaged.

Mobilisation of the thyroid lobe is now complete, and the resection must include the isthmus and pyramidal lobe. The cut surface of the contralateral thyroid lobe is usually sutured to the trachea with vicryl to obtain haemostasis.

The sand bag pillow is removed and the neck space re-examined for bleeding. A valsalva maroeuvre can be useful to unmask occult bleeding. The wound is closed in layers with absorbable material to the muscle layers, and the skin is closed with a subcuticular prolene suture or skin clips, which can be removed at 3 days.

Total thyroidectomy

Total thyroidectomy is usually performed for cancer but occasionally for gross multinodular disease, and the opposite lobe will be mobilised in a similar manner to that described for unilateral lobectomy. If the procedure is for cancer an appropriate lymph node clearance will also be necessary.

Subtotal thyroidectomy

When subtotal thyroidectomy is performed, perhaps for Graves' disease, the principles of identification of the vital structures are the same as those employed in a unilateral total lobectomy. In Graves' disease a small remnant, usually 3–4 g, of tissue is left *in situ* on each side of the trachea and haemostasis secured by suturing the lateral edge of each remnant, without tension, to the anterior surface of the trachea with vicryl. As in unilateral lobectomy, the main trunk of the inferior thyroid artery is not ligated, but individual small bleeding vessels on the surface of the remnant may require ligation. Unilateral total lobectomy and a contralateral resection leaving a larger single remnant may be an acceptable alternative strategy.

Recent minimally invasive endoscopic techniques have been adapted to permit thyroidectomy, usually by performing a unilateral lobectomy for benign disease. The precise role and relevance of this technique in the management of thyroid disease remains to be defined.

Retrosternal goitre

Retrosternal goitres derive their blood supply from the superior and inferior thyroid arteries, and these are usually accessible in the neck. Ligation and division of the superior pole vessels is an essential, preliminary step before mobilisation of the gland is attempted. The retrosternal portion can then be delivered from behind the sternum by gentle traction aided by the introduction of a finger alongside the gland. Placement of traction sutures in the thyroid or the gentle introduction of a dessert spoon alongside the gland may also facilitate delivery. Median sternotomy is rarely necessary to remove a retrosternal thyroid.

Recurrent goitre

Surgery for recurrent thyroid disease is particularly hazardous with respect to damage to the RLN and parathyroid gland, as identification of these structures is likely to be impeded by the presence of scar tissue. A lateral approach to the thyroid lobe to be resected can be gained by dissecting in the plane between the strap muscles and the anterior border of the sternomastoid where there may be fewer adhesions.

Complications of thyroidectomy

The most important complications of thyroidectomy are shown in **Table 2.6**. Those complications relating to damaged individual structures can be kept to a minimum by operating in a bloodless field and performing a meticulous anatomical dissection.

RLN

Damage to the RLN should be extremely rare after routine thyroidectomy,[69] although the risk of damage is increased when performing reoperative thyroid

Recurrent laryngeal nerve injury
External superior laryngeal nerve injury
Hypoparathyroidism
Laryngeal oedema—airway obstruction
Bleeding—haematoma
Hypothyroidism
Hyperthyroidism
Wound infection
Keloid
Suture granuloma

Table 2.6 Complications of thyroid surgery

surgery.[70] Identification of the RLN at surgery is the fundamental step to avoiding damage. When this policy is employed, any nerve damage is likely to be a transient neuropraxia and recovery will be expected, usually after a period of a few weeks or months. If the nerve has not been identified, then paralysis will be permanent in up to one third of patients whose nerves have been injured. Extremely low nerve injury rates have been reported, even when performing extensive surgery for thyroid cancer.[71]

ESLN

Assessment of damage to the ESLN is difficult as the changes may be subtle and easily overlooked. Disability results in changes of voice pitch, range and fatiguability and particularly affects the quality of the signing voice. The nerve is most likely to be damaged at the time of ligation and division of the superior thyroid vessels.[72] To avoid this complication the arterial branches should be individually ligated close to the thyroid and the nerve identified whenever possible.

Hypoparathyroidism

This complication can be avoided by careful identification of the parathyroid glands and preservation of their delicate arterial blood supply. In bilateral subtotal resection for Graves' disease, the incidence of hypoparathyroidism should be no more than 0.5%. The complication is more common after total thyroidectomy for cancer but even in these circumstances the incidence has been reported within the range of only 1–3%.[72]

Hypothyroidism

This sequel of thyroidectomy is most likely to occur after surgery for Graves' disease, with an incidence as high as 50%. This is not a true complication but an acceptable feature of the treatment of hyperthyroidism and is easily managed by the administration of T4.

Recurrent hyperthyroidism

If this occurs after surgery for Graves' disease, it represents a failure of the operation. The incidence is approximately 5% and varies depending on the size of the thyroid remnants left *in situ*, the complex immunological processes taking place in primary hyperthyroidism and iodine intake.

Thyroid crisis

This potentially life-threatening condition is rarely seen but classically occurs in the postoperative period in patients who have undergone surgery for thyrotoxicosis without adequate preoperative preparation. Hormones released by gland manipulation result in an acute postoperative thyrotoxicosis. The condition may also result from stress, infection or other unrelated surgery in the untreated undiagnosed thyrotoxic patient. The clinical picture is one of:

- Extreme distress
- Dyspnoea
- Tachycardia
- Hyperpyrexia
- Restlessness
- Confusion
- Delirium
- Vomiting
- Diarrhoea

Propylthiouracil (200–250 mg) is given every 4 hours, by nasogastric tube if necessary, and Lugol's iodine 0.3 ml p.o. 8 hourly or sodium iodide 1.5 g i.v. over 24 hours should be given, starting an hour later. Adrenergic effects are treated by careful administration of propranolol 1–2 mg i.v. under ECG-monitored control. General supportive measures consist of rehydration with intravenous fluids, cooling with ice packs, the administration of oxygen, digoxin if there is evidence of cardiac failure, appropriate sedation and corticosteroids.

Haemorrhage

Bleeding into the wound is a serious complication of thyroidectomy. When the bleeding and haematoma occur deep to the strap muscles, the situation can rapidly develop into a life-threatening emergency because of associated airway obstruction resulting from laryngeal and subglottic oedema.

Airway obstruction

Although mortality from thyroidectomy is extremely rare today, airway obstruction remains the most potentially dangerous complication. It was once thought that airway obstruction caused by postoperative bleeding was due to compression of the trachea by the expanding haematoma. This is unlikely to be the case except in the rare condition of tracheomalacia. It is subglottic and laryngeal mucosal oedema consequent upon venous and lymphatic obstruction that occludes the airway. It must be appreciated that airway obstruction can occur by this mechanism as a result of operative manipulation of the trachea without any postoperative bleeding or haematoma deep to the strap muscles. It is crucial that early signs of airway obstruction (patient distress and stridor) should be recognised and immediate action taken. If symptoms are mild and there is no haematoma, conservative measures of humidified oxygen and intravenous steroids may suffice. A senior anaesthetist must be consulted immediately, because intubation may subsequently prove necessary to restore an occluding airway. If a skilled anaesthetist is not immediately available, the situation can be retrieved by insertion of a Medicut 12 (blue) needle percutaneously directly into the trachea. Any obvious haematoma should be evacuated, and this should ideally be performed under general anaesthesia with endotracheal intubation in the operating room. Rarely is it necessary to remove sutures on the ward.

Wound complications

The use of absorbable suture material has virtually abolished the complication of suture granuloma after thyroidectomy. Keloid scars may still occur in susceptible individuals.

References

1. Beever K, Bradbury J, Phillips D *et al*. Highly sensitive assays of autoantibodies to thyroglobulin and to thyroid peroxidase. Clin Chem 1989; 35: 1949–54.

2. van Herle AJ, Uller RP. Elevated serum thyroglobulin: a marker of metastases in differentiated thyroid carcinoma. J Clin Invest 1975; 56: 270–7.

3. Doullay F, Ruf J, Codaccioni JL *et al*. Prevalence of autoantibodies to thyroperoxidase in patients with various thyroid and autoimmune diseases. Autoimmunity 1991; 9: 237–44.

4. Rees-Smith B, McLachlan SM, Furmaniak J. Autoantibodies to the thyrotropin receptor. Endocr Rev 1988; 9: 106–21.

5. Melvin KEW, Tashjian AH. The syndrome of excessive thyrocalcitonin produced by medullary carcinoma of the thyroid. Proc Natl Acad Sci USA 1968; 59: 1216–22.

6. Mulligan LM, Kwok JBJ, Healey CS *et al*. Germ-line mutations of the RET proto oncogene in multiple endocrine neoplasia type IIA. Nature 1993; 363: 458–60.

7. Turner JW, Spencer RB. Thyroid carcinoma presenting as a pertechnetate hot nodule without ^{131}I uptake. Case report. J Nucl Med 1976; 17: 22–3.

8. Ochi H, Yamamoto K, Endo K *et al*. A new imaging agent for medullary carcinoma of the thyroid. J Nucl Med 1984; 25: 323–5.

9. Hoefnagal CA, Delprat CC, Marcuse HR *et al*. Role of thallium-201 total-body scintigraphy in follow up of thyroid carcinoma. J Nucl Med 1986; 27: 1854–7.

10. Clarke SEM, Lazarus CR, Wraight P *et al*. Pentavalant (99 mTc) DMSA, ^{131}I MIBG, and (99 mTc) MDP. An evaluation of three imaging techniques in patients with medullary carcinoma of the thyroid. J Nucl Med 1988; 29: 33–8.

11. Rosen IB, Walfish PG, Miskin M. The ultrasound of thyroid masses. Surg Clin North Am 1979; 59: 19–33.

12. Rosen IB, Wallace D, Strawbridge HG *et al*. Re-evaluation of needle aspiration cytology in detection of thyroid cancer. Surgery 1981; 90: 747–56.

13. Miller JH. Needle biopsy of the thyroid: methods and recommendations. Thyroid Today 1982; 5: 1–5.

14. Soderstrom N. Aspiration biopsy punctures of goitres for aspiration and biopsy. Acta Med Scand 1952; 144: 237–44.

 15. **Lowhagen T, Granberg PO, Lundell G et al. Aspiration biopsy cytology (ABC) in nodules of the thyroid gland suspected to be malignant. Surg Clin North Am 1979; 59: 3–18.**

 16. **Grant CS, Hay ID, Gough IR et al. Long term follow up of patients with benign thyroid FNA cytologic diagnosis. Surgery 1989; 106: 980–91.**

17. Gaitin E, Nelson NC, Poole GV. Endemic goitre and endemic thyroid disorders. World J Surg 1991; 15: 205–15.

18. Gaitin E. Aetiology of benign thyroid disease— environmental aspects. In Wheeler MH, Lazarus JH eds. Diseases of the thyroid. Pathophysiology and management. London: Chapman & Hall Medical, 1994: 73–84.

19. Vander JB, Gaston EA, Dawber TR. The significance of non toxic thyroid nodules: final report of a 15 year study of the incidence of thyroid malignancy. Ann Intern Med 1968; 69: 537–40.

20. Hellwig CA. Thyroid gland in Kansas. Am J Clin Pathol 1935; 5: 103–11.

21. Hayles AB, Johnson LM, Beahrs OH et al. Carcinoma of the thyroid in children. Am J Surg 1963; 106: 735–43.

22. Harness JK, Thompson NW, Nishiyama RH. Childhood thyroid carcinoma. Arch Surg 1971; 102: 278–84.

23. Cuello C, Correa P, Eisenberg H. Geographic pathology of thyroid carcinoma. Cancer 1969; 23: 230–9.

24. Williams ED, Doniach I, Bjarnason O et al. Thyroid cancer in an iodine rich area: a histopathological study. Cancer 1977; 39: 215–22.

25. Duffy BJ, Fitzgerald PJ. Cancer of the thyroid in children: a report of 28 cases. J Clin Endocrinol Metab 1950; 10: 1296–1308.

26. DeGroot LJ, Paloyan E. Thyroid carcinoma and radiation: a Chicago endemic. JAMA 1973; 225: 487–91.

27. Naunheim KS, Kaplan EL, Straus FH et al. High dose external radiation to the neck and subsequent thyroid carcinoma. In Kaplan EL (ed). Surgery of the thyroid and parathyroid glands. Edinburgh: Churchill Livingstone, 1983: 51–62.

28. Henry JF, Denizot A, Porcelli A et al. Thyroperoxidase immunodetection for the diagnosis of malignancy on fine-needle aspiration of thyroid nodules. World J Surg 1994; 18: 529–34.

29. Delbridge L, Lean CL, Russell P et al. Proton magnetic resonance and human thyroid neoplasia II: potential avoidance of surgery for benign follicular neoplasms. World J Surg 1994; 18: 512–7.

 30. **Reeve TS, Delbridge L, Cohen A. Total thyroidectomy: the prefered option for multinodular goitre. Ann Surg 1987; 206: 782–6.**

31. Thompson NW, Nishiyama RH, Harness JK. Thyroid carcinoma. Current controversies. Curr Probl Surg 1978; 15: 1–67.

32. Thompson NW. In Johnston IDA, Thompson NW (eds). The thyroid nodule: surgical management in endocrine surgery. London: Butterworths, 1983: 14–24.

33. Reeve TS. Operations for non medullary cancer of the thyroid gland. In Kaplan EL (ed.) Surgery of the thyroid and parathyroid glands. Edinburgh: Churchill Livingstone, 1983: 63–74.

34. Wynford Thomas D. Molecular basis of epithelial tumorigenesis: the thyroid model. Crit Rev Oncogen 1993; 4: 1–23.

35. Lemoine NR, Mayall ES, Wyllie FS et al. High frequency of Ras oncogene activation in all stages of human thyroid tumorigenesis. Oncogene 1989; 4: 159–64.

36. Lemoine NR, Hughes CM, Gullick WJ et al. Abnormalities of the EGF receptor system in human thyroid neoplasia. Int J Cancer 1991; 49: 558–61.

37. Fagin JA, Matsuo K, Karmakar A et al. High prevalence of mutations of the P53 gene in poorly differentiated human thyroid carcinomas. J Clin Invest 1993; 91: 179–84.

38. Lote K, Anderson K, Nordal E et al. Familial occurrence of papillary thyroid carcinoma. Cancer 1980; 46: 1291–7.

39. Pasieka JL, Thompson NW, McLeod MK et al. The incidence of bilateral well differentiated thyroid cancer found at completion thyroidectomy. World J Surg 1992; 16: 711–6.

40. McConahey WM, Hay ID, Woolner LB et al. Papillary thyroid cancer treated at the Mayo Clinic, 1946 through 1970: initial manifestations, pathologic findings, therapy and outcome. Mayo Clin Proc 1986; 61: 978–96.

 41. **Noguchi S, Yamashita H, Murakami N et al. Small carcinomas of the thyroid—a long term follow up of 867 patients. Arch Surg 1996; 131: 187–91.**

42. Thompson NW. Differentiated thyroid carcinoma. In Wheeler MH, Lazarus JH (eds). Diseases of the thyroid, pathophysiology and management. London: Chapman & Hall Medical, 1994: 367–77.

43. Ozaki O, Ito K, Kobayashi K et al. Familial occurrence of differentiated non medullary thyroid carcinoma. World J Surg 1988; 12: 565–71.

44. Thompson NW. Total thyroidectomy in the treatment of thyroid carcinoma. In Endocrine surgical update. New York: Grune & Stratton, 1983: 71–84.

45. Stephenson BM, Wheeler MH, Clark OH. The role of total thyroidectomy in the management of differentiated thyroid cancer. In Daly JM (ed.). Current opinion in general surgery. Philadelphia: Current Science, 1994: 53–9.

46. Hay ID, Grant CS, Taylor WF et al. Ipsilateral lobectomy versus bilateral lobe resection in papillary thyroid carcinoma: a retrospective analysis of surgical outcome using a novel prognostic scoring system. Surgery 1987; 102: 1088–95.

 47. Mazzaferri EL, Young RL. Papillary thyroid carcinoma: a 10 year follow up report of the impact of therapy in 576 patients. Am J Med 1981; 70: 511–8.

48. Spencer CA, Takeuchi M, Kazarosyan M et al. Serum thyroglobulin autoantibodies: prevalence, influence on serum thyroglobulin measurement and prognostic significance in patients with differentiated thyroid carcinoma. J Clin Endocrinol Metab 1998; 83: 1121–7.

49. Vassilopoulou-Sellin R, Kline MJ, Smith TH et al. Pulmonary metastases in children and young adults with differentiated thyroid cancer. Cancer 1993; 71: 1348–52.

50. Backdahl M, Hamberger B, Lowhagen T et al. Anaplastic giant cell thyroid carcinoma. In Wheeler MH, Lazams JH (eds). Diseases of the thyroid. Pathophysiology and management. London: Chapman & Hall, 1994: 379–85.

51. Sirota DK, Segal RL. Primary lymphomas of the thyroid gland. JAMA 1979; 242: 1743–6.

52. Devine RM, Edis AJ, Banks PM. Primary lymphoma of the thyroid: a review of the Mayo Clinic experience through 1978. World J Surg 1981; 5: 33.

53. Hazard JB, Hawk WA, Crile G. Medullary (solid) carcinoma of the thyroid. A clinico-pathologic entity. J Clin Endocrinol Metab 1959; 19: 152–61.

54. Williams ED. Histogenesis of medullary carcinoma of the thyroid. J Clin Pathol 1966; 19: 114–8.

55. Tashjian AH, Howland BG, Melvin KEW et al. Immunoassay of human calcitonin: clinical measurement, relation to serum calcium and studies in patients with medullary carcinoma. N Engl J Med 1970; 283: 890–5.

56. Pyke CM, Hay ID, Goellner JR et al. Prognostic significance of calcitonin immunoreactivity, amyloid staining and flow cytometric DNA measurements in medullary thyroid carcinoma. Surgery 1991; 110: 967–71.

57. Sizemore GW. Medullary carcinoma of the thyroid. Semin Oncol 1987; 14: 306–14.

58. Tunbridge WMG, Evered DC, Hall R et al. The spectrum of thyroid disease in a community: the Wickham survey. Clin Endocrinol 1977; 7: 481–93.

59. Salvatori M, Saletnich I, Rufini V. Severe thyrotoxicosis due to functioning pulmonary metastases of well differentiated thyroid cancer. J Nucl Med 1998; 39: 1202–7.

60. Sheldon J, Reid DJ. Thyrotoxicosis: changing trends in treatment. Ann R Coll Surg Engl 1986; 68: 283–5.

 61. Kendall-Taylor P, Keir MJ, Ross WM. Ablative radioiodine therapy for hyperthyroidism: long term follow up study. BMJ 1984; 289: 361–3.

62. Masiukiewicz US, Burrow GN. Hyperthyroidism in pregnancy: diagnosis and treatment. Thyroid 1999; 9: 647–52.

63. Zimmerman D. Foetal and neonatal hyperthyroidism. Thyroid 1999; 9: 727–33.

64. Furmaniak J, Rees-Smith B. Diagnostic tests of thyroid function and structure—thyroid antibodies. In Wheeler MH, Lazarus JH (eds). Diseases of the thyroid. Pathophysiology and management. London: Chapman & Hall Medical, 1994: 117–30.

65. Few J, Thompson NW, Angelos P et al. Riedels thyroiditis: treatment with taxoxyfen. Surgery 1996; 120: 993–9.

66. Lazarus JH, Othman S. Thyroid disease in relation to pregnancy. Clin Endocrinol 1991; 34: 91–8.

67. Amino N, Miyai K, Onishi T et al. Transient hypothyroidism after delivery in autoimmune thyroiditis. J Clin Endocrinol Metab 1976; 2: 296–301.

68. Stephenson BM, Wheeler MH. Carcinoma of the thyroglossal duct. Aust NZ J Surg 1994; 64: 212.

69. Wade JSH. Vulnerability of the recurrent laryngeal nerves at thyroidectomy. Br J Surg 1955; 43: 164–80.

70. Beahrs OH, Vandertoll DJ. Complications of secondary thyroidectomy. Surg Gynaecol Obstet 1963; 117: 535–9.

71. Clark OH. Total thyroidectomy: the treatment of choice for patients with differentiated thyroid cancer. Ann Surg 1982; 196: 361–70.

72. Lennquist S, Cahlin C, Smeds S. The superior laryngeal nerve in thyroid surgery. Surgery 1987; 102: 999–1008.

3 The adrenal glands

Anthony E. Young
W. James B. Smellie

Adrenal diseases comprise the third commonest group of illness seen by the endocrine surgeon after thyroid and parathyroid disease and as such represent less than 5% of the endocrine surgeon's operative workload. The bulk of the diagnostic preliminaries will have been undertaken by an endocrinologist or general clinician prior to referral, but the complexity of these diseases, the potential for misdiagnosis and the systemic changes that can make surgery dangerous must all be understood by the surgeon, and the communication between surgeon and physician must be of high quality. Surgical adrenal disease essentially falls into two categories:

1. Endocrinologically significant disease of the cortex and medulla, e.g. Conn's syndrome, phaeochromocytoma;
2. Non-functioning tumours; malignant or benign including those incidentally discovered on scanning ('incidentalomas').

These categories will be considered separately, although they are not mutually exclusive. The operative procedure of adrenalectomy is dealt with at the end of the chapter.

The understanding of adrenal endocrine disease is only achievable when the basic physiology of the adrenal cortex and medulla is understood (Figs 3.1–3.3). The knowledge allows a rational testing for endocrine disease and a comprehension of the mechanism of the physical effects that are seen. The adrenal gland consists of two embryologically separate parts. The outer cortex accounts for about 85% of the gland and imparts the characteristically yellow colour seen at operation. It is mesodermal in origin, deriving from coelomic epithelium and is concerned with steroid synthesis and secretion. The inner medulla is derived from neuroectoderm and is responsible for the adrenal component of the sympathoadrenomedullary system.

Figure 3.1
Physiological pathways for the production and control of cortisol secretion.

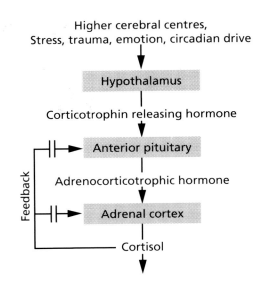

Figure 3.2
Physiological pathways for the production and control of aldosterone secretion.

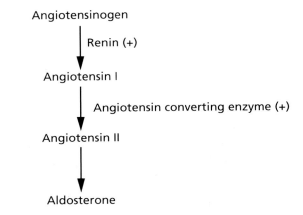

Figure 3.3
Biochemical pathways of the metabolism of adrenaline and noradrenaline.

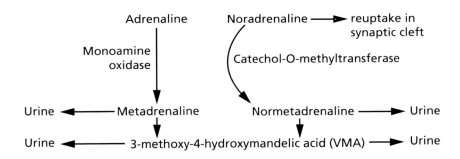

The adrenal cortex

The cortex is separated into three histological layers: the outer zona glomerulosa, which produces mineralocorticoids, e.g. aldosterone; the poorly developed zona fasciculata, which produces glucocorticoids, e.g. cortisol; and the inner zona reticularis, which produces sex steroids. The cortex also contains neuroendocrine fibres responsible for some neural control of endocrine function.

Aldosterone, the predominant mineralocorticoid, is secreted under the control of renin, via angiotensin II. It has the effect of retaining Na^+ and water and causing the loss of K^+ and H^+ from the renal tubules. In the normal adrenal, secretion of the glucocorticoids is under the direct control of adrenocorticotrophic hormone (ACTH). ACTH is secreted from the anterior pituitary gland at a rate determined by the stimulant effect of corticotrophin releasing factor (CRF) and by the inhibitory effect of circulating natural or synthetic glucocorticoids. The rate of release of CRF from the median prominence of the hypothalamus depends on neural stimuli from the brain and is inhibited by glucocorticoids. Glucocorticoids have a wide range of effects on many systems of the body and absence of circulating glucocorticoid is incompatible with life. Adrenal androgen production is under the control of ACTH and possibly a pituitary adrenal androgen-stimulating hormone. The predominant androgen, dehydroepiandrosterone, is weakly androgenic. Another weakly androgenic product, androstenedione, is aromatised outside the adrenal to oestrogen and is an important source of oestrogen in postmenopausal women.

Adrenaline, dopamine and noradrenaline are synthesised in the adrenal medulla from common precursors. The majority of catecholamines are synthesised from dietary tyrosine, although a pathway of conversion of phenylalanine into tyrosine in the liver also exists. The tyrosine is concentrated in the neuroendocrine cells and is converted into dopamine via dihydroxyphenalanine (DOPA) in the ectoplasm. The dopamine is then transported into granulated vesicles and is converted into noradrenaline. Some neurones and adrenal medullary cells contain a further enzyme phenylethanolamine-N-methyltransferase (PNMT) to catalyse the conversion of noradrenaline into adrenaline. The adrenaline is then stored in storage vesicles. Adrenaline and noradrenaline are released in response to direct neural stimuli to the adrenal medulla.

Functioning adrenal abnormalities

These are in the form of benign or malignant tumours or hyperplasia. The categories are as follows.

Cortex

- Cortical tumours; cortisone-secreting tumours leading to Cushing's syndrome; aldosterone-secreting tumours leading to Conn's syndrome; sex hormone-secreting tumours leading to virilisation or feminisation;
- Diffuse hyperplasia either as a primary disease or a consequence of stimulation by trophic hormones leading to hypercortisolism (Cushing's syndrome), hyperaldosteronism (Conn's syndrome), virilisation (adrenogenital syndrome).

Medulla

- Tumours secreting adrenaline/noradrenaline (phaeochromocytoma).

Cushing's syndrome

An excess circulating cortisol concentration leads to physiological and bodily changes, described as Cushing's syndrome. The commonest cause of this is the iatrogenic administration of steroids for the treatment of other disease. This chapter, however, only considers hypercortisolism caused by the following:
Primary adrenal disease

- Adenoma
- Carcinoma
- Primary adrenal hyperplasia—in this rare variant of Cushing's syndrome the hypercortisolism is produced by multiple ACTH independent hyperfunctioning nodules (described as 'macronodular cortical hyperplasia') or by primary pigmented nodular adrenal cortical disease (PPND)

Secondary adrenal disease

- True Cushing's disease, i.e. the disease described by Harvey Cushing in 1932, is adrenocortical hyperplasia due to excess ACTH secretion from a pituitary microadenoma.[1] This is often described as 'pituitary-dependent Cushing's' syndrome;
- Adrenocortical hyperplasia secondary to excess ACTH secretion from a non-pituitary source, 'ectopic ACTH syndrome.'

The incidence of the different causes varies from centre to centre depending on referral patterns, but essentially 50% of Cushing's syndrome is attributable to a primary adrenal source, 25% to primary pituitary disease and 25% to an ectopic source of ACTH.

Clinical presentation

The clinical presentation after iatrogenic administration of steroids is not, in most instances, gross; the patient gains weight, the cheeks become rounded and pink, the patient's appetite increases as does their sense of wellbeing. Slight hirsutism may be noted. Only after long-term high-dose steroid administration do the serious sequelae of muscle weakness, osteoporosis, hypertension and diabetes become problematic. Primary hypercortisolism tends to declare itself late, with the symptoms and signs fully developed. The inexorable slow progression of the signs can often only be appreciated when the family photograph album is produced and the current habitus compared to that of the past. Exceptions to this slow progression are the syndromes produced by an ectopic ACTH source and cortisol-secreting carcinomas when the signs appear rapidly and are severe early. The signs and symptoms of other forms of primary hypercortisolism, together with frequencies, are shown in **Table 3.1**. The detailed changes are complex[2,3] but the overall pattern familiar (**Fig. 3.4**).

Obesity

This may be gross and the patient's body weight may increase by 50%. Weight gain is predominantly truncal, especially in the form of a protuberant abdomen and a 'buffalo hump' on the shoulders. The overall appearances have sometimes been likened to a 'lemon on sticks.' The wasting of the thigh and upper arm muscles and oedema of the ankles contributing to this appearance.

Symptoms	%	Signs	%
Weight gain	71	Obesity	95
Menstrual irregularities	84	Truncal	45
Hirsutism in women	80	Generalised	52
Lethargy/depression	48	Plethora	94
Headache	48	Facial rounding	88
Thirst/frequency	44	Hypertension	84
Backache	41	Bruising	62
Muscular weakness	27	Striae	56
Shortness of breath	26	Buffalo hump	55
Recurrent infections	26	Myopathy	55
Abdominal pain	21	Ankle oedema	47
Fractures	18	Acne	21
Loss of scalp hair	12	Osteoporosis	52

From: Ross EJ, Lynch CD.[3]

Table 3.1 *Presenting symptoms and signs in 70 patients with Cushing's syndrome*

Figure 3.4
The typical stigmata of Cushing's syndrome.

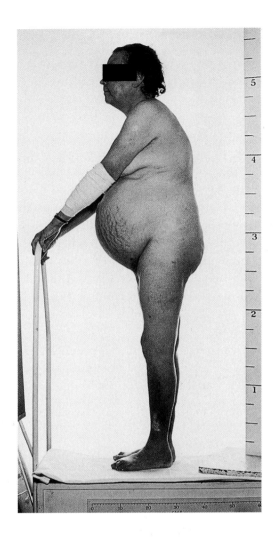

Loss of connective tissue

Thinning of the skin leads to a purple, plethoric face and purple, abdominal striae. The changes in the walls of venules and capillaries allow prompt bleeding in response to trauma, and the lack of subcutaneous connective tissue allows spread of this haemorrhage into large, blotchy haematomas. Blood clotting is normal.

Hirsutism and virilism

In females this is not due to an increased cortisol concentration but to an increase in testosterone concentration. This testosterone originates from excessive synthesis in the adrenal cortex and increased transformation of androstenedione or dehydroepiandrostenedione to testosterone in the periphery. The effect is an increase in the growth of hair, particularly noticeable as facial hair in females. As the disease progresses, the skin becomes oily and acne is prominent. The hair becomes dishevelled and greasy and scalp hair is lost. The typical facies of the patient is one of obesity, plethora, acne, hirsutism and a receding hair line. About 80% of premenopausal women develop menstrual disorders and many develop amenorrhoea.

Whereas plasma testosterone is increased in women, it is decreased in men, as cortisol decreases not only gonadotrophin production but also testicular response to gonadotrophins. Men, therefore, show loss of libido, testicular atrophy and gynaecomastia.

Muscle weakness

Increased protein catabolism occurs predominately in proximal muscle groups, with weakness and loss of muscle bulk. The result is a change in the contour of the body, and the patient has difficulty rising from sitting and difficulty moving around.

Osteoporosis

Cortisol inhibits the development of osteoid and lowers serum calcium concentration, thus producing secondary hyperparathyroidism with increased reabsorption of calcium from bone. This, together with proximal muscle loss, often leads to backache and can even be severe enough to cause crush fractures of vertebrae or spontaneous fractures of other bones.

Hypertension

About 30% of patients with Cushing's syndrome have a degree of hypertension. This is not usually severe, but it may have been present for long enough to lead to a cerebrovascular accident or coronary heart disease.

Glucose intolerance

Glucose intolerance occurs in most patients and may progress to frank diabetes. An increased cortisol concentration reduces the peripheral utilisation of glucose and stimulates gluconeogenesis in the liver. Initially there is a good insulin response, but this eventually fails and the patient becomes frankly diabetic.

Psychological changes

Psychological changes are common and frequently overlooked. They may be interpreted as a natural response to the change in the appearance of the body, to weakness and to malaise. The psychological changes are a genuine, endogenous psychosis in many patients commonly in the form of depression but often with paranoid ideas and even hallucinations. The patient may become retarded and even mimic schizophrenia. Some patients attempt or commit suicide. The usual observation that therapeutic steroids may produce euphoria is not reflected in the patient with overt Cushing's syndrome.

Differential diagnosis

Most fat, plethoric, hairy women with erratic menstrual habits do not have Cushing's syndrome. Biochemical investigation will distinguish those who are simply hypertensive diabetics and those with polycystic ovaries. Greater difficulty may initially be experienced in separating out the depressive who may have an increased cortisol concentration and loss of circadian rhythm or the alcoholic who may also have an increased serum cortisol concentration not suppressible by dexamethasone.

Clinical presentation of ectopic ATCH syndrome

The majority of these patients have a small-cell carcinoma of the lung. The next commonest cause is a carcinoid, usually of the thymus or the lung. Rare causes include medullary carcinoma of the thyroid, and the syndrome has been reported in association with primary carcinomas in most organs of the body. The secretion of corticotrophins is usually high and the symptoms develop rapidly, partly as a consequence of the malignancy and partly because of the Cushing's syndrome. These include weight loss, oedema owing to sodium retention, gross muscle weakness from steroid myopathy combined with paraneoplastic myopathy, pigmentation due to a melanocyte-stimulating hormone-like substance and psychological changes. Investigation usually discloses high circulating cortisol concentrations, glycosuria and marked hypokalaemia.

Occasionally a Cushing's adenoma of the adrenal undergoes spontaneous haemorrhage, and this may be the presenting event (**Fig. 3.5**).

Investigation of Cushing's syndrome

As the clinical presentation does not necessarily define the underlying cause of the Cushing's syndrome, more extensive investigation is usually required. It is important that the surgeon should be involved as early as possible in the diagnostic process. Patients with Cushing's syndrome are often poor candidates for anaesthesia and surgery, and the longer the investigation is allowed to run without a clear treatment plan, the more ill the patient may become. There are three phases to the investigation of a patient with Cushing's syndrome.[4] These are designed to answer three questions:

1. Is it definitely Cushing's syndrome on biochemical testing?
2. Is the primary lesion in the adrenal or pituitary or is it ectopic?
3. What are the anatomical details of the primary lesion?

Figure 3.5
Spontaneous haemorrhage from a large, benign cortisol-producing tumour of the right adrenal. The CT shows not only the tumour but also the haemorrhage filling much of the peritoneal cavity.

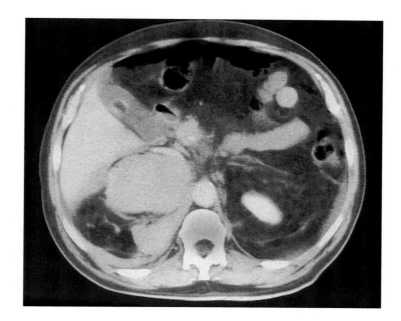

Endocrine investigations

Diagnosis of Cushing's syndrome

The diagnosis of Cushing's syndrome is normally suspected in a patient as a result of the characteristic body habitus and biochemical abnormalities that are associated with the syndrome. A firm diagnosis of Cushing's syndrome depends predominantly on demonstrating a persistent inappropriate increase in serum glucocorticoid concentrations (**Fig. 3.6**). The reason for this increase may be as a result of ACTH-independent hypersecretion of glucocorticoids by the adrenal gland or glands, inappropriately increased ACTH secretion by the pituitary, ACTH secretion from ectopic sources outside the pituitary, inappropriate secretion of CRF or administration of glucocorticoids.

Establishment of the biochemical diagnosis of Cushing's syndrome

Some alternative medicines contain steroids, and it is necessary to take a detailed drug history to exclude exogenous steroid administration. The diagnosis of endogenous Cushing's syndrome depends on demonstrating the loss of normal circadian rhythm as well as a persistent increase in cortisol concentration. It is necessary to take at least three serum samples to demonstrate the loss of rhythm. The mean 24 hour cortisol concentrations can be estimated by collecting and measuring the 24 hour urinary free cortisol (UFC), which gives an integrated measure of the cortisol production. As a screening test, this is 95% accurate.[5,6] Having established the presence of increased serum glucocorticoid concentrations, it is then necessary to establish whether the normal regulation of the hypothalamopituitary–adrenal axis has been disturbed. In a normal individual,

Figure 3.6
Flow chart for the
investigation of
Cushing's syndrome.

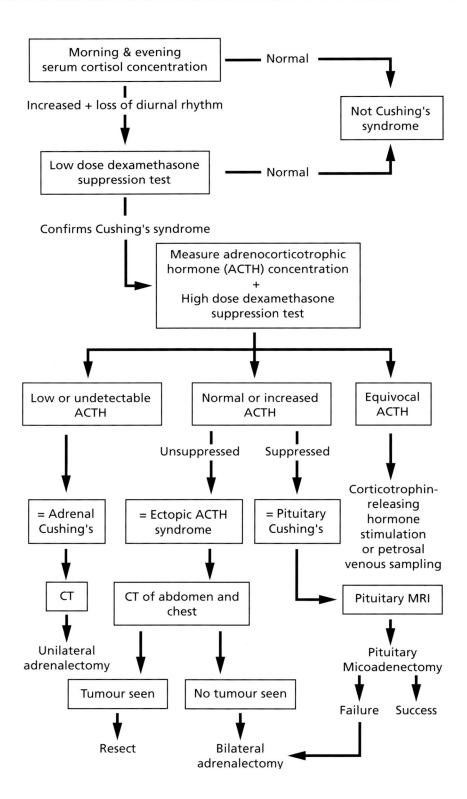

administration of a low dose (1 mg) of dexamethasone results in total suppression of serum cortisol. This suppression is lost in patients with Cushing's syndrome but is normal in patients with obesity in whom an increased UFC has been demonstrated. Patients with psychological depression may also lose cortisol suppression in response to dexamethasone, but the insulin tolerance test will distinguish between these conditions. Patients with Cushing's syndrome are resistant to insulin and therefore do not become hypoglycaemic in response to 0.3 units kg^{-1}. This will usually distinguish between the two conditions. Patients with alcoholic pseudoCushing's syndrome usually have an obvious history and may show deranged liver function tests. The syndrome develops because glucuronation of cortisol is defective owing to liver dysfunction, and hypercortisolism develops secondarily.

Establishment of the cause of Cushing's syndrome

If the ACTH concentration is low, a diagnosis of adrenal disease can be made and the patient imaged to establish the anatomical location of a functioning adrenal neoplasm. If the ACTH concentration is high, a diagnosis of ACTH-dependent adrenal hyperplasia is made and the source of the ACTH must be established. The two tests that are most reliable in determining the source of the ACTH are the corticotrophin-releasing hormone (CRH) test and the high-dose (8 mg) dexamethasone test. Since few ectopic sources of ACTH, e.g. a small-cell carcinoma of the lung, are CRH dependent, the serum ACTH concentration will not increase in patients with an ectopic source after the administration of CRH. Most pituitary adenomas remain CRH dependent, thus patients with Cushing's syndrome (pituitary dependent) will show a rapid increase in serum ACTH concentration in response to CRH. The high-dose dexamethasone test relies on the fact that most patients with pituitary-dependent Cushing's syndrome partially suppress serum cortisol concentrations in response to high doses of exogenous steroids, whereas ectopic sources of ACTH and adrenal tumours do not.

A rare cause of Cushing's syndrome is ectopic CRH production.[7] Nephroblastomas, bronchogenic carcinomas, medullary carcinomas of the thyroid, pancreatic tumours, phaeochromocytomas and pituitary carcinomas can release a peptide with CRH-like activity. These patients seem biochemically as though there is a source of ectopic ACTH.

Primary adrenal hyperplasia is the rarest cause of Cushing's syndrome. The macronodular variant of this hyperplasia is thought to be a result of prolonged stimulation of the glands by ACTH, resulting in the autonomous secretion of cortisol by the adrenal.[8] In PPND there are pigmented micronodules as a result of stimulation by an abnormal immunoglobulin. Carney's syndrome is a cluster of abnormalities, such as mesenchymal tumours, skin pigmentation, peripheral nerve tumours and endocrine abnormalities, including autonomous hypersecreting multinodular adrenal glands.[9]

Imaging in ACTH-dependent Cushing's syndrome

Radiography of the pituitary or chest computed tomography (CT) or magnetic resonance imaging (MRI) of the pituitary or whole body and inferior petrosal venous ACTH assays have been used to localise the source of ACTH.

Anatomical details

Pituitary

Pituitary microadenomas causing Cushing's syndrome are usually small. The overall change in pituitary size cannot, therefore, be seen on conventional skull radiographs even with tomography. CT scanning will identify about 50% of tumours, but the intravenous contrast does not 'light up' microadenomas. Interpretation is confused by the fact that many normal people have non-functioning pituitary microadenomas. Currently the most useful test is MRI with or without gadolinium enhancement. Where there is doubt as to whether high concentrations of ACTH are being secreted by the pituitary or an ectopic source, bilateral inferior petrosal sinus venous sampling may be undertaken.[10] This is, however, technically difficult and very operator dependent. Two catheters must be manipulated by the Seldinger technique from the right femoral vein to the petrosal sinuses and ACTH samples obtained simultaneously from both catheters and from a peripheral vein. These tests are repeated after administration of CRH.

Adrenals

The advent of CT rendered obsolete the assessment of the adrenals by plain radiography with tomography. Ultrasonography is a useful, quick screening test to determine whether there is an adrenal lesion. If this is known early in the investigative process, tests can be targeted to determine if this is the cause of the Cushing's syndrome.

CT is undertaken with contrast and maximum information is obtained if 2 mm slices are taken through the adrenal area (**Fig. 3.7**). A large tumour, with indeterminate edges or areas of necrosis within it, suggests malignancy (**Fig. 3.8**).

MRI is increasingly used to assess the adrenals (**Fig. 3.9**), but is of little additional value over CT when the tumour is small and well circumscribed. It is, however, valuable for very small tumours not clearly defined on CT or in larger tumours where there is a suspicion of malignancy. It is particularly valuable at showing invasion of the vena cava. It has been claimed that there is a higher signal intensity in T2 weighted images with malignant tumours than with benign tumours.

Figure 3.7
CT scan showing an adenoma in the right adrenal gland in association with Cushing's syndrome.

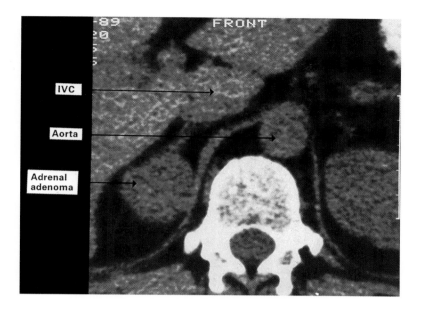

Figure 3.8
CT scan of the abdomen of a patient with gross Cushing's syndrome of rapid onset showing a large tumour of the left adrenal gland with irregular margins and necrosis. This was a malignant tumour.

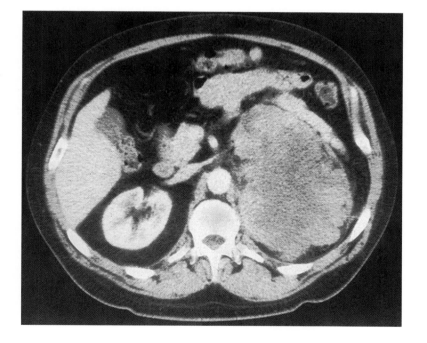

The adrenal cortex can be imaged with scintigraphic cholesterol scans or NP59, but the consequence are a high radiation dose to the adrenals, and the test is best avoided if possible. It is a useful functional test because any nodule will 'light up' on the scintiscan and the other adrenal will be suppressed (Fig. 3.10).

Figure 3.9
MRI scan of a left adrenal tumour showing brightly in relation to surrounding structures.

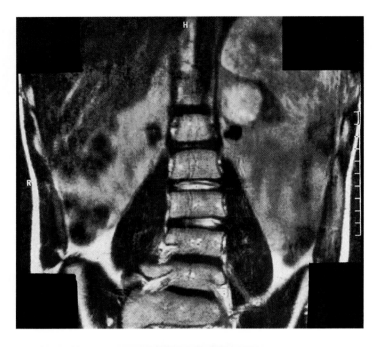

Figure 3.10
Cholesterol scan of the adrenal glands. The bottom left hand image is of the kidneys. The top left image is of the adrenals. The top right scan is of the two other images superimposed to identify the position of the 'hot' spot on the adrenal scan (same patient as Figure 3.7).

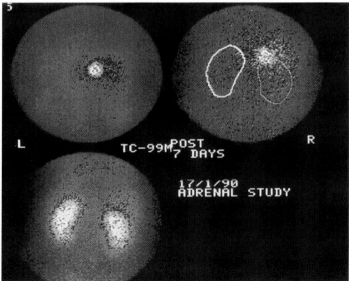

Searching for an ectopic ACTH source

The majority of such tumours will be identifiable on CT of the chest. The smaller ectopic ACTH-producing tumours, particularly carcinoids, may be difficult or impossible to visualise. If a suspicious area is seen on CT or MRI, then angiography, venous sampling or octreotide isotope scanning may help confirm the diagnosis.[11] These tests and results are summarised in **Table 3.2**.

	Serum adrenocorticotrophic hormone (ACTH)	CRH test	High-dose dexamethasone test	CT/MRI of sella	CT/MRI of adrenals	Petrosal sinus sampling	Iodocholesterol scan
Pituitary Cushing's	Normal to mildly increased	+	>50% suppression	+/–	Mild bilateral enlargement or normal	+	+
Ectopic ACTH	Normal to markedly increased	–	No suppression	–	Bilateral enlargement or normal	–	+
Adrenal neoplasms	Undetectable	–	No suppression	–	Unilateral adrenal mass	NA	Adenomas + carcinomas –
Micronodular disease	Undetectable	–	No suppression	–	Minimal diffuse enlargement ('knobby') or normal	–	+/–[a]

[a] At 48 hours, may become positive if studied for longer intervals.
+, positive test; –, negative test; +/–, test may be positive or negative. NA, not applicable.
From Perry et al. Primary adrenal causes of Cushing's syndrome. Ann Surg 1989; 210: 59–68.

Table 3.2 *Results of diagnostic evaluation*

Plan of management

The management of Cushing's disease with a pituitary microadenoma will normally be direct microadenectomy through the trans-sphenoidal route. Larger tumours may require a direct approach through the anterior fossa. Even with good imaging and an experienced operator, the success of microadenectomy may not be greater than 60% even when partial hypophysectomy has been undertaken after failing to identify a microadenoma. It is possible to destroy the pituitary microadenoma by total pituitary ablation surgically or by external or implanted radiotherapy. Nevertheless, the benefit of these radical procedures is far outweighed by the disadvantages of total pituitary loss. Failed microadenectomy is therefore normally best managed by resorting early to bilateral adrenalectomy. The pituitary tumour is left in place and may eventually grow large enough to produce headaches or compromise the optic pathways, in which case further surgery may be required. Normally, the unresected adenoma has few side effects apart from causing the development of hyperpigmentation (Nelson's syndrome). When bilateral adrenalectomy is undertaken for Cushing's syndrome, the route taken will depend on the preference of the surgeon and the habitus of the patient. Bilateral laparoscopic adrenalectomy by the transperitoneal or extraperitoneal route is feasible although time consuming. Using the transperitoneal route in a very fat patient the trocars may not be long enough to penetrate the abdominal wall and the instruments may not be long enough to reach the adrenals! A transperitoneal direct approach through a transverse upper abdominal incision allows easier access, but the wound is long. Some surgeons prefer a bilateral posterior route or even to undertake removal of one adrenal at a time through separate loin approaches (see section on adrenalectomy).

It is important to remember that these patients are often very sick, and even pretreatment with ketoconazole (600–800 mg d^{-1} p.o.), metyrapone or other metabolic blocking agents may not significantly alter their readiness for surgery. At operation, particular care must be directed towards the safe handling of the patient because of their weight, their tissue fragility and spinal osteoporosis. Wounds must be securely sutured in the expectation that healing will be delayed. Prophylactic antibiotics are required as these patients have an impaired resistance to infection. Postoperatively, care should be taken to avoid wound infection, to support good respiratory function, to monitor sugar concentration and electrolyte levels carefully and, most importantly, to replace the cortisol which is now absent from the circulation.

It has been proposed that subtotal adrenalectomy or autologous adrenal autotransplantation might obviate the need for lifelong cortisone replacement after bilateral adrenalectomy, but these techniques should not be employed. Recurrence of Cushing's syndrome is almost invariable after subtotal adrenalectomy, and autotransplantation is rarely successful.[12] Adrenal function should be replaced by the administration of cortisone. To replace adrenal function after bilateral adrenalectomy, all patients should be given 100 mg of hydrocortisone at the time of induction of anaesthesia. The subsequent steroid replacement follows this protocol:

1.   100 mg hydrocortisone sodium succinate in the recovery room and 6 hourly intravenously until the patient is able to take oral medication.
2.   Oral hydrocortisone, 20 mg, with fludrocortisone, 0.1 mg, in the morning and then hydrocortisone, 10 mg, at night. There is no need for mineralo-corticoid supplementation until oral feeding has been recommenced.

Patients who are receiving steroid replacement must be warned of the importance of continuing with therapy, and ideally should wear a bracelet and carry a card with the details of therapy. They should be aware of the need to increase the dose of steroids should intercurrent illness develop and to warn doctors at any hospital to which they are admitted that they are taking steroid medication.

Bilateral adrenalectomy for other causes of Cushing's syndrome

Bilateral adrenalectomy is also required for Cushing's syndrome caused by an ectopic ACTH source (if that source cannot be identified and removed), for PPND and for macronodular adrenal cortical hyperplasia.

Management of Cushing's syndrome due to a solitary adrenal adenoma or carcinoma

Well defined, clearly benign tumours of 10 cm diameter or less may be removed laparoscopically by the transperitoneal or retroperitoneal route. Larger tumours or those in which there is a suspicion of malignancy, should be resected by unilateral adrenalectomy through a loin incision or, if they are very large, through a posterior thoracoabdominal incision. If malignant tumours on the right have invaded the vena cava, the vena cava may need to be opened to remove any tumour that has directly invaded it. In some patients partial removal of the vena cava and its replacement by a polytetrafluoroethylene tube graft may be needed (**Fig. 3.11**). The rare occasion of tumour invasion of the hepatic or suprahepatic veins may require liver transplantation if surgery is contemplated. Large adrenocortical carcinomas on the left may require removal by *en bloc* excision of the adrenal with surrounding organs, such as the spleen, tail of pancreas and kidney.

A unilateral cortisol-secreting tumour will suppress the opposite adrenal, and all such patients require steroid replacement as described above. The patient may subsequently be weaned from the steroid replacement when the pituitary–adrenal axis function is returned to normal (tested using synacthen). This recovery may take 1 year or more.

Figure 3.11
(a) CT showing large malignant right adrenal tumour with no symptoms of caval involvement but (b) a cavagram shows extension of the tumour into the lumen of the vena cava.

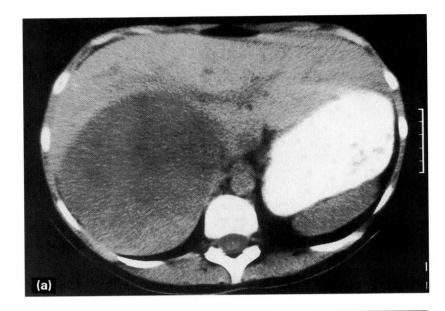

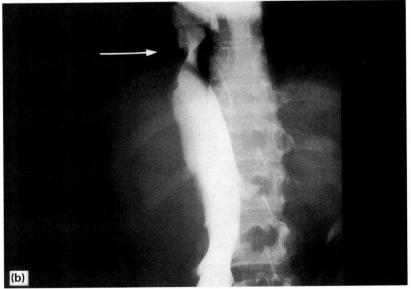

Management of Cushing's syndrome in pregnancy

Patients with Cushing's syndrome rarely become pregnant. When they do the pregnancy is normally complicated and it may be necessary to undertake pituitary surgery or adrenalectomy in the second trimester. For patients with a plasma cortisol concentration greater than 30 μg dl^{-1} there is no evidence that vaginal delivery is contraindicated in the third trimester.[13,14]

Adrenocortical carcinoma

General management of adrenocortical carcinoma

Adrenocortical carcinoma is rare, accounting for 0.02% of cancers. It can occur at any age, with a peak incidence in the fourth and fifth decades. About 60% of such tumours have no important endocrine secretion and vary in tissue type from those closely approximating normal adrenal cortex to the completely undifferentiated. It is sometimes difficult to distinguish between benign and malignant tumours unless there are clear signs of capsular or vascular invasion. Ploidy studies, assessed by flow cytometry, may be helpful in predicting malignancy. Functional and non-functional tumours spread by local invasion and by lymphatic and vascular systems. Non-functioning tumours present by systemic symptoms of weight loss, weakness and occasional fever.

Functional tumours present depending on their type of secretion:

1. Glucocorticoid-secreting tumours present as Cushing's syndrome;
2. Androgen-secreting tumours present as virilisation, hirsutism and amenorrhoea in women and precocious puberty in boys;
3. Oestrogen-secreting tumours are rare and in men are an exceptionally rare cause of gynaecomastia. Such gynaecomastia is associated with testicular atrophy and impotence. Girls show precocious puberty and women show menstrual irregularities;
4. Aldosterone-secreting malignant adrenal tumours are exceptionally rare and the syndrome is identical to that produced by benign tumours.

When possible a surgical resection of adrenocortical malignant tumours must be undertaken, and if there are clear histological margins there is little evidence that radiotherapy to the tumour bed is likely to extend the patient's survival or decrease the risk of recurrence. If recurrence occurs, debulking surgery may be valuable, particularly in hormone-secreting tumours (**Fig. 3.12**).

Chemotherapy has a limited place in the management of adrenocortical tumours and is reserved for recurrence or inoperable or metastatic disease. The agent of choice is mitotane (O′p-DDD). This agent has a specific action in interfering with cortisol synthesis but additionally causes regression of the tumour. It seems to be effective in non-functioning adrenocortical tumours. The starting dose is $1-2$ g d^{-1} increasing gradually to $8-10$ g d^{-1}. During treatment the patient requires maintenance doses of cortisone and may become hypothyroid, requiring treatment. The side effects may be considerable (nausea, vomiting and fatigue) but if they are not marked, it is worth persisting with treatment as good remissions are sometimes obtained.[15] There is only limited experience of the treatment of adrenocortical tumours with other chemotherapeutic agents, but 110 patients from the MD Anderson Cancer Centre had 5-year and 10-year survivals of 23%

Figure 3.12
Survival rates from adrenocortical carcinoma in relation to extent of disease at presentation. Data from Icard P et al. Surgery 1992; 112: 972.

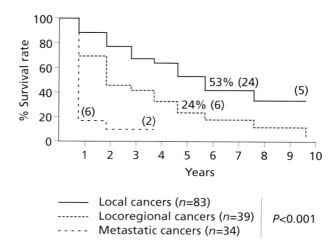

Local cancers (*n*=83)
Locoregional cancers (*n*=39) $P<0.001$
Metastatic cancers (*n*=34)

and 10%, respectively. There is no difference in response between functional and non-functional tumours.[16]

For palliative care, patients with gross Cushing's syndrome should receive blockade with ketoconazole, metyrapone or aminoglutethimide.

Remission of Cushing's syndrome after successful treatment

Almost all the symptoms of Cushing's syndrome regress after correction of the hypercortisolism. The earliest to respond are the psychological changes, which revert to normal within a few days. Within a week of adrenalectomy the blood pressure begins to return to normal, but it may be several months before it reaches its final level. About 80% of patients obtain total remission of hypertension. The cardiac and ECG changes improve at the same rate. The skin changes improve slowly over the first few months. The first sign of improvement is often a scaly desquamation at the margin of the scalp. The excess weight is lost, but dieting may be necessary. The muscles only regain full strength after several months. Facial hair becomes less pronounced but the hirsutism never completely disappears. Of the metabolic changes, the diabetes usually, but not invariably, is cured and the serum electrolytes return to normal within the first few weeks after surgery. Recalcification of the bones takes many months. When seen a year after definitive treatment changes in the patient are usually dramatic, with a near total return to previous physical appearance and function.

Adrenogenital syndrome

Adrenogenital syndrome describes a heterogeneous group of disorders that result in abnormalities of the external genitalia. Most patients have congenital adrenal hyperplasia (CAH) in which there is a congenital deficit in one of the enzymes of steroid production. Any enzyme deficit in the pathway to production of aldosterone or cortisol results in a syndrome characterised by a deficit of the end steroid and overproduction of intermediary steroid metabolites. This is due to increased ACTH production as a result of the deficit in the end steroid. Because the path to production of adrenal androgens shares many steroid intermediates with the corticoid production pathway, any enzyme block to cortisol production increases androgen production and virilisation occurs (**Fig. 3.13**). The clinical presentation of CAH is variable and depends on the site and severity of the block in steroid synthesis.

The most common form is as a result of a deficit in the 21-hydroxylase enzyme, which causes impairment of the production of cortisol and aldosterone. In its mild form the increased secretion of ACTH results in near normal cortisol concentrations with normal or raised aldosterone concentrations. The syndrome includes increased androgen concentrations with ambiguous genitalia and clitoral enlargement in the female and sexual precocity in the male. In its severe form, the deficit of cortisol and aldosterone production results in salt-losing, hypoglycaemic crises that require urgent intervention. The mild forms may only present in adult life and are an important differential diagnosis in women with virilising features and in men with features of excess androgen production.

The treatment of CAH is by replacement of the deficient steroids, which results in a reduction in ACTH concentrations and a reduction of the androgens that cause the virilisation. The adrenal hyperplasia does not require surgical intervention, but the genital manifestations of excess androgen production, particularly in women, may require specialised surgery.[17]

Aldosteronism (Conn's syndrome)

Aldosteronism (excessive secretion of aldosterone) may occur *primarily* due to tumours, nodularity or hyperplasia of the adrenal glands or *secondarily* as a response to excess stimulation by angiotensin. This latter condition occurs as a response to diminished plasma volume in conditions such as cirrhosis, nephrotic syndrome, diuretic therapy and cardiac failure. It also occurs when renin is produced in excess in conditions such as renal artery stenosis and accelerated hypertension and when there is a renin-secreting renal tumour.

In primary aldosteronism one or both adrenals secrete aldosterone in excess, independently of any change in the renin–angiotensin mechanism. Subtypes are:

1.   Hypersecretion from a small, benign 'aldosterone-producing adenoma' (APA) in the cortex of one adrenal; this is the commonest variant of primary hyperaldosteronism;

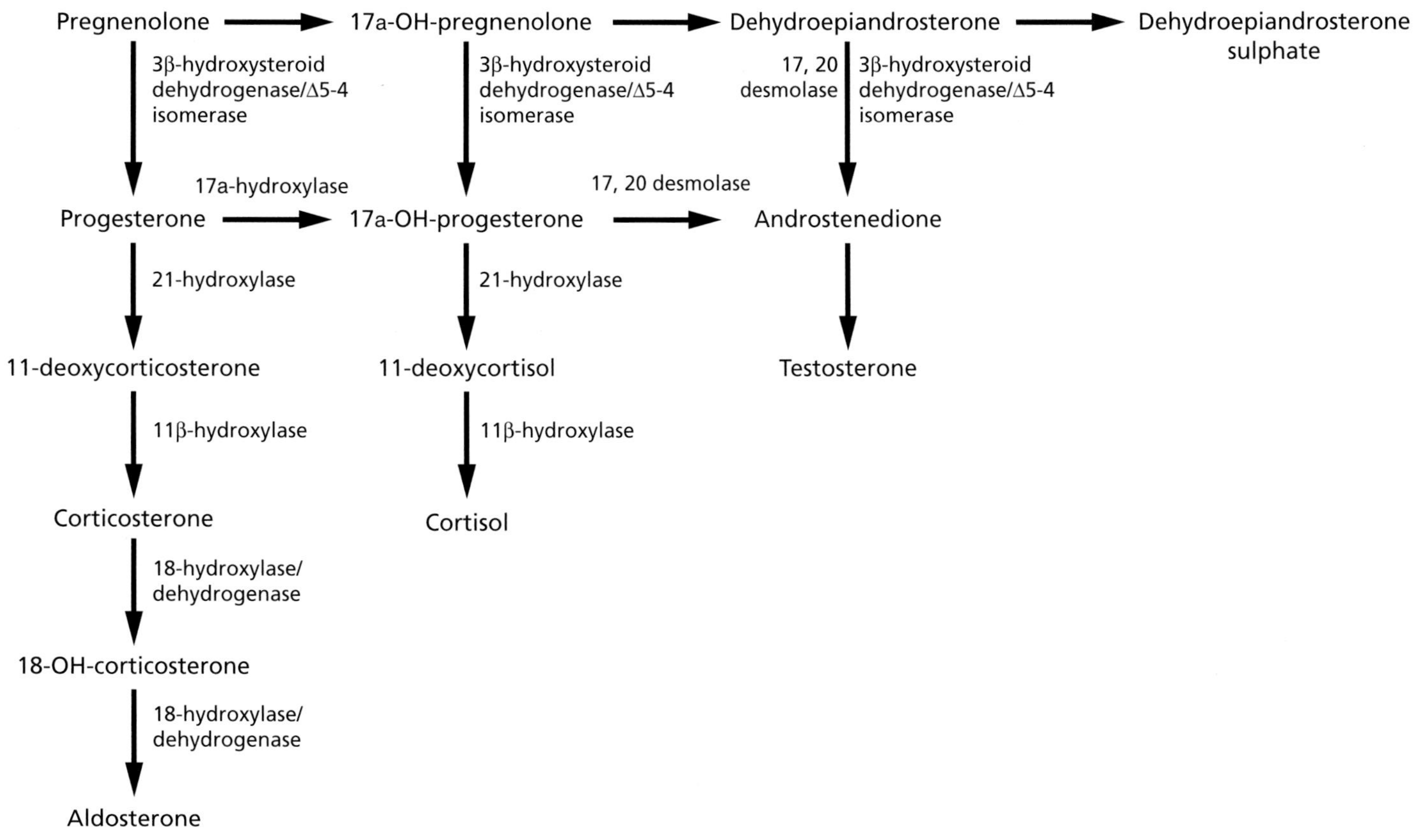

Figure 3.13
Synthetic pathways of steroids in the adrenal cortex.

2. Bilateral micronodular or macronodular hyperplasia of the zona glomerulosa, sometimes described as 'idiopathic hyperaldosteronism' (IHA);

3. Aldosterone-secreting carcinoma; this is rare. Most malignant cortical tumours secrete a range of cortical hormones and related substances. It is rare for such tumours to predominantly produce aldosterone;

4. The dominantly inherited 'familial glucocorticoid suppressible hyperaldosteronism.'

Pathology and pathophysiology

Aldosterone is produced by the zona glomerulosa of the adrenal cortex. It promotes the absorption of sodium by the distal renal tubules via the Na^+/K^+, H^+ channel, and by this mechanism it promotes the retention of water. The normal physiological secretion of aldosterone is controlled primarily by angiotensin II. Angiotensin II is generated as a result of the activity of renin and angiotensin-converting enzyme (ACE) on angiotensinogen. Renin is a hormone secreted from the juxtaglomerular apparatus of the kidney in response to low blood pressure or volume. The secretion of aldosterone is also increased by ACTH and by an increase in serum potassium concentrations. Dopamine, a putative pituitary aldosterone-stimulating factor, serotonin and atrial natriuretic peptide also influence aldosterone secretion. Aldosterone is metabolised by the liver, and plasma concentrations may be pathologically increased as a result of liver impairment. The normal function of aldosterone is to regulate the vascular volume and electrolyte excretion by acting on the renal tubules to increase potassium excretion and encourage water and sodium absorption. Feedback control is by an increasing vascular volume suppressing renin secretion.

Primary hyperaldosteronism is a term that describes an inappropriate secretion of aldosterone that is independent of the influence of renin. The causes are listed in **Table 3.3**.

Low-renin hyperaldosteronism presents with hypertension and hypokalaemic alkalosis owing to the direct effect of the excess aldosterone on the distal renal tubules promoting a loss of K^+ and a retention of Na^+ and water. The retention of Na^+ and water is partly counteracted by increased secretion of atrial natriuretic peptide (ANP), and the sodium concentrations may be normal and water retention is not generally a feature. A low oral Na^+ intake masks the hypokalaemia in many patients.

Incidence

Aldosteronism is twice as common in women as it is in men and rarely occurs in children. It predominantly presents between the ages of 30 and 60 years and

Type	Frequency (%)	Site	Responsiveness		Surgically correctable
			Ang II	ACTH	
Aldosterone-producing adenoma	64	Uni	–	+	+
Idiopathic hyperaldosteronism	32	Bil	+	–	–
Glucocorticoid-suppressible hyperaldosteronism	1	Bil	–	+	–
Primary adrenal hyperplasia	<1	Uni	–	+	+
Aldosterone-producing, angiotensin (Ang) II-responsive adenoma	<1	Uni	+	–	+
Aldosterone-producing carcinoma	<1	Uni	–	–	+

Adapted from reference 19 with permission.
Uni, unilateral pathology; Bil, bilateral pathology; ACTH, adrenocorticotrophic hormone.

Table 3.3 *Causes of primary hyperaldosteronism*

is discovered in 1% of patients investigated for hypertension. Approximately two thirds of patients have an adenoma and the other third idiopathic hyperaldosteronism (IHA). Adenomas are most common on the left side.[18]

Clinical features

There are no specific clinical features, but clinical suspicion should be aroused when hypertension occurs with hypokalaemia. The hypertension is usually moderate or severe and may not have responded satisfactorily to normal medical treatment. The hypokalaemia will usually have been discovered on routine multichannel analysis or only have declared itself as a consequence of diuretic therapy. It may sometimes be marked, with severe symptoms of muscle weakness or cramps, malaise and polyuria and polydypsia and sometimes even episodic paralysis. Women may give a history of toxaemia during pregnancy.

Patients with an aldosterone-producing adenoma as distinct from IHA usually have more severe hypertension, more profound hypokalaemia and higher aldosterone concentrations in the plasma.

Investigations

There are three crucial steps in the diagnostic process. These can be represented as answers to three questions:

1. Is there primary aldosteronism?
2. Is there only one diseased adrenal such that surgery might be appropriate?

3. Is any mass visualized in the adrenal actually the cause of the hyperaldosteronism?

Primary aldosteronism

Investigation to determine primary aldosteronism follows complex algorithms outside the scope of this chapter[20] but one third of patients with primary aldosteronism may have a normal potassium concentration, and hypokalaemia may only be revealed by the prescription of diuretics. Diuretics may, of course, cause hypokalaemia in the absence of any adrenal lesion and it is therefore important when investigating these patients to discontinue the diuretic and replace the deficiency in potassium before retesting. It is also essential to discontinue aldosterone and calcium-channel blocking antihypertensives as these will interfere with the results. The diagnosis of primary hyperaldosteronism is therefore based on the concurrence of hypokalaemia, inappropriately increased urinary potassium excretion and a high plasma aldosterone concentration that is not suppressible by an increased intake of sodium chloride. Glucocorticoid concentrations should be noted as being normal.

Unilateral adrenal pathology

Essentially this is the process of distinguishing APA from IHA. As the glands in IHA may be nodular, this is not always an easy sequence of investigations. If there is a single, significant sized adrenal lesion, CT scanning is the easiest and cheapest way of assessing this. If a high resolution scan with 3 mm contiguous slices is used, approximately 80% of patients with a solitary adenoma will be successfully imaged by CT scan. Contrast enhancement does not improve the value of the films. MRI scanning is equally sensitive but not of any extra value when a single lesion is found. Small equivocal or multiple lesions found on CT or MRI scanning require further evaluation.

Distinction between IHA and APA

One of the best diagnostic tests is to measure blood aldosterone concentrations after recumbency and after subsequent standing, i.e. on waking in the morning and after the patient has been up and about for 3 hours.[21] In normal subjects the plasma concentration of aldosterone increases by a factor of 2–4 when the patient is upright. In patients with IHA this increase is less pronounced but is more than 30% of the concentration after recumbency. Patients with APA show no change in the postural aldosterone concentrations. This test is not always specific.

Is the anatomical abnormality a functioning adenoma?

Incompatibility between preliminary biochemical tests and localisation studies requires additional evaluation such as iodocholesterol isotope scanning with

NP59 or adrenal vein sampling for aldosterone. NP59 scanning provides a functional assessment. Scanning must be carried out for 5 days after the isotope has been given, and the results are more likely to be diagnostic if dexamethasone suppression has been given for 7 days previously and if antihypertensive treatment is discontinued. If only one adrenal gland shows on the NP59 scan then there is a good chance that there is a single, significant functioning adenoma. The accuracy of this test is around 80%. The accuracy of adrenal vein sampling is higher, perhaps up to 95%, but it is technically difficult (especially on the right) and is time consuming. It does not need to be combined with retrograde venography.

Treatment

Unequivocal APA is treated by unilateral adrenalectomy if the patient is fit (**Fig. 3.14**). The tumour is usually small, easily visible and well encapsulated and can be removed laparoscopically or by a posterior approach. The surgery should be preceded by 1–6 weeks of preparation with spironolactone to allow the serum potassium concentration to return to normal. Surgery returns the blood pressure to normal in about 70% of patients. It is important to remember that some adenomas also secrete glucocorticoid, and the opposite adrenal may therefore be suppressed and replacement treatment with cortisone may be necessary.

The treatment of choice for the relatively benign condition of IHA is with spironolactone at a dose of 100 mg d^{-1} increasing to 400 mg d^{-1} until the potassium has normalised and the hypertension is under control. The dose may then be gradually reduced. Spironolactone may not control the hypertension when used alone, and the addition of calcium-channel antagonists, angiotensin converting enzyme inhibitors or diuretics may be required. Spironolactone affects testosterone synthesis, leading to gynaecomastia, reduced libido, impotance and menstrual disorders. It may not be tolerated by the patient and second-line therapy with amiloride or triamterene may be preferable.

Familial bilateral glucocorticoid suppressible hyperaldosteronism is rare. It is ideally treated with spironolactone as this is less physiologically disruptive than the glucocorticoid treatment.

The treatment of aldosterone-producing cortical carcinoma is the same as that for predominantly cortisol-secreting carcinomas described above.

In the rare situation of hyperaldosteronism in pregnancy, surgery is preferred to medical therapy unless there is clearly bilateral disease.[22]

Phaeochromocytoma

Phaeochromocytoma, neuroblastoma (see later), paragangliomas and ganglioneuromas are derived from the neural crest. Phaeochromocytoma may occur

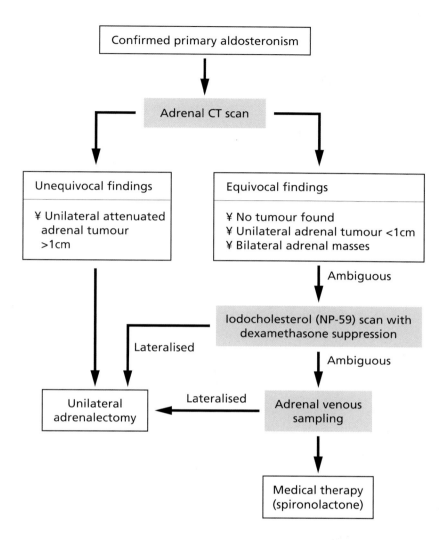

Figure 3.14
Flow chart for selecting patients with primary aldosteronism for unilateral adrenalectomy. From Obara T, Ito Y, Fujimoto Y. Hyperaldosteronism. In: Clark OH, Duh. Q-Y (eds). Textbook of endocrine surgery. Philadelphia: WB Saunders, 1997: p. 485.

wherever neuro–ectodermal tissue is found; hence the occasionally used name chromaffinoma. About 90% are solitary and occur in the adrenal, but 5–10% are bilateral and 10% are extra-adrenal. Extra-adrenal phaeochromocytomas are often described as paraganglionomas and can be found in any of the sites identified in **Fig. 3.15**.

Incidence

The true incidence of phaeochromocytoma is not known, but a phaeochromocytoma was found at 0.3% of autopsies performed at the Mayo Clinic, and the incidence has been calculated at 1–2 per 100 000 adults per year.[23] About 0.1% of patients investigated for hypertension have a phaeochromocytoma. Most

Figure 3.15
(a) Anatomical distribution of extra-adrenal chromaffin tissue in newborn infants. (b) Location of extra-adrenal phaeochromocytomas reported in the literature up to 1965.

Modified from Coupland R. The Natural History of the Chromaffin Cell, Longman Green, 1965.

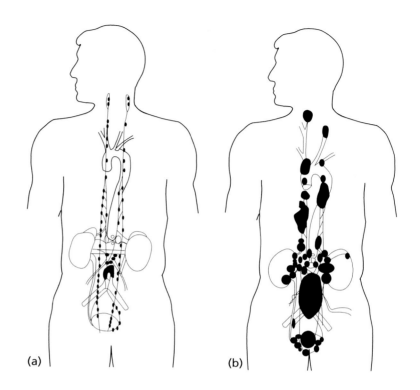

(a)   (b)

phaeochromocytomas are less than 10 cm in diameter when discovered, the average being 5 cm, and they are usually detected early because of physiological catecholamine effects. About 10% of phaeochromocytomas are malignant and these tend to be larger at presentation.

Most phaeochromocytomas secrete predominantly adrenaline but some secrete noradrenaline or dopamine, in which case hypotension may be a presenting sign. A range of other physiologically active agents are released from phaeochromocytomas, including serotonin, ACTH, parathyroid hormone and vasoinhibitory peptide,[24] but the majority of symptoms are attributable to adrenaline and noradrenaline.

Symptomatology

The symptoms are those of excess circulating adrenaline or noradrenaline concentration, but symptoms may be sporadic and paroxysmal against a background of continuing high concentrations of circulating catecholamines and chronic physiological changes such as hypovolaemia.[25] The continuing high background catecholamine concentrations do not produce symptoms as a consequence of tachyphylaxis, the desensitisation of α-adrenergic receptors and β-adrenergic receptors. The presentation of patients with phaeochromocytomas can be dramatic, consisting of severe but transient hypertension, palpitations, tachycardia and sweating with pallor and anxiety. Not all of these may be present, and chest pain and weakness may be associated symptoms in about 50% of patients. The attacks may last for minutes or hours and occur at any frequency of from 1–2 times a year to regularly during an hour. They often occur spontaneously but may be precipitated by vigorous exercise, twisting and bending, alcohol, tobacco and certain specific drugs, such as anaesthetic agents, phenothiazines, β-blockers and tricyclic antidepressants. Occasionally the acute effects of hypertension are so severe that the patient may demonstrate fulminating pulmonary oedema or severe arrhythmias, which may be fatal. In addition to the impressive paroxysmal effects of phaeochromocytoma, there are additional chronic effects, most notably a cardiomyopathy. In some patients the diagnosis is only achieved at autopsy, but a retrospective review of these patients shows that almost all will have had symptoms in life.[27] Some phaeochromocytomas declare themselves during a surgical procedure and a third of sudden deaths attributed to a previously undiagnosed phaeochromocytoma will occur during unrelated minor surgery.[23]

Clinical associations

Multiple endocrine neoplasia type 2

In multiple endocrine neoplasia type 2A (MEN-2A) there is familial occurrence of phaeochromocytoma (which may be bilateral), medullary carcinoma of the thyroid and hyperparathyroidism. Not all patients develop all three abnormalities, but all should be sought in anyone with phaeochromocytoma. In some families only phaeochromocytomas occur and in others there are consistently only medullary carcinomas of the thyroid. In MEN-2B, hyperparathyroidism is uncommon but in addition to phaeochromocytoma and medullary carcinoma of the thyroid mucosal neuromas, a marfanoid habitus and sometimes ganglioneuromas in the gastrointestinal tract are added to the phenotype.[27] All forms of MEN-2 are inherited in an autosomal dominant fashion.

Neurofibromatosis

This is a rare association, but phaeochromocytoma will occur in 10% of patients with neurofibromatosis.

Von Hippel–Lindau syndrome

About 14% of patients with this syndrome (cerebellar haemangioma) have a phaeochromocytoma.[28] Extra-adrenal paragangliomas or phaeochromocytomas may be associated with adrenal phaeochromocytomas in a few patients. These are not always familial and therefore, even in the supposed sporadic patient, should be sought if the biochemistry does not return to normal after excision of the primary adrenal phaeochromocytoma.

Investigations

If phaeochromocytoma is suspected, a basic screen must always be undertaken to establish the clinical diagnosis by assessing (a) urinary vanillylmandelic acid (VMA) concentration in a 24 hour sample of urine; this test, however, has only a 60% sensitivity in diagnosing phaeochromocytoma; and (b) urinary total catecholamines, a more specific test, with 90% sensitivity and specificity. If the 24 hour urinary adrenaline concentration exceeds 35 μg l^{-1} or noradrenaline concentration exceeds 170 μg l^{-1} then phaeochromocytoma must be suspected. Combining the two amines to give values in excess of 100 μg 24 h^{-1} allows a confident diagnosis of phaeochromocytoma. Some laboratories will present the results as a ratio to urinary creatine concentration thus further refining the accuracy of the test. It is possible to measure serum adrenaline and noradrenaline concentrations, but this is technically more difficult and the results are less specific for the diagnosis of phaeochromocytoma. Any of these determinations can be altered by concurrent administration of drugs such as calcium-channel blockers, monoamine oxidase inhibitors, phenothiazines, tricyclic antidepressants, α-blockers, β-blockers and nalidixic acid.[29]

Localisation

Once an abnormal urinary VMA or catecholamine concentration has been confirmed, adrenal CT scanning should be undertaken; this will show 90% of tumours. T2 weighted MRI scans show a characteristic high intensity signal with phaeochromocytomas and give more information about relations with surrounding soft tissues, but MRI is marginally less sensitive at defining the tumour itself. Only rarely will MRI add additional information useful for the surgeon. If an adrenal tumour is discovered, further localisation studies are not needed, particularly if it has a characteristic irregular dark centre on CT scanning. If the patient is pregnant, MRI is the preferred imaging modality. If there is a suspicion that there might be multiple or ectopic phaeochromocytomas or if the patient has a family history of MEN-2 or is under the age of 30, then isotopic scanning is indicated. The agent of choice is meta-iodobenzylguanidine (MIBG) which is highly specific for catecholamine-producing tumours whatever the location. Very few false positives are encountered, but there is a false negative rate of 5–10%, especially with small tumours (**Fig. 3.16**).[30] MIBG scanning is also indicated if the size or CT appearances of the tumour suggest that it might be malignant, as the test can demonstrate metastatic disease.

Occasionally tumours will infarct, perhaps in association with a paroxysm. In these circumstances the MIBG, and indeed the VMA and catecholamine studies, may be negative. The tumour will nonetheless regrow with time.

Figure 3.16
An ectopic phaeochromocytoma. The MIBG scans (a) suggested that the lesion was in the left adrenal gland but the CT scan (b) shows the tumour to be located in ganglionic tissue in the lower chest (arrowed).

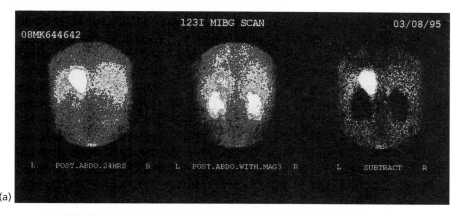

(a)

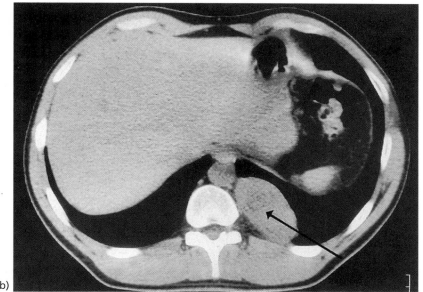

(b)

Management

When a phaeochromocytoma has been identified, the correct treatment is surgical excision. There is no effective medical treatment, but adrenalectomy should not be undertaken without appropriate and adequate preparation of the patient.

Preoperative management of patients with phaeochromocytoma

The anaesthesia of patients with functioning phaeochromocytomas is highly specialised and, even with adequate blockade of catecholamine release, may present major challenges intraoperatively. Close preoperative liasion with the anaesthetist responsible for the perioperative management of the patient is mandatory so that the patient is admitted for surgery in the optimal physiological condition.

The introduction of α-adrenergic blockade with appropriate expansion of the intravascular volume has resulted in a reduction in perioperative mortality from 13–45% to 0–3%. The catecholamine excess associated with the untreated phaeochromocytoma has a wide range of physiological effects. The most obvious are hypertension, caused by the vasoconstrictive action on blood vessels, sweating and tachycardia. In addition phaeochromocytoma causes hyperglycaemia and occasionally cardiomyopathy. Patients must therefore be treated with an α-adrenergic blocking agent before surgery is undertaken. Some patients are sensitive to the α-blockade, so the starting dose should be low and increased until blockade is adequate. Phenoxybenzamine is the agent most frequently used, starting at a dose of 20–60 mg d^{-1} in divided doses. The dose is increased incrementally until hypertension is controlled, orthostatic hypotension becomes a problem or the maximum dose of 160 mg d^{-1} is reached. There are no clear rules to assess when the α-blockade is adequate, but this is likely to be sufficient when sweating and tachycardia cease and when there is a demonstrable increase in the intravascular volume measured by a drop in the haematocrit associated with an increase in body weight. If tachycardia or cardiac arrhythmias develop, a β-blocker may be added *but only once adequate α-blockade has been established*. Pure β-blockade may result in a severe hypertensive crisis.

More selective blockade can be achieved with doxazocin in doses ranging from 2 mg to 5 mg day^{-1}. The advantage of this agent is that it provides more selective α-blockade and the effects are more readily reversed after cessation of therapy. Blocking effects after phenoxybenzamine are prolonged and may cause hypotension in the postoperative period. Phenoxybenzamine affects the α-adrenergic receptor, and reversal of effects must await regeneration of the receptors.

There are no rules as to the duration of treatment with α-blockers prior to surgery, but 2 weeks is probably adequate if there is no evidence of catecholamine-induced cardiomyopathy. If there are ECG abnormalities, e.g. ST-segment elevation, arrhythmias or evidence of global myocardial dysfunction on an echocardiogram, the treatment may have to continue for as long as 6 months. β-Blockade is normally added electively preoperatively if not indicated earlier for control of symptoms. Preoperative preparation with metyrosine (α-methyl-*p*-tyrosine), which interferes with catecholamine synthesis, is worthwhile, but it has little advantage over traditional regimens using α-blockade and β-blockade.

During the operation close liasion between surgeon and anaesthetist is crucial, because manipulation of the gland may result in catecholamine release, and marked hypertension (despite blockade) and devascularisation of the tumour may result in a dramatic drop in concentration of circulating vasoactive catecholamines, with consequent hypotension (**Fig. 3.17**). Intravenous fluids, hypotensive agents (e.g. nitroprusside) and inotropes (e.g. phenylephrine, dopamine) are used to control pressure perioperatively. Continuous monitoring of central venous pressure (CVP)

Figure 3.17
The fluctuations in central venous pressure and blood pressure that may be experienced during operation of a phaeochromocytoma. Good preoperation preparation may blunt the severity of peaks and troughs but unpredictably so.

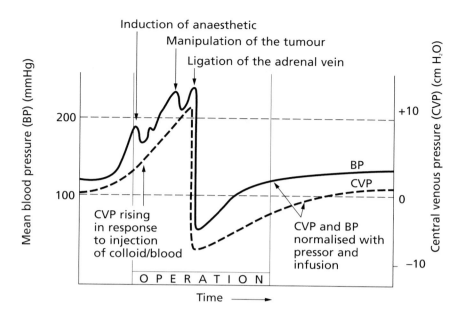

and arterial pressure is mandatory from induction of anaesthesia to the recovery phase. Early in the procedure fluid is given intravenously in a quantity in excess of that dictated from CVP measurements. This deliberate expansion of the circulating blood volume prior to ligation of the adrenal vein and the consequent loss of pressor effect is a valuable prophylaxis against a sudden fall in CVP. This often reduces the need for large doses of pressor agents later in the surgery.[31] If managed well from a pharmacological and circulatory point of view, the patient is usually stable within an hour or so of the end of the operation and does not need prolonged pressor or ventilatory support or monitoring. Overzealous α-blockage prior to the operation, however, may lead to postoperative hypotension.

Phaeochromocytoma in pregnancy

Phaeochromocytoma and pregnancy is a dangerous combination for mother and baby. When the diagnosis is not made, prepartum maternal mortality exceeds 50%. For those where the diagnosis is made during pregnancy, prognosis is better and standard treatment can be undertaken with α-blockade followed in the third trimester by synchronous adrenalectomy and caesarean section. Vaginal delivery is contraindicated.[32,33]

Malignant phaeochromocytoma

Malignant phaeochromocytomas are rare and account for less than 10% of phaeochromocytomas. Malignancy is more common in extra-adrenal phaeochromocytoma (paraganglionoma), where 50% may be malignant, and in familial forms. As with many other endocrine tumours, the histology of the primary lesion may not distinguish benign from malignant, even when ploidy studies are added. The presence of metastases is the only true indicator of malignancy. Many phaeochromocytomas are poorly encapsulated and may seem at operation to be invading local structures. They are, nevertheless, usually benign. Metastases normally take up MIGB, which can be used in localisation and in therapeutic doses that may be palliative. The value of radiotherapy is unproven, but a 50% response rate to a chemotherapeutic regimen of cyclophosphamide, vincristine and dacarbazine has been reported.[34]

Adrenal neuroblastomas

Adrenal neuroblastomas are tumours of the developing neuroendocrine system. Such tumours may develop in neonates and infants wherever such tissue exists. Overall, 40% occur in the adrenal gland and a further 40% in the nearby paraspinal sympathetic tissue. They are the commonest solid tumour of infancy. Neuroblastomas normally present as adrenal masses and are often very large. In children over 3 years of age there are usually metastases in liver, bone, lung or subcutaneous nodules at the time of presentation. The diagnosis is made by CT scan, and primary tumour and metastases may be identified by isotope MIBG or octreotide scans. Urinary catecholamine concentrations are increased in most patients.

Treatment

The treatment depends on the type and stage, but for most patients it consists of surgical resection of the adrenal tumour or debulking, followed by chemotherapy. This combination produces a complete remission in most patients, but many recur later. In some infants where the primary tumour is completely resected and metastases are limited to the liver, skin or bone marrow (stage IVS), spontaneous remission may occur after resection of the primary tumour, and chemotherapy may not then be needed. In this special subset of children there is an 85% long-term survival rate. For most others survival is worse. Quantification of the *N-myc* oncogene provides prognostic information, and when there is a single copy of the oncogene, a 98% long-term survival rate may be expected. Patients with tumours with more than 10 copies of the gene have an exceptionally poor prognosis regardless of treatment. Neuroblastoma is a complex condition requiring treatment in a specialist centre.[35,36]

Incidentaloma

About 7% of autopsies uncover an unsuspected adrenal tumour, and an adrenal mass is an incidental finding in 1–4% of abdominal CT scans. The term 'incidentaloma' is now in common usage for such tumours discovered coincidentally. When found they should be assessed objectively because they are a potential source of unnecessary and possibly harmful surgery.

About 5% of such tumours are found to be primary adrenal cancers, and a further 5% are metastases from an occult primary tumour. About 50% are, however, metastases from known primary tumours. A further 30% are cortical adenomas and may have potential or actual endocrine significance. About 5% will be phaeochromocytomas only half of which will have displayed symptoms.[37] The remainder consist of haematomas, cysts and myelolipomas (**Fig. 3.18**). This last group, however, can normally be diagnosed on CT scan and may not require further evaluation. Cysts are normally simple and not associated with malignancy. Haematomas are occasionally a result of trauma but can occur spontaneously in an underlying primary or metastatic tumour. Myelolipomas are benign, non-functioning tumours, which only require excision if significant growth occurs.

Those patients who have no obvious CT diagnosis and no known malignancy elsewhere require investigation to exclude endocrine disease. It is sufficient to undertake a urinary VMA or catecholamine assay to exclude phaeochromocytoma, a serum potassium test to exclude Conn's syndrome and a serum cortisol test to exclude Cushing's syndrome. If any one of these screening tests is abnormal, then further testing is indicated. If each is normal then the decision whether

Figure 3.18
Myelolipoma. (a) CT scan showing a right adrenal tumour with typical features of myelolipoma. The tumour consists of areas of dark fatty tissue divided by thick bands; (b, c) MRI scans of same tumour. MRI adds little in terms of detail about the surgical anatomy of the tumour. The tumour has not been removed but will be followed with CT scans.

Figures (b) and (c), see overleaf.

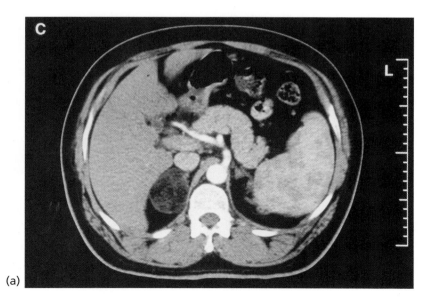

(a)

Figure 3.18
Continued.

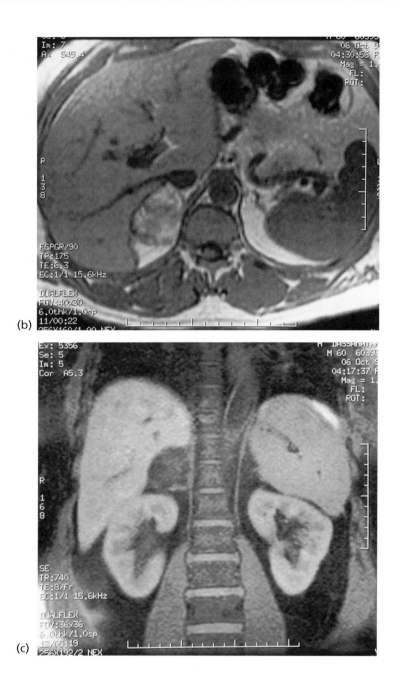

(b)

(c)

to remove the adrenal lesion or merely to watch it with serial CT scans is based on the size of the tumour and its CT appearance (**Fig. 3.19**). CT evidence of irregular contour, invasion of adjacent structures and metastases to retroperitoneal nodes are indications for surgery. In the absence of such signs, size is the best determinant of malignancy; MRI scanning and isotope scanning do not

Figure 3.19
CT scan of a small incidentaloma. It is important that sequential CT measurements are made at the same level and with the same axes for measurement.

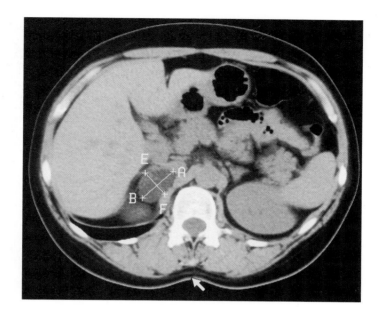

significantly improve the diagnostic power of the CT scan, although claims have been made that by using T2 weighted MRI scans ratios can be calculated between the adrenal tumour and the adjacent liver. Phaeochromocytomas are said to have a 'bright' image, with a ratio of greater than 3. Adenomas are less bright, with a ratio of 0.7–1.4 and primary or metastatic malignancies an intermediate figure with a ratio between 1.4 and 3.[38] In practice, however, most clinicians base their judgements on tumour size as documented by CT scanning. Tumours less than 3 cm in diameter can normally be watched with serial CT scans. Tumours larger than 6 cm must be excised. If the patient is unfit or unwilling to undergo adrenalectomy then the diagnosis may be improved with CT-guided biopsy (**Fig. 3.20**). This form of biopsy is, however, dangerous in an unsuspected phaeochromocytoma and is unable to distinguish between cortical adenomas and carcinomas.[39] Its best use is in identifying the incidentaloma as a metastasis. There is debate about the management of tumours measured on CT at between 3 and 6 cm. Although the negative predictive value of an adrenal tumour of less than 6 cm being malignant is 99%, the Mayo Clinic recommend that lesions of 4 cm or greater should be excised and smaller tumours re-scanned after 3 months.[40] Age should be taken into account and younger patients more readily considered for surgery. There are some who have averred that the arrival of laparoscopic surgery means that 'nearly all' incidentalomas should be removed.[41] The present authors disagree. Any form of surgery is more risky than no surgery, and the fascination of laparoscopic adrenalectomy is not an indication for inappropriate surgery and should not encourage departure from the management plan outlined above.[42]

Figure 3.20
CT-guided biopsy of an incidentally discovered non-functioning adrenal tumour.

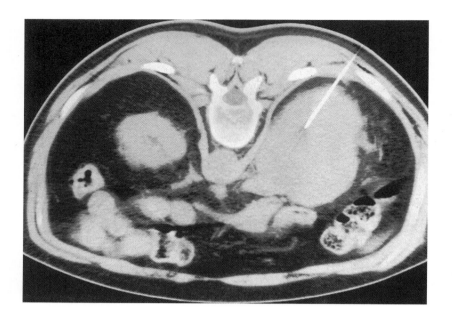

The operation of adrenalectomy

Regardless of the size of the tumour, the normal procedure is to undertake total removal of the gland on the affected side. During bilateral adrenalectomy the implantation of part of the residual normal adrenal gland into a muscle (as in parathyroid autotransplantation) has only rarely been shown to be successful at retaining adrenal cortical function and should not normally be attempted. The routes by which the adrenal may be removed are:

1. Open
    (a) the posterior approach
    (b) the posterolateral or loin approach
    (c) the transperitoneal anterior approach
2. Laparoscopic
    (a) transperitoneal anterior
    (b) transperitoneal lateral
    (c) retroperitoneal

Open methods

The posterior approach described in 1936 by Hugh Young[43] is the most direct route to the adrenals (**Figs 3.21 and 3.22**). It involves a nearly vertical posterior incision in the lumbar muscles, with division of the neck of the 12th rib. Both

Figure 3.21
Posterior surgical approaches to the adrenal gland. On the left side of the illustration the semivertical curved incision over the necks of the 11th and 12th ribs made in the true posterior (Hugo Young) approach. On the right an incision along the 12th rib. When undertaken with the patient in the side-up position, this incision begins more laterally, continues more anteriorly and extends beyond the tip of the 12th rib.

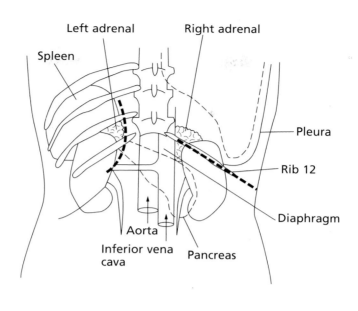

Figure 3.22
The three anterior incisions for approach to the adrenal gland. The choice of incision depends on the size and habitus of the patient.

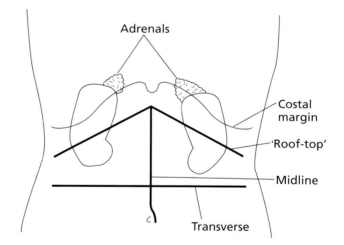

adrenals can be approached synchronously through two parallel incisions, with the patient prone. This can be technically difficult, especially in obese patients and those with Cushing's syndrome. The posterolateral loin approach is perhaps the most popular open approach and is familiar as a standard approach to the kidney.

The patient is positioned with the affected side up and the table 'broken' (**Fig. 3.23**). The incision approaches the adrenal via the bed of the 12th rib or, in thin patients, below it. The approach is extraperitoneal, although the peritoneum can be opened if necessary. Large right-sided tumours may be better approached

Figure 3.23
Positioning of patient for left adrenalectomy via the posterolateral approach, either open or laparoscopic.

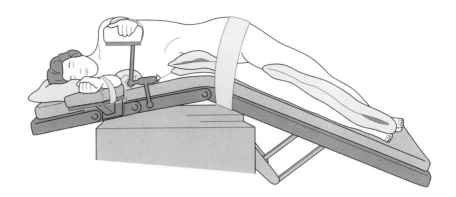

through the bed of the 11th rib, but this greatly increases the risk of opening the pleura. If the tumour is very large and invasive, a higher thoracoabdominal incision can be used, although this is rarely needed. The open transperitoneal approach is normally only used for bilateral adrenalectomy in Cushing's syndrome when pituitary surgery has failed. A transverse, or 'roof-top', incision allows good access in all but the most obese of patients. The open transperitoneal approach was traditionally employed when operating for phaeochromocytoma to allow the abdomen to be explored for a second or ectopic phaeochromocytoma. Modern preoperative imaging renders this unnecessary.[44] The full technical details of adrenalectomy are outside the scope of this chapter, but the following 'tips' are offered in relation to open adrenalectomy.

1. A right adrenalectomy is more difficult than a left.
2. The kidney is invaluable as a retractor and the plane between it and the adrenal should be left undissected until the cranial extremity of the adrenal is freed.
3. The right adrenal vein emerges from the *posterior* aspect of the inferior vena cava, and in anterior approaches careful rotation of the cava by an assistant helps to identify the adrenal vein.
4. The clipping or ligature of the short right adrenal vein must be absolutely secure; a slipped ligature or clip may leave an alarmingly large hole in the side of the inferior vena cava. A small Satinsky vascular clamp should always be at hand to deal with this eventuality.
5. A dangerous pitfall is the extra or ectopic right adrenal vein arising from the hepatic veins and entering the cranial aspect of the adrenal. These veins are easily torn during mobilisation.
6. When using the transperitoneal route for a left adrenalectomy it is easier to approach from the side after reflecting the splenic flexure of the colon, the spleen and the tail of the pancreas medially than it is to reach the adrenal by way of the lesser sac.

7. Accessory veins on the left may arise from the ascending phrenic vein but are easily controlled.

8. Loin approaches risk the development of intractable postoperative pain if the intercostal nerve is traumatised or caught up in the closure. Postoperative pain is reduced if the nerve is formally blocked with bupivacaine either by the anaesthetist or peroperatively by the surgeon.

9. Regardless of how carefully a flank approach to the adrenal is performed and the wound closed, some such wounds develop a bulge postoperatively, which may be interpreted as an incisional hernia. In fact it is normally simply attenuated muscle and does not require repair.

Laparoscopic route

 Laparoscopic adrenalectomy should by now be the standard technique being less traumatic, more cosmetic and allowing earlier discharge from hospital.[45]

The techniques of laparoscopic adrenalectomy are still being developed. It can be used in preference to the open approach for non-malignant tumours less than 10 cm in diameter although 6 cm is the more usual size, above which an open approach is preferred. The necessary expertise must, however, be available and many centres have found the combination of two surgeons, one skilled in laparoscopy and the other skilled in open adrenalectomy, to be a safe and effective team. Experience is gradually shortening operating time for these procedures, and an eventual expected average operating time will probably be about 90 to 120 minutes for a single adrenal. The proportion requiring conversion to open operation will also probably be less than 10%. Reported operating times are, however, still sometimes very long, one series reporting average times in excess of 350 minutes.[46]

The transperitoneal approach is the route most commonly used and can be undertaken with the patient supine or more usually in the same flank–up position as is used for the standard open loin approach (**Fig. 3.23**). Four or more 10 mm ports will be needed, and crucial implements include an articulated liver retractor, multifire clip applicator and a suction irrigator. There is, as yet, no available instrument suitable for holding the gland effectively without rupturing delicate adenomas or crushing functioning phaeochromocytomas. The laparoscopic approach should probably not be used for operations where malignancy is suspected but seems to be safe for phaeochromocytoma as there is minimal manipulation of the gland prior to clipping of the adrenal vein. There may be less manipulation than is applied during open procedures. When bilateral adrenalectomy is required, it is best undertaken as separate procedures with the patient turned and redraped between the two.

Technique of laparoscopic left adrenalectomy

The patient is positioned as shown in Fig. 3.23 and the team arranged as shown in **Figure 3.24**. The Veress needle is inserted via the midline or subcostally. When the pneumoperitoneum has been induced three medial ports are inserted as shown in **Figure 3.25**. The next step is to mobilize the splenic flexure of the colon down and medially to expose the lower margin of the spleen and the upper pole of the kidney. The next and most important phase of the procedure is to divide the lieno renal peritoneal ligament just lateral to the spleen along the full length of the spleen from the lower pole to the diaphragm. The lateral decubitus position now allows gravity to help the spleen fall medially, exposing the retroperitoneal space and the left adrenal gland. The adrenal should now be sought in the perirenal fat and mobilisation begun at its lateral or inferior border.

Figure 3.24
Position of patient and operating team for laparoscopic left adrenalectomy using the posterolateral approach.

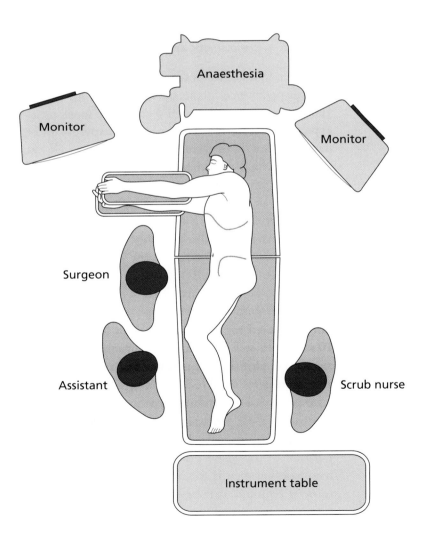

Figure 3.25
Trocar sites for left adrenalectomy.

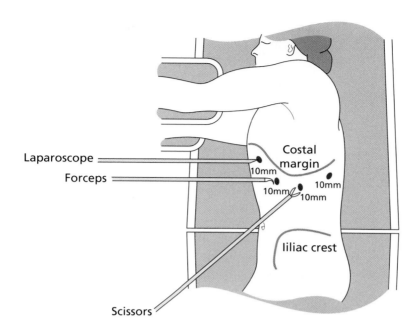

To achieve this it may be necessary to insert a fourth port laterally allowing a retractor to be inserted so that the spleen may be retracted more medially. The capsule of the adrenal is followed inferomedially until the adrenal vein is reached. Its junction with the renal vein is defined and two titanium clips applied about 1 cm from the renal vein. After division of the adrenal vein, mobilisation of the gland can proceed straightforwardly as described for the right adrenal. Other adrenal veins are often encountered arising from the phrenic vein between the adrenal and the aorta. Once freed, the adrenal is manipulated into a plastic bag and extracted through an enlarged port site without rupturing the bag or allowing any contents to spill into the peritoneum

Technique of laparoscopic right adrenalectomy

The patient is settled in the lateral decubitus position with the table 'broken.' The Veress needle may be inserted in the familiar midline site or 2 cm below the costal margin in the anterior axillary line, care being taken not to puncture the liver. When the pneumoperitoneum has been established, the ports may be inserted as shown in **Figure 3.26**, using normal safe laparoscopic practice. Surgeons vary in their preference as to which port to use for which instrument, but in general the most anterior port is best reserved for the liver retractor and the two lateral ports reserved for the dissection. The first stage of the operation is to take down any subhepatic adhesions and mobilise the hepatic flexure of the colon if necessary. The right triangular ligament may have to be divided to allow adequate retraction. The liver retractor is now inserted via the anterior port and

Figure 3.26
Trocar sites for right adrenalectomy.

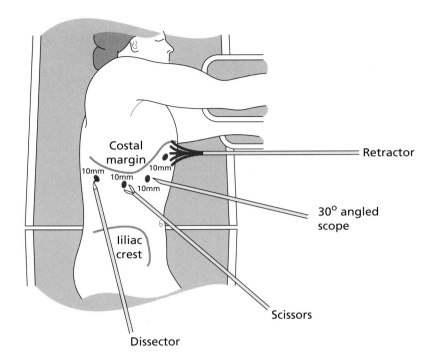

the right lobe of the liver carefully lifted and retracted medially. There is now sufficient exposure to allow incision of the posterior peritoneum just below the liver so as to open a curved space between the adrenal and the liver superiorly and the adrenal and the inferior vena cava medially. In most patients the adrenal is now readily identified by its characteristic golden colour, but in the obese Cushingoid patient quite extensive exploratory dissection may be needed to identify its site. If the tumour is small the plane between the adrenal and the inferior vena cava can now be deepened and extended and the adrenal vein iden-tified. The vein is now clipped, leaving, if possible, a generous stub on the caval side to avoid tearing the friable caval wall. At least two clips must be on the caval end of the vein. When the vein has been divided the gland is dissected out with the dissection as close to the gland surface as possible. Most of the dissection can be done with the hook or diathermy scissors, but the adrenal arteries emerging from behind the inferior vena cava and any aberrant adrenal veins may need to be clipped. The same careful technique for removal of the gland is used as for the left adrenal.

Larger tumours require modification of this technique, and the tumour and gland may need to be mobilised from laterally and cranially before access to the adrenal vein can be achieved.

An alternative laparoscopic approach is to operate with the patient supine, three trocars being inserted in the midline and one subcostally. Using this approach the left adrenal is more difficult to visualise because gravity cannot be used to retract the spleen medially. The details of this technique are described and illustrated on the internet at www.laparoscopy.net.

Publications of large series of laparoscopic adrenalectomies are now appearing in the literature from many centres, attesting to the straightforwardness of laparoscopy in trained hands. Operating time seems invariably longer than for the open methods but postoperative discomfort is less and the hospital stay down to 3–5 days. The procedure is particularly useful for the small tumours encountered in hyperaldosteronism, and it is valuable for Cushing's syndrome where wound healing is impaired and where the large loin or abdominal wound of an open operation is more likely to lead to postoperative respiratory complications.

Although most surgeons are currently employing the transperitoneal approach, the alternative laparoscopic approach involves the creation of a retroperitoneal space beside the kidney and adrenal gland using an inflatable balloon (**Fig. 3.27**). The operating space that becomes available is smaller than that with the transperitoneal route, bleeding points are more difficult to control and the risks of subcutaneous emphysema greater. It has, however, been claimed that the retroperitoneal

Figure 3.27
Technique of laparoscopic retroperitoneal adrenalectomy showing the use of a balloon to establish an extraperitoneal space adjacent to the adrenal. This technique is currently less commonly used than the straightforward anterior transperitoneal laparoscopic approach. Modified from reference 42.

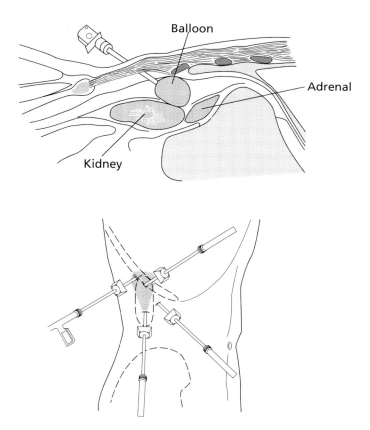

route is associated with a shorter postoperative hospital stay and less pain.[46] Each technique has its protagonists, but there are not yet sufficient data from randomised studies to determine whether one technique is superior to the other or whether both techniques have a place but in different circumstances. In addition to standard techniques using 10–12 mm ports, there are now reports of 'needle-scopic' adrenalectomies performed using two 2 mm ports, one 5 mm and one umbilical 10/12 mm port for specimen extraction. This minimalist technique is reported as allowing laparoscopic adrenalectomy to be undertaken with a one night stay in hospital.[47]

References

1. Cushing HW. The basophil adenomas of the pituitary body and their clinical manifestations. Bull Johns Hopkins Hosp 1932; 50: 137–95.

 2. Yanovski JA, Cutler GB. Glucocorticoid action and the clinical features of Cushing's syndrome. Endocrinol Metab Clin North Am 1994; 23: 487–509.

3. Ross EJ, Lynch CD. Cushing's syndrome: killing disease. Lancet 1982; ii: 64–9.

4. Perry RR, Neiman LK, Cutler GB *et al.* Primary adrenal causes of Cushing's syndrome. Ann Surg 1989; 210: 59–68.

5. Crapo L. Cushing's syndrome: a review of diagnostic tests. Metab Clin Exp 1979; 28: 955–77.

6. Bouloux P-MG, Rees LH (eds). Diagnostic tests in endocrinology and diabetes. London: Chapman & Hall Medical, 1994.

7. Upton GV, Amatruda TT. Evidence for the presence of tumour peptides with corticotrophin-releasing-factor-like activity in the ectopic ACTH syndrome. N Engl J Med 1971; 285: 419–24.

8. Samuels MH, Loriaux DL. Cushings syndrome and the nodular adrenal gland. Endocrinol Metab Clin North Am 1994; 23: 555–69.

9. Grant CS, Carney JA *et al.* Primary pigmented nodular adrenocortical disease: diagnosis and management. Surgery 1986; 100: 1178–84.

10. Zovickian J, Oldfield EH, Doppman JL *et al.* Usefulness of inferior petrosal sinus venous endocrine markers in Cushing's disease. J Neurosurg 1988; 68: 205–10.

 11. Becker MB, Aron DC. Ectopic ACTH syndrome and CRH mediated Cushing's syndrome. Endocrinol Metab Clin North Am 1994; 23: 585–606.

12. Negesser SK, Kievit J, Derksen J *et al.* Autologous adrenal transplantation for Cushing's disease. In: Clark

OH, Duh Q-Y (eds). Textbook of endocrine surgery. Philadelphia: WB Saunders, 1997; pp. 506–11.

13. Watanabe Y, Izumi Y, Yagugi T. Pregnancy in Cushing's syndrome. Folia Endocrinol Japon 1992; 68: 1130–49.

14. Percapio B, Knowlton AH. Radiation therapy of adrenal cortical carcinoma. Acta Radiol Ther Phys 1976; 15: 288–92.

15. Hogan TF, Citrin DL, Johnson BM *et al.* o'p-DDD (Mitotane) therapy of adrenal cortical carcinoma. Cancer 1978; 42: 2177–81.

16. Venkatesh S, Hickey RC, Sellin RV *et al.* Adrenal cortical carcinoma. Cancer 1989; 64: 765–9.

17. Young MB, Hughes IA. Response to treatment of congenital adrenal hyperplasia in infancy. Arch Dis Child 1990; 65: 441.

 18. Young Jr WFJ, Klee G. Primary aldosteronism. Endocrinol Metab Clin North Am 1988; 17: 367–95.

19. Bouloux LH, Rees LJ (eds). Diagnostic tests in endocrinology and diabetes. London: Chapman & Hall, 1994; pp. 166.

20. Young WF, Hogan MJ, Klee GG *et al.* Primary aldosteronism: diagnostic treatment. Mayo Clin Proc 1990; 65: 96–110.

21. Gleason PT, Weinberger MH, Pratt JH *et al.* Evaluation of diagnostic tests in the differential diagnosis of primary aldosteronism. J Urol 1993; 150: 1365–8.

22. Aboud E, De Suriet M, Gordon H. Primary aldosteronism in pregnancy—should it be treated surgically? Irish J Med Sci 1995; 764: 279–80.

23. St John Sutton MG, Sheps SG, Lei JT. Prevalence of clinically unsuspected phaeochromocytoma: review of a 50-year autopsy series. Mayo Clin Proc 1981; 56: 354–60.

24. Bravo EL, Gifford RW, Manger WM. Adrenal medullary tumours; phaeochromocytoma in endocrine tumours. In: Mazzaferri EL, Samaan NA (eds). Endocrine tumours. Boston: Blackwell, 1993; pp. 426–47.

25. Johns VJ, Brunjes S. Phaeochromocytoma. Am J Cardiol 1962; 9: 120–5.

26. Kran NN. Clinically unsuspected phaeochromocytomas: experience at Henry Ford Hospital and a review of the literature. Arch Intern Med 1986; 146: 54–7.

27. O'Riordain DS, O'Brien T, Crotty TB et al. Multiple endocrine neoplasia type 2B: more than an endocrine disorder. Surgery 1995; 118: 926–42.

28. Richard D, Beigelman C, Duclas J-M et al. Phaeochromocytoma as the first manifestations of Von Hippel–Lindau disease. Surgery 1994; 116: 1076–108.

29. Sheps SG, Jiang N, Klee GG et al. Recent developments in the diagnosis and treatment of phaeochromocytoma. Mayo Clin Proc 1990; 65: 88–95.

30. Peplinski GR, Norton JA. The predictive value of diagnostic tests for phaeochromocytoma. Surgery 1994; 116: 1101–10.

31. Deoreo GA, Stewart BH, Tarazi RC et al. Preoperative blood transfusion in the safe surgical management of phaeochromocytoma. J Urol 194; 111: 715–21.

32. Scheker JC, Chowers I. Phaeochromocytoma and pregnancy. Review of 89 cases. Obstet Gynecol Surg 1971; 26: 729–47.

33. Dreier DT, Thompson NW. Phaeochromocytoma and pregnancy: the epitome of high risk. Surgery 1993; 114: 1148–52.

34. Averbuch SD, Steakley CS, Young RC et al. Malignant phaeochromocytoma. Ann Intern Med 1988; 109: 267–73.

35. O'Dorisio MS, Qualman SJ. Neuroblastoma. In: Mazzaferri EL, Samaan NA (eds). Endocrine tumours. Boston: Blackwell, 1993.

36. Rosen EM, Cassady JR, Frantz CN et al. Neuroblastoma. J Clin Oncol 1984; 2: 719–32.

37. Mantero F, Arnaldi G. Investigation protocol: adrenal enlargement. Clin Endocrinol 1999; 50: 141–6.

38. Reining JW, Doppman JL, Dwyer AJ et al. Adrenal masses differentiated by MR. Radiology 1986; 158: 81.

39. Silverman SG, Mueller PR, Pinkey LP et al. Predictive value of image guided adrenal biopsy: analysis of results of 101 biopsis. Radiology 1993; 187: 715.

40. Herrera MF, Grant CS, Van-Heerden JA et al. Incidentally discovered adrenal tumours; an institutional perspective. Surgery 1991; 110: 1014–21.

41. Linos DA. Adrenaloma (incidentaloma). In: Clark OH and Duh Q-Y (eds). Textbook of endocrine surgery. Philadelphia: WB Saunders 1997; pp. 475–82.

42. Gairai H, Young AE. Adrenal incidentalomas. Br J Surg 1993; 80: 422–6.

43. Young HH. A technique for simultaneous exposure and operation on the adrenals. Surg Gynecol Obstet 1936; 63: 179–88.

44. Orchard T, Grant CS, Van-Heerden JA, Weaver A. Phaeochromocytoma, continuing evolution of surgical therapy. Surgery 1993; 114: 1153–9.

45. Dudley NE, Harrison BJ. Comparison of open posterior versus transperitoneal laparoscopic adrenalectomy. Br J Surg 1999; 86: 656–60.

46. Miyake O, Yoshimura K, Yoshioka T et al. Laparoscopic adrenalectomy. Comparison of the transperitoneal and retroperitoneal approach. Eur Urol 1998; 33: 303–7.

47. Gill IS, Soble JJ, Sung GT et al. Needlescopic adrenalectomy—the initial series: comparison with conventional laparoscopic adrenalectomy. Urology 1998; 52: 180–6.

4 Familial endocrine disease—genetics and early treatment

Radu Mihai
John R. Farndon

Familial endocrine diseases form a group of rare conditions producing much clinical and scientific interest. Recent development of genetic tests allows less invasive screening and this has a major impact on the management of such patients. It is hoped that early detection may translate into more effective therapy.

This chapter focuses on several endocrine diseases, each with an inherited pattern:

- Multiple endocrine neoplasia syndrome type 1 (MEN-1 syndrome)
- MEN-2 syndromes and familial medullary thyroid carcinoma
- Familial papillary carcinoma of the thyroid
- Familial hyperparathyroidism syndromes
- Phaeochromocytoma as part of von Recklinghausen and von Hippel–Lindau syndromes
- Familial primary hyperaldosteronism
- Carney syndrome

MEN-1

MEN-1 is a rare condition, inherited as an autosomal dominant disease with high penetrance and no special geographical, racial or ethnic preferences. Patients present with tumours of the parathyroid glands, pancreatic islets and anterior pituitary. Considerable insight into the genetics and management of this syndrome has been achieved since 1954 when Wermer reported the first family recognised with the condition.[1]

Incidence

The true incidence of MEN-1 is unknown, because there are no long-term, population-based studies. The disease prevalence is estimated to be in the range of 20 to 200 per million but this may be an underestimate of the real penetrance because of the lack of recognition of the syndrome.

The largest known genealogy of a kindred with MEN-1 dates back to 1840 and has been constructed in Tasmania. An initial study of over 600 descendants of one English migrant suggested that, overall, one quarter of all family members and one half of those over the age of 40 manifest one or more endocrine tumours.[2] In the majority, the diagnosis was not suspected until the practitioner was informed of the family history, since symptoms were vague, sometimes bizarre and overlapped with those of common disorders. More detailed analysis of nearly 2000 descendants of this English immigrant found MEN-1 to be highly probable in 130 and moderately probable in 22.[3] Another 242 children and siblings were 50% likely to have inherited the dominant gene. In all age groups, especially elderly relatives, most affected members had symptoms of only one endocrine disorder or were asymptomatic. In teenagers the most common presentation was pituitary lesions then insulinomas, and these often developed before hyperparathyroidism. An increased concentration of gastrin, usually associated with hypercalcaemia, was rarely seen in patients younger than 25 years. These data confirm that the familial specificity of the clinical picture varies and that the classic presentation (i.e. with symptoms of multiple endocrinopathy) may represent only a small fraction of patients with MEN-1 in the community.

Morbidity and mortality

Few data are available on the natural history of untreated MEN-1 syndrome. When the cause of death was determined in a large MEN-1 kindred (159 patients) in a retrospective study of recorded medical data from 1861 to 1991,[4] 46 patients were classified as 'highly probable' of having MEN-1 and 20 died of a recognised complication of MEN-1 (12 of malignant neoplasma, six of renal calculi and two of peptic ulcer). The mean age of death (51 years) was significantly younger than that of other family members. It was concluded that MEN-1 leads to premature death, malignant neoplasms being the main cause.[4]

Early diagnosis through prospective screening and the current therapeutic approach should improve the quality of life and decrease the morbidity and mortality associated with MEN-1 tumours.

Aetiology

In 1997 the gene for MEN-1 was cloned by two independent groups.[5,6] This represented a major breakthrough in the understanding of the disease.

It has been known for the past 10 years that the predisposing genetic defect for MEN-1 is located on the long arm of chromosome 11 (11q13 locus),[7] loss of heterozygosity at this site being detected for all typical MEN-1 families. In affected patients, inactivation of the wild-type MEN-1 allele inherited from the unaffected parent by variable extensive deletions unmasks a constitutional mutation (inherited from the affected parent) in a putative gene with tumour suppressor function.[8] According to this model for tumorigenesis, congenital abnormality of one allele of this gene is carried in the germ line of parathyroid, pituitary and pancreatic cells, and tumour growth is initiated by a secondary, somatic mutation, affecting the normal allele. Each tumour in MEN-1 is thus monoclonal but apparently arises in a background of polyclonal hyperplasia, and the patients are prone to have multiple synchronous or asynchronous lesions. Because the secondary mutation occurs randomly, sometimes with an appreciable time lag, the patients may present a variable number of microscopic and macroscopic tumours. Before the *MEN-1* gene was cloned, the MEN-1 locus was estimated to be one tenth of chromosome 11, with about 30 candidate genes.

An additional tumorigenesis mechanism was suggested by the presence of a mitogenic factor with structural analogy with basic fibroblast growth factor (bFGF) in plasma of patients with MEN-1. The *bFGF*-related gene was known to be localised at 11q13 and mitogenic activity seemed to be high in known gene carriers, to precede overt endocrine hyperfunction and to correlate with parathyroid (but not pancreatic or pituitary) function.[9] Even if genetic studies ruled out this *bFGF*-like gene as the *MEN-1* gene, it can be speculated that a phase of polyclonal expansion, triggered or sustained by this growth factor, may precede the monoclonal expansion of the parathyroid clone precursor.

The *MEN-1* gene encodes a ubiquitously expressed 610-amino acid protein product, referred to as *MENIN*.[5,6] MENIN is principally a nuclear protein, the role of which remains to be elucidated, because it does not have homologies to other proteins known to be involved in cell proliferation and control of cell cycle. Over 40 mutations of the *MEN-1* gene have been identified so far,[10] but correlation between the mutations and the clinical manifestations of MEN-1 could not be established either between families or even within the families. The majority of such mutations are nonsense mutations, frameshift deletions or insertions that are likely to inactivate MENIN function.[10] These recent findings are consistent with the proposal that MEN-1 is due to inactivating mutations of a tumour-suppressor gene. Such a mechanism is in contrast with the related disorder MEN-2, where activating mutations of the *RET* oncogene are responsible (see below).

In addition to the classic form of MEN-1, a related syndrome was first described in the Burin peninsula (MEN-1$_{burin}$), which links hyperparathyroidism, prolactinoma and carcinoids and a lower frequency of pancreatic endocrine tumours. All the five families identified in Newfoundland and the Pacific Northwest have the same PYCM allele and flanking polymorphic markers of the *MEN*-1 gene.[11]

Presentation

The mode of presentation of patients with MEN-1 varies according to the index lesion and the nature/quantity of its secreted hormones.

Any clinical components of MEN-1 can be the presenting manifestation, but there is a propensity for specific patterns of organ involvement or peptide over-production, with distinct and identifiable family-specific syndromes.[12] Unlike sporadic patients (non-familial), MEN-1 tumours are often multicentric, are commonly associated with hyperplasia and have a higher rate of recurrence.

Clinical diagnosis within probands requires identification of at least two lesions classically associated with MEN-1, although only one is sufficient in members of established kindreds. Some tumours, although associated with hormonal excess over long periods, produce no symptoms.

Because of age-dependent penetrance, most individuals carrying the MEN-1 predisposing genetic defect do not develop clinical manifestations until the third decade of life, and by the time the clinically overt syndrome appears, most patients are in the fourth decade. The advent of efficient prospective biochemical screening programmes has reduced the age at first diagnosis by two decades, to a mean of 14–18 years.

Hyperparathyroidism

Hyperparathyroidism (HPT) is the most common lesion in MEN-1, with an estimated 90% prevalence in necropsy and screening studies. It is usually the first abnormality detected on screening, and parathyroid glands are almost always hyperfunctional by the time islet cell or pituitary involvement becomes clinically evident. Patients are first detected in their teens, and by age 40 more than 95% of patients have hypercalcaemia. The onset is gradual and clinically subtle, and patients become symptomatic relatively late. The clinical picture is similar to sporadic HPT (see Chapter 1), apart from a greater incidence of peptic ulcer in patients with MEN-1 (due to occurrence of gastrinomas). Characteristically, multiglandular hyperplasia is found, with possible adenomatous transformation, but one or more glands can be macroscopically and microscopically normal (**Fig. 4.1**).

Although monoclonality has been described in parathyroid adenomas and hyperplasia in MEN-1,[13] it does not correlate with the heterogeneous reduced expression and function of a putative calcium-sensing protein regulating parathyroid hormone release.[14]

Figure 4.1
One of the four enlarged hyperplastic parathyroid glands from a patient with MEN-1 syndrome.

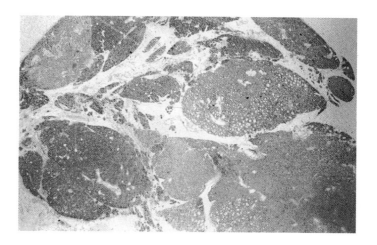

Pancreatic islet cell tumours

Pancreatic islet cell tumours have a prevalence of 30–75%, assessed by clinical screening techniques, and 80% in necropsy studies.[15] They are characteristically multicentric, slow growing and range from nesidioblastosis through adenomas to carcinomas. Multiple peptides might be secreted by a tumour, although usually only one predominates, and this pattern can vary from one sibling to another.

Most pancreatic tumours are detected by screening or imaging of the pancreas or liver. Some present after the development of specific symptoms owing to hypersecretion of one or more peptide hormones or from mechanical effects of a non-functional tumour. A spectrum of islet cell tumours has been associated with the MEN-1 syndrome, from the most frequently encountered insulinoma and gastrinomas to vasoactive intestinal polypeptide secreting adenoma (VIPoma), glucagonoma, somatostatinoma, pancreatic polypeptide (PP)-secreting and ectopic adrenocorticotrophic (ACTH)-secreting tumours.

Gastrinoma

Gastrinomas occur in 30–60% of patients with MEN-1. Increased serum gastrin concentrations induce gastric acid hypersecretion, which causes recurrent and multiple peptic ulcers, severe reflux oesophagitis and diarrhoea (Zollinger–Ellison syndrome; ZES). Many patients with ZES have small (1–2 mm) gastrinomas arising within the duodenal wall, which metastasise to the peripancreatic and periduodenal lymph nodes and rarely to the liver (10% of patients).[16]

Insulinoma

Insulinomas occur in up to 35% of patients with MEN-1 and in 10–15% represent the only functional component of pancreatic neuroendocrine disease. They tend to be multiple, but multiple tumours in these patients are not always insulinomas unless proven by immunocytochemistry. Only a minority of these tumours metastasise.

Other pancreatic islet cell tumours

Glucagonomas cause hyperglycaemia and a characteristic rash, necrolytic migratory erythema. VIPoma is recognised by the association of watery diarrhoea, achlorhydria and hypokalaemia (Verner Morrison syndrome). Human pancreatic polypeptide (hPP) secretion by pancreatic tumours is often detected biochemically but is clinically silent.

Pituitary adenomas

These can be detected in 15–40% of patients, although necropsy studies report up to 65% prevalence. Anterior pituitary hyperfunction is most commonly recognised during the fourth decade and manifests as hyperprolactinaemia (prolactinomas) and less commonly as acromegaly (growth hormone (GH)-secreting adenoma) or Cushing's syndrome (ACTH hypersecretion). Hyperthyroidism due to secretion of thyroid stimulating hormone (TSH) is extremely rare. Sometimes the first sign of a pituitary tumour is impaired vision due to compression of the optic chiasma by suprasellar extension of a pituitary adenoma. The recurrence rate is higher than for sporadic tumours.

The differential diagnosis of a pituitary lesion should include ectopic secretion from pancreatic tumours inducing acromegaly (ectopic GH-RH) or Cushing's syndrome (ectopic ACTH) or corticotrophin-releasing hormone (CRH).

Other clinical manifestations

- Neuroendocrine carcinoid-like tumours of the duodenum have been reported with high prevalence and can secrete serotonin, somatostatin or gastrin (causing ZES). Carcinoid tumours may occur in the thymus, lungs and foregut. Carcinoid tumours are more common in the Tasmanian kindreds.
- Thyroid neoplasia (adenomas or differentiated carcinomas) are identified with increased frequency.
- Adrenocortical adenomas and/or macronodular hyperplasia are discovered in one third of patients with MEN-1 either radiologically or at necropsy (compared with 10% of the general population), the majority of such tumours being hormonally silent and without an aggressive course.[17] The presence of adrenal lesions seems to correlate with the extent of pancreatic disease: an ultrasonographic analysis of a large Tasmanian MEN-1 kindred identified adrenal disease in 75% of patients with pancreatic lesions and in 10% of those with pancreatic lesions and hepatic metastases, whereas none of the patients without pancreatic lesions had adrenal abnormalities.[18] The

pathogenic mechanism for adrenal lesions in MEN-1 is not understood because there is no hypothalamic–pituitary–adrenal dysfunction, and the role of pancreatic hormonal hypersecretion is still hypothetical (i.e. similar to Cushing's syndrome, secondary to excess secretion of gastrin-inhibitory polypeptide).

- Lipomas are more common than in the general population.
- Spinal cord ependymomas and pinealomas are further possible associations.
- Recently, collagenomas and multiple angiofibromas of the dermis have been recognised as frequent associations.

Screening for MEN-1 syndrome

Signs and symptoms of MEN-1 usually appear in the fourth decade of life, but biochemical testing can identify affected individuals at 14–18 years of age and DNA analysis at any age. Presymptomatic detection and identification of gene carriers should, therefore, be the screening strategy. Although prospective screening studies in affected families have lowered the age of detectable onset to the mid-teens and most patients are detected before 25 years, there is still no clearly demonstrated reduction in mortality by early diagnosis (in contrast to the effects on survival after screening for MEN-2 syndrome). A consensus regarding the optimal and cost-effective MEN-1 screening programme design is still lacking. The impact of genetic testing for MENIN mutations is yet to be evaluated.

Genetic screening

Because MEN-1 is an autosomal dominant inheritance, one copy of the predisposing genetic defect is sufficient to cause the disease. Consequently, a child with one affected parent has a 50% chance of inheriting the disease. DNA-based methods are now employed to distinguish gene carriers in MEN-1 families because the risk estimated for carrying the defective gene is greater than 99.5%.[19] Non-carriers can therefore be excluded from repeated biochemical testing whereas gene carriers are subjected to annual biochemical investigation from the onset of adolescence (over 10–15 years of age). Identification of gene-carrier status at an early age makes it possible for family members to make informed decisions regarding childbearing.

Before the *MEN-1* gene was isolated, direct mutation analysis was not possible, and the diagnosis relied on demonstrating the presence or absence of the allele (MEN-1 locus) identified in at least two affected members of the same family. A panel of flanking polymorphic DNA markers segregating with *MEN-1* in a given family were used for linkage analysis and restriction fragment length polymorphism to identify gene carriers with great accuracy (for a review see Reference 20).

The recent studies involving characterisation of the *MEN-1* gene showed that it has a high penetrance after the age of 5 years and is 52% and 100% penetrant by the ages of 20 years and 60 years, respectively.[10] An additional important finding is that more than 10% of the mutations are *de novo*,[10] and the development of MEN-1 tumours in a patient without a family history of the disorder does not necessarily imply that the siblings are at risk. In addition, the subsequent inheritance of such *de novo* mutation places the children at risk and in need of clinical/biochemical/genetic evaluation.

Biochemical screening

Thorough screening studies have demonstrated that the MEN-1 trait is biochemically detectable about 20 years before overt disease. Screening includes measurement of serum concentrations of calcium (ionised or total corrected for albumin) and intact PTH for the parathyroids, prolactin and insulin growth factor 1 (IGF-1) for pituitary lesions and serum glucose, insulin, pancreatic polypeptide, gastrin and chromogranin A for duodenal/pancreatic tumours. Because an optimal interval between screening investigations has not been identified, some groups recommend annual investigations. More extensive screening is recommended by other groups (**Table 4.1**),[15] but compliance is greater if screening tests are kept simple and regular. On the other hand, measurements of serum gastrin, prolactin and calcitonin concentrations are needless screening

Test	Comments
Plasma calcium (ionised/albumin corrected)	Measuring parathyroid hormone (PTH) with ionised plasma calcium allows earlier detection than albumin-corrected plasma calcium levels
PTH	Biterminal assays for intact PTH
Prolactin	
Gastrin	Consider stimulation tests
Glucose	
Insulin-like growth factor	
Insulin	Fast for up to 3 days and consider stimulation tests
Proinsulin	
Glucagon	
Pancreatic polypeptide (pp)	
Meal test with PP and gastrin measurements	PP increased to twice the reference range after a test meal indicates the necessity for surveillance of tumour development

Table 4.1 *Biochemical screening profile for patients with MEN-1*

determinations in patients undergoing surgery for primary HPT with no symptoms of MEN-1 syndromes.[21]

Biochemical evaluation of individual tumours

- HPT is diagnosed by using the same criteria as in those with sporadic disease, with hypercalcaemia accompanied by increased/non-suppressed plasma PTH concentrations.
- Basal gastrin concentrations as a sole marker would reveal only 20% of gastrinomas at the time of diagnosis. Increased basal concentrations are, however, not normally found in MEN-1 microadenomas and should be regarded as an indicator of a large pancreatic tumour (with a 50% risk of malignancy) or a duodenal carcinoid. Hypergastrinaemia (fasting concentration >1000 pg ml^{-1}) and gastric acid hypersecretion (basal acid output >15 mmol h^{-1}) confirms the diagnosis of gastrinoma. Less convincing biochemical values can be confirmed by provocative tests, demonstrating an increase in gastrin concentrations by 50% or 200 pg ml^{-1} after a rapid infusion of calcium and secretin.[22]

  Changes to serum gastrin and pancreatic polypeptide (PP) concentrations with a meal stimulation test are advocated to improve the sensitivity of the diagnosis; a 560 kcal meal rich in carbohydrates and low in proteins is recommended.[23] A meal-stimulated response twice the normal basal values for gastrin and exceeding by two standard deviations the mean serum PP concentrations in a control group should lead to enhanced observation and additional investigation. Exaggerated serum gastrin responses appear in approximately one half of patients and serum PP responses in all patients with verified pancreatic tumours. This test is described as being equally useful in the diagnosis of gastrinomas, PPomas, VIPomas, somatostatinomas, glucagonomas and non-functional pancreatic tumours.
- In patients suspected of having an insulinoma, blood samples for glucose, insulin and proinsulin concentrations should be obtained during episodes of symptomatic hypoglycaemia. Hypoglycaemia and hyperinsulinaemia (and high C-peptide concentrations, to exclude factitious hypoglycaemia) during symptomatic episodes and an increased ratio of serum proinsulin to insulin are diagnostic. Simultaneous measurement of plasma glucose and insulin concentrations during a fasting period (up to 7 hours) is widely used as a 'provocative' test. A rapid calcium infusion (2 mg kg^{-1} min^{-1}) is also a potent insulin secretagogue in patients with insulinoma.[24]
- Extended investigations, including chromogranins, human chorionic gonadotrophin subunits, VIP, calcitonin, ACTH, somatostatin and serotonin should be reserved for patients with positive radiology but normal/equivocal increased routine screening markers. After surgery for pancreatic tumours, it

is important to include these markers in the follow-up criteria as relapse or liver metastases could produce hormones different from those secreted by the initial tumour.

● Pituitary tumours are most readily diagnosed by prolactin and somatomedin C determinations and pituitary imaging (MRI) every 5 years. Since pancreatic tumours can be the source of ectopic CRH or CRH/ACTH secretion, plasma concentrations of releasing hormones should also be measured in patients with acromegaly or Cushing's syndrome.

Radiological screening

Imaging studies for parathyroid tumours are not worthwhile unless HPT recurs and re-exploration is anticipated (see Chapter 1).

Pancreatic tumours are not easy to localise. A multicentre study found that none of the localising techniques have satisfactory accuracy rates: computed tomography (CT) (33.3%), ultrasonography (39.2%) and arteriography (61.6%) being less sensitive than the more invasive percutaneous transhepatic portography (88.7%).[25] Recently, endoscopic and intraoperative ultrasonography have been used (**Fig. 4.2**), but intraoperative palpation sometimes remains the best method to localise pancreatic tumours. It is suggested that all patients with biochemically proven pancreatic tumours should have adrenal imaging because of the frequent association of the two lesions.

Figure 4.2
Endoscopic ultrasound image of a pancreatic gastrinoma. The transducer is located in the stomach and is scanning the pancreas through the posterior gastric wall, demonstrating a 7 mm neuroendocrine tumour in the pancreatic body (between marks). (Courtesy of Dr S. Norton, Bristol Royal Infirmary.)

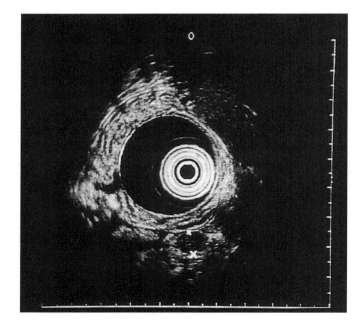

Other diagnostic techniques

- Intraoperative pancreatic ultrasonography.
- Portal venous sampling for pancreatic tumours. Sequential injection of secretin into the coeliac axis with subsequent hepatic vein sampling for gastrin concentration has been reported to localise pancreatic gastrinomas better than angiography alone and to have less morbidity than transhepatic portal venous sampling.[26]
- Selective arterial catheterisation with calcium injection (as an insulin secretagogue) may be helpful for localising insulinomas.[27] Percutaneous transhepatic selective venous sampling of insulin concentration for insulinomas is no longer considered to be necessary.
- Intraoperative selective intra-arterial secretin test with rapid radio-immunoassay for gastrin concentration may be useful to determine whether an operation for ZES was curative.[28] If the rapid test is not available, fasting gastrin concentrations of less than 100 pg ml^{-1} or an increase to less than 200 pg ml^{-1} after a secretin test is used as a biochemical test for cure.

Management options

Parathyroid tumours

HPT usually begins in a subtle or non-aggressive fashion, and early surgical treatment is not required. Some advocate early parathyroidectomy because hypercalcaemia is progressive and potentiates pancreatic (and possibly pituitary) disease. All parathyroid tissue should be located and removed because of the high incidence of recurrence: when 50 such patients were followed-up 2 to 27 years, persistent or recurrent HPT was found in 66% and 20% of patients after subtotal and total parathyroidectomy, respectively.[29] Therefore total parathyroidectomy plus autologous grafting in the forearm is preferred. Several weeks might be required until the graft functions sufficiently to maintain normocalcaemia and the immediately postoperative hypoparathyroidism is corrected with oral calcitriol and calcium supplements. Parathyroid tissue from patients with MEN-1 can be cryopreserved for genetic testing or further autotransplantation (if the first failed).

Pancreatic tumours

The objective in all patients is to detect and excise tumours before any malignant potential is declared by hepatic metastases. Surgical treatment can be life saving for patients with some tumours (insulinoma, VIPoma) and can eliminate the need for expensive daily drug therapy (gastrinoma). Patients with functional hormonal syndromes have one or more discrete tumours rather than islet cell hyperplasia and microadenomatosis and therefore can be effectively treated by tumour excision without the need of extensive pancreatectomy.

The development of efficient antisecretory drugs (H_2-blockers and proton pump inhibitors) allows effective medical management of ZES without the need for total gastrectomy for acute complications of peptic ulcer disease or unremitting symptoms. The disadvantages of medical therapy include life-long dependency, the possible progression of localised malignancy to lymph nodes and liver and the possible development of multiple enterochromaffin-like tumours, especially within the stomach.[30]

Enucleation should be attempted for lesions in the pancreatic head or duodenum. Distal pancreatectomy is performed for gastrinomas in the tail and body of the pancreas. Total pancreatectomy is reserved for patients with family members who have demonstrated aggressive tumour behaviour. Other surgical strategies include:

- Duodenotomy and palpation of the wall circumferentially from the pylorus to the third part. Small gastrinomas (<0.5 cm) are locally excised and larger gastrinomas are excised with a full-thickness margin of duodenal wall;
- Excision of peripancreatic lymph nodes, including those along the common bile duct and within the porta hepatis, medial to the coeliac axis;
- Full mobilisation of the head and uncinate process and enucleation of palpable or ultrasonographically identified pancreatic tumours;
- Distal pancreatectomy (neck, body and tail), preserving the spleen when feasible.

Recurrent and/or metastatic disease occurs in 50% of patients.[31] Large pancreatic tumours are predictive of the development of metachronous liver metastases, and surgery does not seem to prevent them.[32] Symptomatic therapy includes H_2-blockers, proton pump inhibitory drugs and octreotide. Partial hepatectomy and hepatic transplantation are palliative options in patients with hepatic involvement.

Enucleation of the insulinoma is the best option. Blind 'subtotal pancreatectomy' is not advisable. Inoperable metastatic insulinomas or recurrent disease can be treated with diazoxide and chemotherapy (streptozocin, dacarbazine and 5-fluorouracil). Octreotide is effective in blocking pancreatic secretion and reduces the incidence of postoperative complications.

Pituitary tumours

Hypophysectomy plus external beam radiation may be curative for pituitary tumours, but medical treatment is extremely efficient for prolactinomas (bromocriptine) and can be considered for acromegaly.

Other tumours

Carcinoids can usually be totally excised. Octreotide has been successfully used, but interferon and palliative chemotherapy (methotrexate, cyclophosphamide, streptozocin, 5-fluorouracil) are of unproven efficacy.

Research interests in MEN-1 syndrome

Now that the *MEN-1* gene has been cloned, studies are being undertaken to understand its role in tumour development. This is even more challenging because *MEN-1* gene abnormalities have been demonstrated in non-familial tumours, such as parathyroid adenomas (see Chapter 1). It is also important to determine its role in the diagnosis in younger patients at risk to assess the value of identifying or excluding the presence of a mutation before the onset of symptoms. The better understanding of the molecular basis of this disorder should allow the development of better therapeutic strategies.

Multiple endocrine neoplasia type 2

Multiple endocrine neoplasia type 2 (MEN-2) is an autosomal dominant syndrome with incomplete penetrance, so that 30% of patients have no symptoms, even by the age of 70.[33] Three different forms of MEN-2 are identified:

1. MEN-2A refers to patients with medullary thyroid carcinoma (MTC) associated with phaeochromocytoma (50% of patients) and hyperparathyroidism (HPT) (15% of patients). This association was first recognised by Sipple in 1961[34] and represents up to 90% of patients in recent series.
2. MEN-2B is the association of MTC, phaeochromocytomas, a general (not absolute) lack of parathyroid disease and a specific phenotype consisting of marfanoid body habitus, mucosal neuromas and intestinal ganglioneuromatosis. It accounts for approximately 5% of all patients with MEN-2.
3. Familial MTC (FMTC) refers to patients having inherited MTC without other endocrinopathy.

Aetiology

Initial evidence suggested that MEN-2 is a familial cancer syndrome arising from a mutation in chromosome 10 (region 10p11.2–q11.2). Based on the frequent allele losses on several other chromosomes, it was suggested that several genes contribute to tumour development in MEN-2: an initiating locus on chromosome 10 and additional loci on chromosomes 1p, 3p, 9q, 13q, 17 and 22q.[35]

Recent studies have shown that germ-line point mutations in the RET proto-oncogene segregate with the disease phenotype in MEN-2 and FMTC.[36,37] Multiple mutations have been described and are currently being collected by a *RET Mutation Consortium* for confirmation of a predicted genotype–phenotype correlation.[38]

The RET proto-oncogene is located on chromosome 10 and encodes a cell-surface glycoprotein related to the family of receptor tyrosine kinases that is expressed in derivatives of neural crest cells and whose ligand is still unknown (for a review see reference 39). Alterations in one of its three functional domains are implicated in the development of MTC, and rearranged versions of RET have also been described in up to 30% of papillary thyroid carcinomas.[40]

Point mutations affecting the RET-extracellular domain (codon 609, 611, 618, 620 in exon 10 and 634 in exon 11) are found in 97% of patients with MEN-2A and 96% of patients with isolated familial MTC. The catalytic core region of the tyrosine kinase domain is affected in almost all patients with MEN-2B owing to changing of a highly conserved methionine ($Met^{918}Thr$, in exon 16). Mutations within the intracellular domain of RET ($Glu^{768}Asp$ in exon 13 and $Leu^{804}Val$ in exon 14) have been identified in a family with FMTC.

A challenging issue concerns the relationship between genetic mechanisms for MEN-2 and Hirschsprung's disease. A point mutation in the *RET* gene ($Cys^{618}Ser$) was described in two large unrelated MEN-2A kindreds in which Hirschsprung's disease cosegregated.[41] It is suggested that specific mutations in cysteine codons 618 and 620 not only result in MEN-2A or FMTC but can also predispose to Hirschsprung's disease, with low penetrance.[42]

Mechanisms

C-cells of the thyroid, adrenal medullary cells and cells of the autonomic plexus and ganglia of the alimentary tract all arise from the neural crest. A molecular abnormality affecting cells of this lineage could, therefore, readily account for all the dominant features of MEN-2. The RET proto-oncogene is normally expressed in C-cells, chromaffin and parathyroid cells.[43] Expression of an activated RET receptor in these cell types results in initiation of transformation, but it seems likely that these mutations represent only the first step in the oncogenetic pathway.

The incidence of each *RET* gene mutation varies. In families with MEN-2A and FMTC, 80–90% of patients have a mutated codon 634; mutations of codon 620 account for 6–8% of patients, and less than 5% of patients have mutations in other codons. When codon 634 is affected, mutation of a single base changes a highly conserved cysteine (encoded by TGC sequence) to another amino acid—arginine (CGC), serine (AGC), tyrosine (TAC), phenylalanine (TTC), tryptophan (TGG)—and has major functional implications.

RET is a proto-oncogene, which means that a single activating mutation of only one allele should be sufficient to cause neoplastic transformation. All *RET* gene mutations identified result in oncogenic activity of the RET protein. Mutations affecting the five cysteine residues of the extracellular domain (i.e. codon 634) activate the RET receptor and cause receptor monomers to dimerise, thereby mimicking the effects caused by the binding of a ligand to the receptor and inducing enhanced phosphorylation and constitutive activation of the tyrosine-kinase domain.

In families with MEN-2B, a single mutation in exon 16 of the RET proto-oncogene (Met^{918}Thr) is present in 95% of patients.[44] Codon 918 is part of the encoding for the pocket that recognises the substrate for the receptor tyrosine-kinase; the mutated receptor is not only constitutively activated but also causes enhanced phosphorylation of a different set of substrate proteins (such as *c-src* and *c-abl*) resulting in cellular transformation. Although it is rare, the absence of this particular mutation of the RET proto-oncogene does not always exclude the diagnosis of MEN-2B, and in families with this syndrome routine biochemical screening for MTC and phaeochromocytoma must be maintained for all individuals at genetic risk.[45] Some patients with MEN-2B occur *de novo*,[46] and the high incidence of newly discovered mutations could be owing to the low reproductive rates of patients with MEN-2B (increased mortality, low marriage rates, impotence due to neurological problems).

Further evidence for the role of RET mutations in tumorigenesis was obtained by transfecting cell lines with the MEN-2A (Cys^{634}Arg) and MEN-2B (Met^{918}Thr) RET constructs. The Ret-MEN-2A and Ret-MEN-2B proteins were found to be constitutively phosphorylated and their *in vitro* kinase activity was significantly higher than that of the wild-type protein.[47]

The mechanism for development of HPT in MEN-2A is not obvious. It is not caused by increased concentrations of calcitonin because it is not associated with sporadic MTC or MEN-2B syndromes. The role of RET in parathyroid development and pathogenesis of HPT remains unclear.

Presentation

Because of a near complete penetrance of the *MEN-2* gene, all gene carriers are likely to be affected. Clinical expression of each individual component of the syndrome in affected families is variable, and not all the components of the syndrome must be present in each member of one family. Changes in the glands seem to be causally and temporally independent of each other, and the timelag between the development of each component of the syndrome varies. The first clinical manifestation of disease may occur during the second decade or even later. Once the diagnosis of an endocrine tumour known to be associated with

MEN-2 is achieved in a young patient, this should stimulate a search for other tumours in the patient and family because, if diagnosed early, all MEN-2 lesions are treatable and curable.

Clinical presentation of MEN-2A

MTC

MTC is the most common manifestation of MEN-2A and its hallmark. It occurs in 95% of gene carriers during life and can be lethal.

MTC originates from the thyroid parafollicular cells (C-cells), which synthesise, store and secrete calcitonin. These cells derive from the embryonic neuroectoderm and are more numerous in the lateral upper two thirds of the thyroid (the usual location for MTC). In hereditary MTC, tumours are multicentric and bilateral and occur in a background of diffuse or nodular C-cell hyperplasia. C-cell hyperplasia is thought of as the precursor lesion for macroscopic tumours and is frequently found as the sole pathology in screen-detected disease (especially through genetic tests).

The age distribution depends on the method of detection, but the age at diagnosis of FMTC (third decade for MEN-2A and second decade for MEN-2B) is earlier than that for sporadic MTC or phaeochromocytoma. **Figure 4.3** shows the percentage of cases not yet diagnosed, as a function of age, in 30 patients with

Figure 4.3
Age and the diagnostic evolution of medullary thyroid carcinoma and phaeochromocytoma in familial patients.

From Endocrine Surgery, Johnston, IDA, NE Thompson (eds), Butterworths International Medical Reviews, 1983, pp. 189–202.

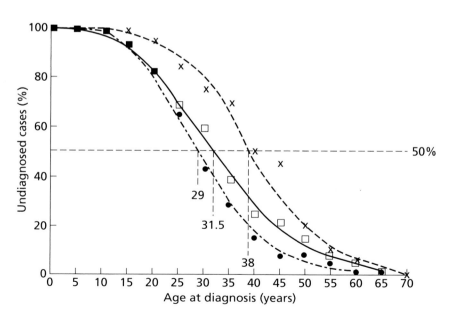

(●) Medullary thyroid carcinoma in MEN-2.
(□) Phaeochromocytoma in MEN-2.
(X) Sporadic, non-familial phaeochromocytoma.

MEN-2 syndrome and 20 patients with sporadic, non-familial phaeochromo-cytoma. This time-course of diagnosis suggests that MTC appears before phaeochromocytoma but it has not been shown whether these data reflect a different biological expression of each tumour or are affected by the ability to screen/detect each tumour (i.e. the calcitonin provocation test may be a more incisive and accurate test than measurement of urinary catecholamine concentrations). Genetic testing skews the curves further to the left.

Clinically apparent cases are identified when a unilateral or bilateral thyroid nodules are found incidentally during a routine examination. A fine needle biopsy shows characteristic changes of MTC, which can be further confirmed by immunocytochemical staining for calcitonin. Metastases to cervical lymph nodes are present in half the patients with palpable nodules, but distant metastases (lung, liver, bone) occur late in the course of disease.

Diarrhoea is relatively common in patients with widespread tumours but can also be present at the time of first presentation. The causative humoral factor has not yet been identified.

Other peptides are secreted by tumoral C-cells, including calcitonin-gene related peptide (CGRP), chromogranin A, somatostatin, ACTH and CRH. Their clinical importance is not well understood apart from the possibility of developing ectopic Cushing's syndrome due to excess ACTH/CRH concentrations.

Phaeochromocytoma

Phaeochromocytoma was the cause of death of the first patient reported in Sipple's original description of MEN-2. As a result of regular family screening, diffuse or nodular hyperplasia of the adrenal medulla are now diagnosed and recognised as precursors of phaeochromocytomas. The symptoms are subtle and may include intermittent headaches, palpitations and nervousness, whereas paroxysmal hypertension is rather uncommon. Although the clinical presentation seems not to be severe, this is still a life-threatening condition.

Phaeochromocytomas are frequently bilateral. When unilateral, they are usually associated with diffuse/nodular enlargement on the other side. Bilateral involvement of the adrenals varies between families. Asynchronous tumour development has been reported, and malignant tumours are rare. The incidence of phaeochromocytoma varies between kindreds.

Although often presenting later than the MTC, phaeochromocytoma needs to be excluded before an operation on a patient known to have RET mutations.

Hyperparathyroidism

Hypercalcaemia and increased serum PTH concentrations occur in 10–25% of patients with MEN-2A. If symptomatic, the clinical presentation does not differ from sporadic cases (see Chapter 1). The median age at diagnosis is about 38 years, and the vast majority of patients are asymptomatic.[48] Asymmetrical parathyroid hyperplasia is the most common histological abnormality.

Cutaneous lichen amyloidosis

Bilateral or unilateral pruritic and lichenoid skin lesions located over the upper portion of the back have been described in five families with MEN-2A and are considered to be a variant of this syndrome. It is due to deposition of amyloid at the dermis–epidermis interface in the affected areas. Because in most patients it precedes the development of MTC, it could serve as a phenotypic marker of MEN-2A. The molecular mechanism is not established.

Clinical presentation of MEN-2B

Distinctive clinical features are pathognomonic for MEN-2B syndrome and usually recognised in early life, making it possible to diagnose MTC by identification of the phenotype.

Marfanoid habitus

Marfanoid habitus can be identified in up to 90% of patients and consists of a tall slender body, high arched palate and long extremities. Arachnodactyly, joint laxity and skeletal deformities (pes cavus, slipped femoral capital epiphysis, kyphosis, scoliosis, lordosis) are less frequent. A minority of patients have peripheral neuropathy, xerophthalmia, xerostomia, facial hyperhidrosis and dental abnormalities. In contrast with true Marfan's syndrome, no patients with MEN-2B have been reported to have ectopia lentis or cardiac/aortic abnormalities.

Ganglioneuroma phenotype

The ganglioneuroma phenotype is also evident in most patients with MEN-2B. Neuromas of the anterior one third of the tongue are most characteristic but can also be identified on the lips, buccal mucosa, conjunctiva and eyelids.

Neuromas of ocular structures can be shown by slit lamp examination, and prominent corneal nerves, thickened eyelids and subconjunctival neuromas can be seen.

Gastrointestinal symptoms

Gastrointestinal (GI) symptoms occur in 90% of patients and are a major feature of the syndrome. Marked hypertrophy of nerve fibres and an increased number of ganglion cells are present throughout the GI tract, and this diffuse intestinal ganglioneuromatosis causes colonic motility dysfunction. Severe chronic constipation and diarrhoea, abdominal distension and crampy abdominal pain appear early in life and precede detection of endocrine disease. Megacolon and severe colonic diverticulosis are reported.[49]

Although the colonic pathology in MEN-2B (ganglioneuromatosis) is different from that in Hirschsprung's disease (aganglionosis), it is of interest that both diseases are related to similar genetic abnormalities in the intracellular tyrosine kinase domain of the RET proto-oncogene.

MTC

MTC in patients with MEN-2B presents at a younger age—as early as the first year of life—and the mean age at diagnosis is 16 years. It is associated with more extensive disease within the thyroid gland, has a higher incidence of metastatic disease (which remains the main cause of death of patients with MEN-2B) and is much less amenable to surgical cure.[50]

It seems that the aggressiveness of MTC covers a spectrum, decreasing from the most severe forms in MEN-2B, to sporadic to MEN-2A and least aggressive in FMTC. Some suggest that the natural course of MTC in MEN-2B is comparable to that found in MEN-2A and that the major reason for difference in prognosis results from the earlier age of development of MTC in patients with MEN-2B.

Phaeochromocytoma

Phaeochromocytoma occurs later than MTC, but 50% of patients after 25 years of age will also have phaeochromocytomas. Its real incidence depends on the duration and intensity of follow-up. Often there are bilateral tumours or adrenal medullary hyperplasia.

Hyperparathyroidism

HPT is less common than in MEN-2A.

Other associated problems related to health also occur with MEN-2B syndrome. The threat of cancer at any early age, the trauma of multiple surgical procedures, the persistent GI symptoms, the skeletal and phenotypic abnormalities have disruptive effects on the psychological wellbeing and quality of life of patients and their families.

Investigative techniques

Clinical examination is the best method of identifying the pathognomonic signs of the MEN-2B syndrome. For patients with MEN-2A, annual assessment for phaeochromocytoma includes a careful history plus physical examination (supine and erect blood pressure). Thickening of corneal nerves was suggested as a useful screening test for MEN-2A, but there is no relationship between prominent nerves and either the evolution of the disease or the occurrence of phaeochromocytomas.[51]

Screening for MEN-2A and MEN-2B

The need for screening programmes is evident because the penetrance of the gene is incomplete and a negative family history in a patient presenting with MTC or phaeochromocytoma is not a reliable exclusion of familial disease. If a high index of suspicion is maintained, new families with MEN-2A are discovered regularly. At least 10% of consecutive, unselected patients with apparently sporadic MTC are in fact familial, and bilateral phaeochromocytomas should certainly prompt screening.

The reproductive rate of patients with MEN-2B is low, possibly because of increased mortality, impotence due to neurological problems, infertility and low marriage rates. This implies that new mutations cause a high proportion of MEN-2B.

Genetic screening

The initial use of molecular linkage techniques allowed identification of the primary genetic defect in the centromeric region of chromosome 10, with up to 95% accuracy when DNA extracted from two affected patients was compared with DNA from family members. The identification of point mutations of the RET proto-oncogene now allows identification of gene carriers with 100% certainty in such families. Mutations are present in approximately 97% of families with MEN-2A[35–38] and in more than 93% of families with MEN-2B.[40] Identification of a mutation in a family enables certain determination of members who carry the mutations and those who do not. Non-carriers are discharged from further regular biochemical screening tests, their risk being no greater than the normal population.

Genetic screening allows early identification of children at risk before any biochemical abnormality becomes evident[52] and allows total thyroidectomy to be discussed for affected children prior to the age of 4.

Genetic DNA is extracted from peripheral blood white cells of at least one affected family member and from those at risk. Millions of DNA copies of a selected portion of the RET proto-oncogene are made by polymerase chain reaction (PCR) starting from small fragments that are complementary to the RET gene (oligonucleotide primers) in the region of interest (exons 10, 11, 13, 16). The amplified DNA serves as the starting material for subsequent mutational analysis techniques.[53] At least five methods are currently available to identify RET mutations, and some details about each of them are summarised in **Table 4.2**.

Technique	Principle	Advantages	Disadvantages
Direct DNA sequencing	The codons in exon 11 (634) and 10 (609, 611, 618, 620) are sequenced from both alleles of the RET gene	The only methodology capable of identifying previously non-reported mutations	Technically complex Not easily automated
Restriction enzyme analysis	80% of reported mutations create or destroy a restriction site. Gel electrophoresis is used to prove that the mutant allele is digested differently by one of a multitude of restriction enzymes available	Can be used as a sole technique to identify a mutation in a family with a known DNA sequence abnormality	
Single-strand conformational polymorphism analysis	A single nucleotide change results in a conformational change that alters DNA mobility on a non-denaturing polyacrylamide gel	Simple, cost-effective method to identify patients with sequence abnormalities	Does not identify a specific mutation
Denaturing gradient gel electrophoresis analysis	The DNA denaturation is sequence-dependent; therefore, a single nucleotide change generates a specific denaturation pattern		Uncertainty regarding the specificity of the result
Allele-specific oligonucleotide hybridisation analysis	Oligonucleotides containing a normal codon 634 sequence or four mutant codons identified are dotted and immobilised on a membrane. Only perfectly matched DNA sequence from the PCR amplification will hybridise with a probe.	Simple and rapid to perform Ability to identify specifically the causative mutation Useful for screening of families in which a specific mutation has been identified by other techniques	It makes it necessary to synthesise and dot oligonucleotides with all possible mutations A previously undetected or unreported mutation will be missed

Table 4.2 *Methodologies for detection of a single nucleotide mutation of the RET proto-oncogene*[45]

Although rare, there are recognised sources of error in genetic testing: sample mix-up (can occur as frequently as 5%), contamination during laboratory evaluation with DNA from patients with known RET mutations and failure to amplify or copy both RET alleles (resulting in the possibility of a false negative result if only the normal allele is included in the analysis). To minimise the impact of such errors on patient care, each analysis can be repeated (whether positive or negative) in a different laboratory on a sample obtained independently.

Biochemical screening

Before DNA-based predictive testing was available, all clinically unaffected first degree relatives were screened annually for MTC, phaeochromocytomas and HPT, from the age of 6 to the age of 35. Calcitonin concentration after stimulation with calcium plus pentagastrin, 24-hour excretion of catecholamines and serum concentrations of calcium and PTH were measured.

Figure 4.4
Age at which clinical evidence of MEN-2A is detected by examination or biochemical screening in MEN-2A gene carriers.

Adapted from Ponder et al. Risk estimations and screening in families of patients with medullary thyroid carcinoma. Lancet 1988; 1: 397–401.

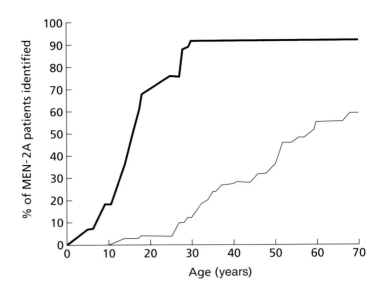

Basal concentrations of calcitonin are not increased in the early subclinical stages of MTC (premalignant C-cell hyperplasia and microscopic carcinoma), but these patients have an abnormal increase of calcitonin concentrations during stimulation tests with two secretagogues—calcium and pentagastrin. Because by the age of 30 nearly all gene carriers (95%) have a positive test result,[33] (**Fig. 4.4**) and because lifelong annual testing is associated with low compliance and high costs, calcitonin screening is stopped in adulthood.

Serum calcitonin concentrations in response to stimulation with pentagastrin (bolus injection of 0.5 $\mu g\ kg^{-1}$ body weight) are measured at 0, 1, 2, 5 and 10 minutes postinjection. A 1-minute calcium infusion (2 mg kg^{-1} body weight) can be associated with the pentagastrin injection. Because normal subjects also have detectable basal calcitonin concentrations and a response to provocative tests (higher in men than in women), interpretation of the results should be adapted to individual laboratories. C-cell hyperplasia (as seen occasionally adjacent to benign or follicular thyroid tumours and in Hashimoto's thyroiditis) can cause a false positive result with a pentagastrin test. As with many other screening tests, overlap between normal and early abnormal tests can exist, and family members with borderline values should be retested after 3–6 months.

Because there is considerable overlap between pentagastrin test results in individuals who are positive for a RET mutation and those who are negative, a coupling of pentagastrin test results and RET proto-oncogene analysis for all individuals at risk of developing MEN-2A or FMTC was thought to be necessary for the decision to proceed with thyroidectomy.[54] However, the increasing specificity and accuracy of genetic testing makes it sufficient in modern practice.

The importance of early diagnosis is apparent. C-cell hyperplasia has been found in children as young as 1.5 years, and MTC was documented in a child aged 2.8 with MEN-2B syndrome. If the only evidence of MTC is a minimally increased (over basal values) peripheral plasma calcitonin concentration (between 250 and 1000 pg ml^{-1}) after provocative testing, the chance of curing the patient (postoperative stimulated plasma calcitonin concentration <200 pg ml^{-1}) by total thyroidectomy is approximately 95%. Even if the preoperative stimulated plasma calcitonin concentration is between 1000 and 5000 pg ml^{-1}, surgery is curative in approximately 90% of patients. Conversely, when the preoperative stimulated plasma calcitonin concentration exceeds 10 000 the cure rate falls to 40%.[55]

Urinary catecholamine and metanephrine concentration have high sensitivity and specificity for the diagnosis of phaeochromocytoma. In contrast with sporadic cases, a predominance of adrenaline over noradrenaline secretion can be documented. Because most tumours are evaluated while still small, repeated measurements are necessary to uncover the abnormal secretion of catecholamines, preferably on days when suggestive symptoms are present. Even if the urinary catecholamine concentrations are within the normal range, any operation on a patient with a proven RET mutation should be considered to carry the risk of a possible phaeochromocytoma. Pharmacological provocative tests are potentially hazardous and therefore frequently avoided, but physical exercise coupled with the calculation of adrenaline:dopamine ratio has been proposed as an alternative stimulation test for patients with MEN-2A.

Annual determination of serum calcium concentration is sufficient to exclude HPT in patients with MEN-2. If the calcium concentration is increased, measurement of intact PTH concentrations is indicated.

Radiological screening

Localisation of MTC recurrence can be determined using radionuclide scanning with ^{201}Thallium, ^{99m}Tc-DMSA, ^{99m}Tc-sestamibi, ^{131}I-metaiodobenzylguanidine (MIBG), CT and MRI. Radiolabelled monoclonal antibodies and labelled somatostatin receptors are being evaluated.

Imaging of the adrenals using ^{123}I- or ^{131}I-MIBG has a good sensitivity (up to 100%) and detects unilateral or bilateral phaeochromocytomas but should not be used as a screening test (either at diagnosis or during follow-up).[56] CT scans and T2 weighted MR images are important options in the balance between sensitivity, specificity, radiation exposure and cost.

Management options

A comparison between a screening approach or pentagastrin testing provides convincing cost-efficiency savings. Genetic testing currently costs approximately

$250 per sample (possibly twice as much if the test is repeated) and needs to be carried out once only. A pentagastrin test with four calcitonin measurements costs $500 per test and needs repeating annually. Considering that biochemical testing will start at the age of 6 years and a mean age of 10 years for conversion of the pentagastrin test in a gene-carrier child, at least $2000 will be spent to identify a gene carrier. The costs will be much higher for non-carriers tested from age 6 to 35 years.[57]

MTC

The application of genetic screening to the management of hereditary MTC is advantageous because early thyroidectomy might be curative for MTC, is well tolerated and has no major long-term impact on quality of life.

Long-term follow-up studies of families screened biochemically in which a decision for thyroidectomy relied on the presence of abnormal calcitonin concentrations (basal or stimulated) reported an 85% and higher 15–20-year cure rate. The ability to determine gene-carrier status in affected families provides an opportunity to improve on this cure rate. Two paradigms for clinical management of children with confirmed RET mutations have recently evolved. The first is to perform pentagastrin testing only in children with RET mutations and to perform total thyroidectomy at the time the test converts to abnormal (a similar approach as the previous screening protocols). The second is to perform total thyroidectomy at between 5 and 7 years of age in all children with RET mutations.[58] The 50% of family members without RET mutations are excluded from further screening in both paradigms. Most would favour the second paradigm because almost half the thyroidectomy specimens from RET-positive children with a normal pentagastrin test have microscopic MTC.[59] Up to 50% of children who convert from a normal to an abnormal pentagastrin test result are found to have microscopic MTC.

Because surgery of MTC in the preclinical phase has a high probability of curing patients, genetic screening soon after birth and total thyroidectomy in gene carriers as early as possible should improve the prognosis.[60] Metastases of MTC have been described within the first year of life, and this is considered a supplementary reason to perform thyroidectomy as soon as possible (ideally in the first year of life) in children clinically suspected for MEN-2B and confirmed by a codon 918 mutation analysis.[61] High incidence of lymph node metastases at the time of first operation for clinically apparent MTC oblige complete total thyroidectomy with routine dissection of the central compartment and removal of lymph nodes in the lateral neck compartment and upper mediastinum. Radical neck dissection does not give an improvement in long-term outcome.

Screening for MTC recurrence relies on determination of calcitonin concentration, and debulking of macroscopic recurrence is still the best treatment option. None of the chemotherapeutic regimens has proved effective. Doxorubicin is the most effective single agent, but only 30% of patients will have partial responses. Palliative radiotherapy is used for bone pain and octreotide for symptomatic treatment.

Phaeochromocytomas

Because this is a generally late manifestation of MEN-2 and is rarely associated with malignant transformation, annual or biannual biochemical screening for individuals with RET mutations should suffice. If the diagnosis of phaeochromocytoma is made, surgery is performed 2–3 weeks after α-receptor blockade. Bilateral adrenalectomy need not be carried out if one adrenal is normal, but continued surveillance is required.

HPT

The parathyroid disease is of secondary importance during neck exploration for MTC. Resection of enlarged parathyroid glands is sufficient for patients with no family history of HPT.

Research interests

Apart from a major impact of genetic diagnosis on the management of the MEN-2 syndrome, genotype–phenotype correlation studies in patients with identified RET mutations could define the RET signal transduction pathway and its role in the development of neural crest derivatives. Understanding the functions of the RET proto-oncogene and its complex involvement in development and oncogenesis may allow new approaches to treatment, which might reverse or prevent tumour formation.

Fimilial medullary thyroid carcinoma

The occurrence of MTC with a familial inheritance but without the other endocrine or phenotypic manifestations of MEN-2A or MEN-2B has been reported. In an evaluation of 213 patients from 15 kindreds with FMTC, 41 such patients were identified.[62] Its course is more benign than that of MEN-2A or MEN-2B, and the prognosis is good.[62] There were no differences in the peak stimulated plasma calcitonin concentrations at the time of diagnosis or the incidence of regional lymph node metastases when compared with patients with MEN-2A, but the mean age at diagnosis was significantly higher in patients with FMTC than in those with MEN-2A (43.1 years vs. 21.1 years), suggesting that MTC developed at a later age or grew more slowly.

In addition to RET mutations common with the MEN-2A syndrome, germline mutations in exons 13 (Glu^{768} ASP) and 14 (Val^{804} Leu) of the RET proto-oncogene have been described recently in four families with FMTC.[63] Both mutations segregated with the disease in these families and support the idea that FMTC is a different condition from that of MEN-2A.

A unique kindred presenting with MTC and corneal nerve thickening without other aspects of the MEN syndrome has been described.[64] Of 11 family members spanning four generations, seven have corneal nerve thickening, and DNA sequence analysis for the RET proto-oncogene showed that none of the affected individuals have mutations characteristic of families with MEN-2A or MEN-2B syndrome. Linkage analysis showed cosegregation of alleles, with the presence of both corneal nerve thickening and MTC/C-cell hyperplasia. This kindred seems to represent a true clinical overlap syndrome, the genetic basis of which may be distinct from the other syndromes.

Familial papillary carcinoma of the thyroid

Papillary carcinoma of the thyroid is usually sporadic but occasionally may be familial. In an analysis of 226 consecutive patients with papillary carcinoma, 3.5–6% were identified as having an affected relative. In a French series, 7 of 53 patients with papillary carcinomas (13%) were considered to be familial, suggesting that when two or more family members have papillary carcinoma, all first-degree and second-degree relatives should be clinically evaluated.[65] Because familial papillary carcinoma is often multifocal, total thyroidectomy is recommended.[66] Because some of the affected patients might be diagnosed as having only a nodular goitre, thyroidectomy should be performed if a family history of papillary carcinoma is certain.

Gardner's syndrome (familial adenomatous polyposis)

Gardner's syndrome seems to be associated with a higher risk of thyroid carcinoma. It is an autosomal dominant syndrome consisting of multiple adenomatous polyps, after in conjunction with osteomas, epidermoid cysts, desmoid tumours, retinal pigmentation and, more rarely, with hepatoblastomas and adenomas in the upper GI tract and pancreas. Some have reported about 160 times enhancement of risk for thyroid cancer in young female patients when compared with normal subjects. Up to 9% of lesions were papillary carcinomas, the rest being follicular neoplasms. Gardner's syndrome predominates in women (approximately 1:16 male to female ratio), appears at a relatively young age (20s) and is often multicentric, with relatively low aggressiveness but with a significant risk of recurrence. These data suggest that close clinical observation for thyroid neoplasia is important in patients who have a personal or family history of familial adenomatous polyposis.

Cowden's syndrome

Cowden's syndrome is characterised by multiple mucocutaneous hamartomas, keratoses on hands, feet and mouth, GI polyps, fibrocystic disease of the breast or bilateral breast cancer and benign and malignant thyroid tumours.[67] In a review of Cowden's syndrome, 8 of 26 patients had thyroid carcinoma (most commonly well differentiated), but little is known about the pathological characteristics and outcome of the thyroid lesion in these patients. The locus for Cowden's syndrome was mapped to chromosome 10q22–23.[68] Mutations at this locus do not account for susceptibility to hereditary tumours outside families affected by the syndrome.

Familial isolated hyperparathyroidism

Familial isolated hyperparathyroidism (FIHPT) is a rare syndrome inherited as an autosomal dominant disorder and characterised by hypercalcaemia, inappropriately high PTH concentrations and isolated parathyroid tumours, with no evidence of hyperfunction of any other endocrine tissues.

A study of 19 family members of a large kindred over four generations has shown no linkage between FIHP and the MEN-1 and MEN-2A syndromes. In one individual, a parathyroid carcinoma was found after recurrence of hypercalcaemia. This report suggests that FIHP is a distinct autosomal dominant syndrome with an increased risk of malignant parathyroid transformation.[69] The same conclusion was supported by the lack of any clinical, biochemical or genetic evidence of MEN syndromes in 37 members of a similar family.[70]

The relationship between MEN-1 and FIHP is still unresolved. Although the presentation of individual families seems to represent a distinct disease entity, it remains possible that FIHP is a variant or partial expression of MEN-1.

The association of hereditary HPT and jaw fibroma is a rare condition.[71–72] In such patients HPT is due to multigland disease. They also present cementifying and ossifying fibromas of the mandible and/or maxilla which are different from 'brown tumours of the bone' usually seen in patients with primary HPT. This disease is clinically and genetically different from MEN syndromes and results from mutations on the long arm of chromosome 1, where a dominant oncogene (HRPT2) maps in the 1q21–31 region.[73]

Several familial syndromes with parathyroid hyperfunction have been described, but some are documented only by individual case reports (see **Table 4.3**).[74]

Dominant disorders	Recessive or uncertain transmission
Cystic parathyroid adenomas with/without jaw tumours Familial parathyroid hyperplasia	Parathyroid hyperplasia associated with: Parathyroid carcinoma Nephropathy and neural deafness Colonic neoplasms Carcinoid tumours of the foregut

Table 4.3 *Familial syndromes with parathyroid function*

Phaechromocytoma as part of other familial diseases

In 10% of patients with phaeochromocytoma, the adrenal tumour is part of a familial disorder (i.e. MEN syndromes, von Recklinghausen disease, von Hippel–Lindau syndrome).

Von Recklinghausen disease

Von Recklinghausen disease is the eponym for type 1 neurofibromatosis (NF1), an autosomal dominant disorder produced by somatic mutations in the *NF1* gene on chromosome 17. Because of its variable expression, it is estimated that 1 in 3000 people have at least a minor variety of this disease, but only 11% of these patients also have a phaeochromocytoma. Two or more of the following clinical criteria are necessary for the diagnosis of NF1 and could raise the suspicion of a concomitant phaeochromocytoma:

- Six or more café-au-lait spots (larger than 5 mm in prepubertal patients and 15 mm in postpubertal patients);
- Two or more neurofibromas of any type or one plexiform neurofibroma; freckling in the axillary/inguinal region;
- Optic glioma;
- Two or more Lisch nodules (pigmented hamartomas of the iris);
- Distinctive osseous lesions (sphenoid dysplasia or thinning of long bone cortex and pseudoarthritis);
- A first-degree relative with NF1.

Patients with type 2 neurofibromatosis do not have phaeochromocytomas.

Von Hippel–Lindau syndrome

Von Hippel–Lindau syndrome (VHL) includes retinal angiomatosis, haemangioblastoma of the central nervous system, renal cysts and carcinoma, pancreatic cysts and epididymal cystadenoma. In the adrenal glands, VHL may be associated with phaeochromocytomas, which occur more frequently in some families than in others but are quite common in families that have adrenal involvement. They are rarely malignant (less than 1%).

Patients with VHL are screened yearly for a phaeochromocytoma. Recent data indicate that adrenal tumours are as much as four times more common among people with VHL than previously thought, and that traditional blood and urine tests are inadequate for detection. Clinical examination, ophthalmoscopy, fluorescein angiography and CT of the brain are used to identify other possible lesions. It is anticipated that DNA screening for a specific gene on the short arm of chromosome will become available.

Familial primary aldosteronism

Primary aldosteronism due to adrenocortical hyperplasia, adenoma or carcinoma can occur as part of the MEN syndromes. 'Isolated' familial primary aldosteronism can occur in two familial forms: familial hyperaldosteronism types I and familial hyperaldosteronism type II.

1. *Familial hyperaldosteronism type I* is an ACTH-dependent and glucocorticoid-suppressible form, attributed to adrenal hyperplasia and not, as yet, associated with tumours. Recently, a 'hybrid' gene between 11-β-hydroxylase and aldosterone-synthase has been detected by PCR, allowing genetic screening of such families.[75]
2. *Familial hyperaldosteronism type II* is an autosomal dominant form, not suppressible by glucocorticoids and often associated with aldosterone-producing adenomas. The genetic defect is different from that of families with the type I form, but is yet to be exactly described.[76]

The morphology of adrenocortical hyperplasia causing primary aldosteronism ranges from glomerulosa-like (idiopathic hyperplasia of the adrenals, responsive to angiotensin II) to fasciculata-like (glucocorticoid-suppressible hyperaldosteronism, unresponsive to angiotensin II). Both subtypes can be found in a single family.[77]

Carney syndrome

In 1995 JA Carney and colleagues described a group of 40 patients presenting with autosomal dominant familial association of myxomas, spotty pigmentation and endocrine hyperactivity.[78] A further detailed clinical evaluation of 101 patients from 11 families with Carney complex confirmed the presence of myxomas (cardiac, breast and cutaneous), pigmented skin lesions, and ACTH-independent Cushing's syndrome due to primary pigmented nodular adrenal hyperplasia. Other endocrine tumours included pituitary somatotroph adenomas leading to acromegaly and Sertoli cell testicular tumours leading to precociuous puberty.[79]

Mutation on chromosome 17q and 2p have been identified in affected patients. Very recently, the mechanism for Carney complex has been show to involve a susceptibility gene on chromosome 17 that encodes a regulatory subunit of protein kinase A (protein kinase A type I-a regulatory subunit, *PPKARIA*). In affected tissues *PPAKRIA* is absent or diminished, and this leads to increased sensitivity of protein-kinase A-dependent cellular processes (such as hormone secretion and cell proliferation). The susceptibility gene mapped on chromosome 2 is yet to be identified (reviewed in reference 80).

References

 1. Wermer P. Genetic aspects of adenomatosis of endocrine glands. Am J Med 1954; 16: 363–7.

2. Shepherd JJ. Latent familial multiple endocrine neoplasia in Tasmania. Med J Aust 1985; 142: 395–7.

3. Shepherd JJ. The natural history of multiple endocrine neoplasia type 1: highly uncommon or highly unrecognized? Arch Surg 1991; 126: 935–52.

 4. Wilkinson S, Teh BT, Daey KR. Cause of death in multiple endocrine neoplasia type 1. Arch Surg 1993; 128: 683–90.

5. Chandrasekharappa SC, Guru SC, Manickam P *et al*. Positional cloning of the gene for multiple endocrine neoplasia-type 1. Science 1997; 276: 404–8.

6. The European Consortium on MEN-1. Identification of the multiple endocrine neoplasia type 1 (MEN-1) gene. Hum Mol Genet 1997; 6: 1117–1183.

7. Weber G, Friedman E *et al*. The phospholipase C beta 3 gene located in the MEN-1 region shows loss of expression in endocrine tumours. Hum Mol Genet 1994; 3: 1775–81.

8. Beckers A, Abs R, Reyniers E *et al*. Variable regions of chromosome 11 loss in different pathological tissues of a patient with MEN-1 syndrome. J Clin Endocrinol Metab 1994; 79: 1498–502.

9. Marx SJ, Sakaguci K, Green J III *et al*. Mitogenic activity on parathyroid cells in plasma from members of a large kindred with multiple endocrine neoplasia type 1. J Clin Endocrinol Metab 1988; 67: 149.

 10. Bassett JH, Forbes SA, Pannett AAJ *et al*. Characterisation of mutations in patients with multiple endocrine neoplasia type 1. Am J Hum Genet 1998; 62: 232–44.

11. Petty EM, Green JS, Marx SJ. Mapping the gene for hereditary hyperparathyroidism and prolactinoma (MEN-1 burin) to chromosome 11: evidence for a founder effect in patients from Newfoundland. Am J Hum Genet 1994; 54: 1060–6.

12. Skogseid B, Eriksson B, Lundqvist G *et al*. Multiple endocrine neoplasia type I: a 10-year prospective screening study in four kindreds. J Clin Endocrinol Metab 1991; 75: 76–81.

13. Friedman E, Sakaguci K, Bale AE *et al*. Clonality of parathyroid tumours in familial MEN type 1. N Engl J Med 1989; 321: 213–8.

14. Carling T, Rastad J, Ridefelt P *et al*. Hyperparathyroidism of multiple endocrine neoplasia type 1: candidate gene and parathyroid calcium sensing protein expression. Surgery 1995; 118: 924–31.

 15. Vasen HF, Lamers CB, Lips CB. Screening for the multiple endocrine neoplasia syndrome type 1: a study of 11 kindreds in The Netherland. Arch Intern Med 1989; 149: 2717–22.

16. Thompson NW. Surgical management of MEN-1. J Intern Med 1995; 238: 269–80.

17. Skogseid B, Rastad J, Gobl A. Adrenal lesion in multiple endocrine neoplasia type 1. Surgery 1995; 118: 1077–82.

18. Burgess JR, Harle RA, Tucker P *et al*. Adrenal lesions in a large kindred with multiple endocrine neoplasia type 1. Arch Surg 1996; 131: 699–702.

19. Larsson C, Shepherd J, Nakamura Y *et al*. Predictive testing for multiple endocrine neoplasia type 1 using DNA polymorphism. J Clin Invest 1992; 89: 1344–9.

20. Larsson C, Calender A, Grimmond S *et al*. Molecular tools for presymptomatic testing in multiple endocrine neoplasia type 1. J Intern Med 1995; 238: 239–44.

 21. Farndon JR, Geraghty JM, Dilley WG *et al*. Serum gastrin, calcitonin, and prolactin as markers of multiple endocrine neoplasia syndromes in patients

with primary hyperparathyroidism. World J Surg 1987; 11: 253–7.

22. Farndon JR. Gastrin and gastrinomas. Br J Surg 1990; 77: 1–2.

23. Skogseid B, Rastad J, Oberg K. Multiple endocrine neoplasia type I: clinical features and screening. Endocr Metab Clin North Am 1994; 27: 1–17.

24. Brunt LM, Dilley WG, Farndon JR. Evaluation of calcium as an insulin secretagogue in patients with insulinoma. Surg Forum 1984; 35: 49–52.

25. Rothmund M, Angelini L, Brunt LM *et al.* Surgery for benign insulinoma—an international review. World J Surg 1990; 14: 393–9.

26. Fraker DL, Norton JA. Controversy in surgical therapy for APUDomas. Semin Surg Oncol 1993; 9: 437–42.

27. Zeiger MA, Shawker TH, Norton JA. Use of intraoperative ultrasonography to localise islet cell tumours. World J Surg 1993; 17: 448–54.

28. Imamura M, Takahashi K. Use of selective intraarterial secretin injection test to guide surgery in patients with Zollinger–Ellison syndrome. World J Surg 1993; 17: 433–8.

29. Hellman P, Skogseid B, Oberg K *et al.* Primary and reoperative parathyroid operations in hyperparathyroidism of multiple endocrine neoplasia type 1. Surgery 1998; 124: 993–9.

30. Solcia E, Cappela C, Fiocca R *et al.* Gastric argyrophil carcinoids in patients with Zollinger Ellison syndrome due to type I multiple endocrine neoplasia. Am J Surg Pathol 1990; 14: 503–13.

31. Grama D, Skogseid B, Wilander E *et al.* Pancreatic tumours in multiple endocrine neoplasia type 1: clinical presentation and surgical treatment. World J Surg 1992; 16: 611–8.

32. Cadiot G, Vuagnat A, Doukhan I *et al.* Prognostic factors in patients with Zollinger–Ellison syndrome and multiple endocrine neoplasia type 1. Gastroenterology 1999; 116: 286–93.

33. Ponder BA, Ponder MA, Coffey R *et al.* Risk estimation and screening in families of patients with medullary thyroid carcinoma. Lancet 1988; 1: 397–401.

34. Sipple JH. The association of phaeochromocytoma with carcinoma of the thyroid gland. Am J Med 1961; 31: 163–6.

35. Mulligan LM, Gardner E, Smith BA *et al.* Genetic events in tumour initiation and progression in multiple endocrine neoplasia type 2. Genes Chromosomes Cancer 1993; 6: 166–77.

36. Donis-Keller H, Shenshen D, Chi D *et al.* Mutations in the RET protooncogene are associated with MEN2A and FMTC. Hum Mol Genet 1993; 2: 851–6.

37. Mulligan LM, Kwok JBJ, Healey CS *et al.* Germline mutations of the RET proto-oncogene in multiple endocrine neoplasia type 2A. Nature 1993; 363: 458–60.

38. Mulligan LM, Marsh DJ, Robinson BG *et al.* Genotype–phenotype correlation in MEN 2: report of the international RET mutations consortium. J Intern Med 1995; 238: 343–6.

39. Pasini B, Ceccherini I, Romeo G. RET mutations in human disease. Trends Genet 1996; 12: 138–44.

40. Carlson KM, Dou S, Chi D *et al.* Single missense mutation in the tyrosine kinase catalytic domain of the RET protooncogene is associated with multiple endocrine neoplasia type 2B. Proc Natl Acad Sci USA 1994; 91: 1579–83.

41. Borst MJ, VanCamp JM, Peacock ML *et al.* Mutational analysis of multiple endocrine neoplasia type 2A associated with Hirschsprung's disease. Surgery 1995; 117: 386–91.

42. Mulligan LM, Eng C, Attie T *et al.* Diverse phenotypes associated with exon 10 mutations of the RET protooncogene. Hum Mol Genet 1994; 3: 2163–7.

43. Pausova Z, Soliman E, Amizuka N *et al.* Expression of the RET protooncogene in hyperparathyroid tissues: implications for the pathogenesis of the parathyroid disease in MEN2A. J Bone Miner Res 1995; 10(suppl 1): 249.

44. Eng C, Mulligan LM, Smith DP *et al.* Mutation of the RET protooncogene in sporadic medullary thyroid carcinoma. Genes Chromosomes Cancer 1995; 12: 209–12.

45. Toogood AA, Eng C, Smith DP *et al.* No mutation at codon 918 of the RET gene in a family with multiple endocrine neoplasia type 2B. Clin Endocrinol 1995; 43: 759–62.

46. Carlson KM, Bracamontes J, Jackson CE *et al.* Parent of origin effects in multiple endocrine neoplasia type 2B. Am J Hum Genet 1994; 55: 1076–8.

47. Borrello MG, Smith DP, Pasini B *et al.* RET activation by germline MEN-2A and MEN-2B mutations. Oncogene 1995; 11: 2419–27.

48. Raue E, Kraimps JL, Dralle H *et al.* Primary hyperparathyroidism in multiple endocrine neoplasia type 2A. J Intern Med 1995; 238: 369–73.

49. O'Riordain DS, O'Brien T, Crotty TB *et al.* Multiple endocrine neoplasia type 2B: more than an endocrine disorder. Surgery 1995; 118: 936–42.

50. O'Riordain DS, O'Brien T, Hay ID *et al.* Medullary thyroid carcinoma in multiple endocrine neoplasia type 2A and 2B. Surgery 1994; 116: 1017–23.

51. Dupond JL, De Wazieres B, Fest T *et al.* Prominent corneal nerves in multiple endocrine neoplasia type 2A: another sign for familial screening? Eur J Intern Med 1995; 6: 177–8.

52. Frilling A, Dralle H, Eng C *et al.* Presymptomatic DNA screening in families with multiple endocrine neoplasia type 2 and familial medullary thyroid carcinoma. Surgery 1995; 118: 1099–104.

53. Wohllk N, Cote GJ, Evans DB et al. Application of genetic screening information to the management of medullary thyroid carcinoma and multiple endocrine neoplasia type 2. Endocrinol Metab Clin North Am 1996; 25: 1–25.

54. Marsh DJ, McDowall D, Hyland VJ et al. The identification of false positive responses to the pentagastrin stimulation test in RET mutation negative members of MEN 2A families. Clin Endocrinol 1996; 44: 213–20.

55. Wells SA, Dilley WG, Farndon JR et al. Early diagnosis and treatment of medullary thyroid carcinoma. Arch Intern Med 1985; 145: 1248–52.

56. Bonnin F, Lumbroso J, Schlumberger M et al. Interest of MIBG scintigraphy in screening for pheochromocytoma in patients with medullary thyroid carcinoma. Med Nucl 1995; 19: 177–2.

57. Gagel RF, Cote GJ, Martin Bughalo MJG et al. Clinical use of molecular information in the management of multiple endocrine neoplasia type A. J Intern Med 1995; 238: 333–41.

58. Wells SA, Chi DD, Toshima K et al. Predictive DNA testing and prophylactic thyroidectomy in patients at risk for multiple endocrine neoplasia type 2. Ann Surg 1994; 220: 237–50.

59. Cote CI, Wohhlk N, Evans D et al. RET protooncogene mutations in multiple endocrine neoplasia type 2 and medullary thyroid carcinoma. Baillière's Clin Endocrinol Metab 1995; 9: 609–30.

60. Pacini F, Romei C, Miccoli P et al. Early treatment of hereditary medullary thyroid carcinoma after attribution of multiple endocrine neoplasia type 2 gene carrier status by screening for ret gene mutations. Surgery 1995; 118: 1031–5.

61. Samaan NA, Draznin MB, Halpin RE et al. Multiple endocrine syndrome type IIB in early childhood. Cancer 1991; 68: 1832–4.

62. Farndon JR, Leight GS, Dilley WG et al. Familial medullary thyroid carcinoma without associated endocrinopathies: a distinct clinical entity. Br J Surg 1986; 73: 278–81.

63. Bolino A, Schuffenecker I, Luo Y et al. RET mutations in exons 13 and 14 of FMTC patients. Oncogene 1995; 10: 2415–9.

64. Kane LA, Tsai MS, Gharib H et al. Familial medullary thyroid cancer and prominent corneal nerves: clinical and genetic analysis. J Clin Endocrinol Metab 1995; 80: 289–93.

65. Stoffer SS, Van Dyke DL, Bach JV et al. Familial papillary carcinoma of the thyroid. Am J Med Genet 1986; 25: 775–82.

66. Kraimps JL, Fieuzal S, Margerit D et al. Familial papillary thyroid cancers: coincidence or genetic cause? Lyon Chir 1994; 90: 16–8.

67. Hanssen AMN, Fryns JP. Cowden syndrome. J Med Genet 1995; 32: 117–9.

68. Nelen MR, van Staveren WC, Peeters EA et al. Germline mutations in the PTEN/NMAC1 gene in patients with Cowden disease. Hum Mol Genet 1997; 6: 1383–7.

69. Wassif WS, Moniz CF, Friedman E et al. Familial isolated hyperparathyroidism: a distinct genetic entity with an increased risk of parathyroid cancer. J Clin Endocrinol Metab 1993; 77: 1485–9.

70. Kassem M, Zhang X, Brask S et al. Familial isolated primary hyperparathyroidism. Clin Endocrinol 1994; 41: 415–20.

71. Jackson CE, Norum RA, Boyd SB et al. Hereditary hyperparathyroidism and multiple ossifying jaw fibromas: a clinically and genetically distinct syndrome. Surgery 1990; 108: 1006–13.

72. Inoue H, Miki H, Oshimo K et al. Familial hyperparathyroidism associated with jaw fibroma: case report and literature review. Clin Endocrinol 1995; 43: 225–9.

73. Szabo J, Heath B, Hill VM et al. Hereditary hyperparathyroidism—jaw tumor syndrome: the endocrine tumor gene HRPT2 maps to chromosome 1q21–31. Am J Hum Genet 1995; 56: 944–50.

74. Mallette LE. Management of hyperparathyroidism in the multiple endocrine neoplasia syndromes and other familial endocrinopathies. Endocrinol Metab Clin North Am 1994; 23: 19–36.

75. Stowasser M, Gartside MG, Gordon RD. A PCR-based method of screening individuals of all ages, from neonates to the elderly, for familial hyperaldosteronism type I. Aust NZ J Med 1997; 27: 685–90.

76. Torpy DJ, Gordon RD, Lin JP et al. Familial hyperaldosteronism type II: description of a large kindred and exclusion of the aldosterone synthase (CYP11B2) gene. J Clin Endocrinol Metab 1998; 83: 3214–8.

77. Gordon RD, Stowasser M, Klemm SA et al. Primary aldosteronism—some genetic, morphological, and biochemical aspects of subtypes. Steroids 1995; 60: 35–41.

78. Carney JA, Gordon H, Carpenter PC, Shenoy BV, Go VLW. The complex of myxomas, spotty pigmentation and endocrine overactivity. Medicine 1985; 64:270–83.

79. Stratakis CA, Carney JA, Lin J-P. Carney complex, a familial multiple neoplasia and lentiginous syndrome: analysis of 11 kindreds and linkage to the short arm of chromosome 2. J Clin Endocrinol metab 1996; 97:699–705.

80. Malchoff CD. Carney complex – clarity and complexity. J Clin Endocrinol Metab 2000; 85(11):4010–13.

5 Endocrine tumours of the pancreas

Jade S. Hiramoto
Gary R. Peplinski
Jeffrey A. Norton

Introduction

Pancreatic endocrine neoplasms consist predominantly of gastrinomas and insulinomas, but a variety of other more rare tumours may occur as well. All of these tumours arise from neuroendocrine cells, display characteristic ultrastructural features and biochemically consist of amine precursor uptake and decarboxylation cells (APUDomas). Pancreatic endocrine tumours, as a group, are different from most other neoplasms because they commonly produce physiologically uncontrolled levels of hormones, each of which may cause a clinical syndrome. The clinical syndrome identified and the detection of hormone proteins produced allow the classification of pancreatic endocrine tumours into specific types. Potentially life-threatening situations caused by hormone overproduction are a major reason to identify and resect these neoplasms. Some tumours may not secrete any immunohistochemically detectable or clinically relevant peptides and only cause symptoms by mass effect. Additionally, except for insulinomas, pancreatic endocrine neoplasms are malignant in most cases.

Insulinoma

In 1927, endogenous hyperinsulinism was first described and was the first syndrome of excessive pancreatic hormone production to be recognised.[1] Hyperinsulinaemia and consequent hypoglycaemia are the major cause of morbidity and potential mortality associated with insulinoma, a neoplasm arising from the pancreatic insulin-producing β cells. Insulinoma occurs in approximately 1 person per million population per year (**Table 5.1**).[1] The hyperinsulinaemic hypoglycaemia is not well controlled by medical therapy, and surgery has

Tumour	Incidence (people/million/year)	Hormone secreted	Signs or symptoms	Diagnosis	Location (%) Duodenum	Location (%) Pancreas	Malignant (%)	MEN-1 (%)
Gastrinoma	0.1–3	Gastrin	Ulcer pain, diarrhoea, oesophagitis	Fasting serum gastrin >100 pg ml^{-1} Basal acid output >15 mEq h^{-1}	38	62	60–90	20
Insulinoma	0.8	Insulin	Hypoglycaemia	Standard fasting test	0	>99	5	5–10
VIPoma		Vasoactive polypeptide (VIP)	Watery diarrhoea, hypokalaemia, hypochlorhydria	Fasting plasma VIP >250 pg ml^{-1}	15	85	60	<5
Glucagonoma		Glucagon	Rash, weight loss, malnutrition, diabetes	Fasting plasma glucagon >500 pg ml^{-1}	0	>99	70	<5
Somatostatinoma		Somatostatin	Diabetes, cholelithiasis, steatorrhoea	Increased fasting plasma somatostatin concentration	50	50	70	<5
GRFoma	0.2	Growth hormone-releasing factor (GRF)	Acromegaly	Increased fasting plasma GRF concentration	0	100	30	30
ACTHoma		Adrenocorticotrophic hormone (ACTH)	Cushing's syndrome	24-hour urinary free cortisol >100 µg, plasma ACTH >50 pg ml^{-1}, no dexamethasone suppression, no CRH suppression	0	100	100	<5
PTH-like-oma		Parathyroid hormone (PTH)-like factor	Hypercalcaemia, bone pain	Serum calcium >11mg dl^{-1}, serum PTH undetectable, increased serum PTH-like factor	0	100	100	<5
Neurotensinoma		Neurotensin	Tachycardia, hypotension, hypokalaemia	Increased fasting plasma neurotensin concentration	0	100	>80	<5
Non-functioning (PPoma)		Pancreatic polypeptide (PP) neurone-specific enolase	Pain, bleeding mass	Increased plasma PP concentration, increased neurone-specific enolase concentration	0	>99	>60	80–100

Table 5.1 Features of endocrine tumours of the pancreas

remained the cornerstone of treatment over the past 70 years. Insulinomas are unique among pancreatic endocrine tumours because 90% of insulinomas are benign, solitary growths that occur uniformly throughout and almost exclusively within the pancreatic parenchyma, with no evidence of local invasion or locoregional lymph node metastases.[2] However, the tumour may be as small as 6 mm in diameter and is usually less than 2 cm in size, which makes localisation difficult in many cases.[3]

Patient presentation

Excessive and physiologically uncontrolled secretion of insulin by the tumour causes periods of acute, symptomatic hypoglycaemia, which results in patient presentation for medical evaluation. Acute neuroglycopenia induces anxiety, dizziness, obtundation, confusion, unconsciousness, personality changes and seizures.[3] Symptoms commonly occur during early morning hours, when glucose reserves are low after a period of overnight fasting and endogenous insulin overproduction continues. Patients may present when food intake is decreased to reduce weight, as most patients (80%) experience major weight gain. A majority (60–75%) of patients are women and many have undergone extensive psychiatric evaluation. Many patients will have been diagnosed with a neurological condition such as seizure disorders, cerebrovascular accidents or transient ischaemic attacks.[4] Potentially life-threatening symptoms may be present for several years before the correct diagnosis is considered.[3] In a recent review of 59 patients with insulinoma, the interval from the onset of symptoms to the time of diagnosis ranged from 1 month to 30 years, with the median time to diagnosis being 2 years.[4] Because insulinoma is rare and neuroglycopenic symptoms are relatively non-specific, a high index of suspicion for insulinoma is necessary when other explanations for these symptoms are not evident. The recognition of symptomatic patients and the liberal use of simple and precise biochemical tests results in accurate diagnosis of insulinoma prior to life-threatening sequelae. Approximately 5–10% of patients with insulinoma also have multiple endocrine neoplasia type 1 (MEN-1; **Table 5.1**).

Screening for MEN-1

About 5–10% of patients with insulinoma have MEN-1, and these patients must be recognised because they frequently have multiple pancreatic tumours and this greatly influences operative management.[5] MEN-1 is inherited as an autosomal dominant disease, and tumours develop in several endocrine organs. Virtually all patients have four-gland parathyroid hyperplasia, up to 75% develop pancreatic islet cell tumours, and pituitary tumours (usually prolactinomas) occur in less than 50% of patients. Functional pancreatic tumours are most commonly gastrinomas, with insulinomas occurring second in frequency.[1] Islet cell tumours of different types may occur simultaneously in a patient with MEN-1. Patients may also have thyroid adenomas, adrenocortical tumours, carcinoid tumours and lipomas.

Questions should be directed at other possible manifestations of the syndrome and a family history of endocrine tumours. If the clinical history is equivocal or suspicious for MEN-1, then the measurement of serum concentrations of calcium, prolactin, chromogranin A and pancreatic polypeptide may help to confirm or exclude MEN-1. Screening of other family members for features of MEN-1 is indicated when a patient is suspected to have MEN-1. The *MEN-1* gene has been cloned and mapped to the long arm of chromosome 11 (locus 11q13) and encodes a 610 amino acid protein termed MENIN.[6,7] Early studies have shown MENIN to be a nuclear protein.[8] The exact functional role of MENIN has not been confirmed, but recent research supports a tumour suppressor function of *MEN-1*, and germline *MEN-1* mutations have been identified in most MEN-1 families.[8,9] Genetic counselling and screening should be provided to family members to identify those individuals who are carriers of the mutant gene and have a high risk of developing the disease. These patients should enter a clinical screening programme, which can enable earlier detection and treatment of MEN-1-associated tumours and prompt treatment of hyperparathyroidism.[9,10]

Diagnosis

The classic diagnostic triad, proposed by Whipple in 1935 based on his observations in 32 patients, consists of symptoms of hypoglycaemia during a fast, a concomitant blood glucose concentration less than 3 mmol l^{-1} and relief of the hypoglycaemic symptoms after glucose administration.[1] Symptomatic patients with suspected insulinoma may first be instructed to undergo an overnight fast in an outpatient setting, during which time the development of any symptoms can be recorded and the serum glucose and insulin concentrations measured. The development of symptoms during fasting hypoglycaemia strongly suggests an insulinoma.

'Factitious hypoglycaemia,' in which exogenous insulin or oral hypoglycaemic drugs are administered clandestinely, may present with exactly the same symptoms as an insulinoma and may lead to an inappropriate diagnosis.[11] Factitious hypoglycaemia may be suspected more often in a patient with relatives who are diabetic or in a young woman associated with the medical profession, such as a nurse. The diagnosis of insulinoma must be reached (excluding factitious hypoglycaemia) in each patient by using the 72-hour supervised standard fasting test in a hospital setting with appropriate biochemical measurements prior to tumour localisation or surgery. Urinary sulphonylurea concentrations (to exclude oral hypoglycaemic drugs) should be measured by gas chromatography-mass spectroscopy; they are undetectable in patients with insulinoma. Anti–insulin antibodies should not be detectable in those with insulinoma and C–peptide concentrations are increased in equimolar concentrations with insulin.

Supervised standard fasting test

The standard fasting test is carried out in a hospital setting and begins with a baseline examination in which recent memory, calculations and coordination are documented. An intravenous catheter with a heparin lock is then placed, and the patient is allowed to drink only non–caloric beverages. Close observation is necessary. Blood is collected every 6 hours for measurement of serum glucose and immunoreactive insulin concentrations. As the blood glucose level falls below 3 mmol l^{-1}, blood samples are collected more frequently (every hour or less), and the patient is observed more closely. When neuroglycopenic symptoms appear, blood is collected immediately for determination of serum insulin, glucose, C–peptide, and proinsulin concentrations. Glucose is then administered, and the fast is terminated. If a patient remains symptom–free for the entire 72 hours, the test is terminated and the above blood concentrations are measured.

Neuroglycopenic symptoms manifest in approximately 60% of patients with insulinomas within 24 hours after fasting begins,[1] and nearly all patients with insulinomas have symptoms by 72 hours.[12] Approximately 16% of patients with insulinoma develop symptoms when the blood glucose concentration is greater than 2.5 mmol l^{-1}.[3] The blood glucose concentration eventually decreases below 2.5 mmol l^{-1} in approximately 85% of patients with insulinomas during the 72-hour fast (**Table 5.2, Fig. 5.1**). The most definitive diagnostic biochemical test for insulinoma is an inappropriately increased plasma immunoreactive insulin concentration above 5 µU ml^{-1} at the time of documented hypoglycaemia and symptoms.[12] The plasma insulin concentration is usually greater than 10 µU ml^{-1} in most patients (**Fig. 5.1**).[3] Although prolonged maximal stimulation of insulin

Blood measurement	Fasting normal range	Result with insulinoma	Result with factitious hypoglycaemia	Test sensitivity (%)
Glucose	90–150 mg/dl	<40 mg/dl	<40 mg/dl	99
Immunoreactive insulin (IRI)	<5 µU ml^{-1}	Increased	Increased (usually >10 µU ml^{-1})	100
C-peptide	<1.7 ng ml^{-1}	Increased	Normal range	78
Direct proinsulin-like component (PLC)	<0.2 ng ml^{-1}	Increased	Normal range	85
PLC/total IRI	<25%	Increased	Normal range	87

Table 5.2 *Standard fasting test results and the differentiation of insulinoma from factitious hypoglycaemia*

Figure 5.1
Serum glucose and insulin concentrations at time of development of neuroglycopenic symptoms and termination of fast in 25 patients with insulinoma. Each number represents a patient. All patients had a serum insulin concentration >5 uU ml⁻¹, whereas 21 patients had a serum glucose concentration of <49 mg dl⁻¹. Each patient had an insulinoma resected. Data are from Reference 3, with permission.

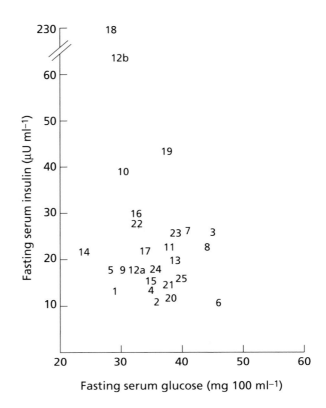

secretion in normal subjects does not cause the release of the insulin precursor molecule, proinsulin, some insulinomas secrete large amounts of uncleaved proinsulin. Patients with high proinsulin-producing tumours may remain euglycaemic and asymptomatic for longer periods during the fast because proinsulin is not biologically active. The proinsulin-like component (PLC) is measured at the time of symptomatic hypoglycaemia and termination of the fast. A value greater than 25% or an increased PLC:total immunoreactive insulin ratio are abnormal and consistent with the diagnosis of insulinoma.[3,12] Some data suggest that an increased PLC value may also be an indication of malignancy,[12] but this has not been substantiated by other groups. Hypersecretion of endogenous insulin also results in increases of the circulating concentration of C-peptide, a biologically inactive byproduct of enzymatic insulin cleavage from the precursor proinsulin molecule. Most patients with insulinomas have C-peptide concentrations greater than 1.7 ng ml⁻¹ (**Fig. 5.2**).[3]

To exclude definitively factitious hypoglycaemia, sulphonylurea concentrations in the blood from oral hypoglycaemic drugs should be measured. Human antibodies to animal insulin are detectable if the patient is not receiving recombinant human insulin. Increased serum concentrations of proinsulin or C-peptides during hypoglycaemia effectively excludes the diagnosis of factitious

Figure 5.2
Serum C-peptide concentrations at time of development of neuroglycopenic symptoms and termination of fast in 25 patients with insulinoma. Shaded area is normal range. Twenty-three of 25 patients had increased concentrations. Data are from Reference 3, with permission.

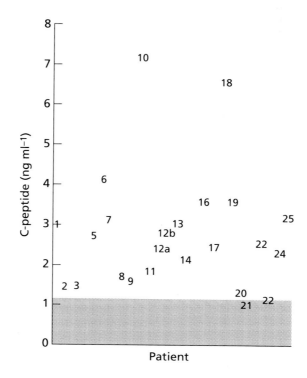

hypoglycaemia because exogenously administered insulin does not contain these proteins and actually suppresses their endogenous production. However, approximately 13–22% of patients with insulinoma do not have increased serum proinsulin or C-peptide concentrations, and a supervised fast prohibiting exogenous insulin administration remains the best test to diagnose insulinoma and conclusively exclude factitious hypoglycaemia. The biochemical parameters measured during the standard fasting test cannot discriminate between patients with MEN-1 or these with sporadic insulinoma.[12]

Nesidioblastosis

Because the surgical managements are different, insulinoma must also be distinguished from nesidioblastosis, a congenital islet cell dysmaturation or malregulation that occurs in infants and causes hyperinsulinaemic hypoglycaemia. Age at the time of presentation is the most important distinguishing factor. Nesidioblastosis occurs most commonly in children under the age of 18 months. Although the existence of adult nesidioblastosis remains plausible,[13] the diagnosis of nesidioblastosis in an adult should be critically suspect because islet cell hyperplasia may be present in the pancreas of patients with insulinoma and an occult insulinoma may be missed in this situation.[1,14] In a review of over 300 cases of hyperinsulinaemic hypoglycaemia at the Mayo Clinic since 1927, only five adult patients had a reasonably confirmed diagnosis of nesidioblastosis.[15]

Biochemical tests (blood glucose, immunoreactive insulin and C-peptide) do not reliably distinguish hyperinsulinaemic hypoglycaemia caused by an insulinoma from that attributed to nesidioblastosis. Thus, children symptomatic after age 18 months must be evaluated to exclude an insulinoma, which must be localised and resected as for an adult. Approximately half of infants with nesidioblastosis require a spleen-preserving near-total pancreatectomy, in which 95% of the pancreas is removed, because this disorder affects the entire pancreas diffusely.[16,17]

Medical management of hypoglycaemia

Medical management should prevent hypoglycaemia caused by the hyperinsulinism so that symptoms and life-threatening sequelae are avoided. In patients with acute hypoglycaemia, blood glucose concentrations are normalised initially with an intravenous glucose infusion. To prevent hypoglycaemic episodes during diagnosis, tumour localisation and the preoperative period, euglycaemia is maintained by giving frequent feeds of a high carbohydrate diet, including a night meal. Cornstarch may be added to food for prolonged slow absorption. For patients who continue to become hypoglycaemic between feedings, diazoxide may be added to the treatment regimen at a dose of 400–600 mg orally each day. Diazoxide inhibits insulin release in approximately 50% of patients with insulinoma; however, side effects of oedema, weight gain and hirsutism occur in 50% of patients and nausea occurs in over 10%.[15] Diazoxide should be discontinued 1 week prior to surgery to avoid intraoperative hypotension. Calcium-channel blockers or phenytoin may also suppress insulin production in some patients. The short-term use of octreotide preoperatively may be beneficial if the patient is not responding well to traditional medical management and surgery is delayed for tumour localisation. Long-term control of hypoglycaemic symptoms with medical management has generally been ineffective for patients with insulinoma. Knowledge of the patient's response to medical management is important for the surgeon so that the urgency and potential benefits of surgery can be determined.[18]

Octreotide is a synthetic, long-acting (half life >100 minutes) analogue of the naturally occurring hormone somatostatin.[18] Octreotide binds to and activates somatostatin receptors on cells expressing them, inhibiting the secretion of many gastrointestinal peptides. Octreotide may be useful for treating symptoms caused by VIPomas and carcinoid tumours but is not recommended for insulinomas because its efficacy in inhibiting insulin release is unpredictable.[19,20] The usefulness of radiolabelled octreotide in imaging insulinomas and in treating metastatic islet cell tumours has been equally disappointing.[21] Therefore, long-term medical management of hypoglycaemia in patients with insulinomas generally is reserved for the few patients (<5%) with unlocalised, unresected tumours after thorough preoperative testing and exploratory laparotomy and for patients with metastatic, unresectable malignant insulinoma.[20] Patients with malignant insulinomas and refractory hypoglycaemia may even require the placement of implantable glucose pumps for continuous glucose infusions.[15]

Preoperative tumour localisation

After definitive diagnosis the tumour must be localised and the presence of unresectable metastatic disease excluded. Accurate tumour localisation is the most difficult aspect of management because the tumours are usually very small and solitary.

Non-invasive imaging studies

An initial attempt should be made to localise the tumour and identify metastatic disease by using non-invasive tests. The least expensive and invasive imaging modality for the pancreas is transabdominal ultrasonography in which an insulinoma appears as a sonolucent mass on a background of 'echodense' normal pancreas. However, the ability to image the pancreas is severely limited by obesity and overlying bowel gas and overall test sensitivity is only 0–25% in most studies (**Table 5.3**).[3,22–24]

Study	Insulinoma	Gastrinoma			
		Overall	Pancreas	Duodenum	Liver metastases
Preoperative					
Non-invasive					
Transabdominal ultrasonography	0–25	20–30			14
Abdominal computed tomography	11–40	50	80	35	50
Abdominal magnetic resonance imaging	11–43	25			83
Octreoscan	0–50	88			
Invasive					
Endoscopic ultrasonography	70–90	85	88–100	<5	<5
Selective arteriography	40–70	68		34	86
+ calcium stimulation	88–94	–	–	–	–
+ secretin injection	–	90–100			
Portal venous sampling	67–80	70–90			
Unlocalised primary tumour	10–20	15			
Intraoperative					
Palpation	65	65	91	60	
Intraoperative ultrasonography	75–100	83	95	58	
Endoscopic transillumination	–	–	–	70	
Duodenotomy	–	–	–	100	
Unlocalised primary tumour	1	5			

Table 5.3   *Sensitivities of localisation studies for insulinomas and gastrinomas*

Computed tomography (CT) and magnetic resonance imaging (MRI; Table 5.3) are able to identify pancreatic tumours as small as 1 cm in diameter. For CT, oral contrast should be administered to differentiate bowel and to define more clearly the pancreas, and thin slices of the peripancreatic area—at most 5 mm apart—should be obtained.[25] The administration of intravenous contrast may cause a tumour blush owing to increased vascularity. The sensitivity of CT for insulinoma ranges between 11 and 40% in most series.[3,22–24,26] MRI may image an islet cell tumour based on increased signal intensity (brightness) on T2 weighted images. The sensitivity of MRI is equivalent to that of CT[3,22,23] and, as expected, the accuracy of both CT and MRI increase with larger tumour size, achieving a sensitivity of 100% as tumour size is increased to 6 cm.[27]

Malignant insulinomas are almost always very large (>4 cm) and are easily imaged by CT or MRI. The extent of bulky metastatic tumour deposits and hepatic metastases are also usually readily identifiable by CT or MRI. Metastases should be identified preoperatively so that the operative approach can be planned, or, in the case of unresectability, unnecessary surgery is avoided.

Somatostatin receptor scintigraphy (SRS), or octreoscan, is a relatively new modality, which utilises octreotide, a somatostatin analogue, labelled with a radioactive tracer and given intravenously (**Table 5.3**). The radiolabelled octreotide binds to tumours with somatostatin receptors, causing the tumour to appear as a 'hot spot' on whole-body gamma camera scintigraphy.[28] Thus, the SRS depends on the ability of a particular islet cell tumour to express somatostatin receptors.[29] Some islet cell tumours, such as gastrinomas, express somatostatin receptors and are nearly always (80%) imaged by labelled octreotide. However, less than 50% of insulinomas are imaged by SRS[28,29] because they do not consistently express high levels of somatostatin receptors. Thus SRS is not recommended for localising insulinomas. Radioiodinated vasoactive intestinal polypeptide (VIP) scanning[30] may be useful but experience is presently too limited to consistently recommend its use.

Invasive localising procedures

Approximately 50% of patients have small (<2 cm) insulinomas that are not detected by non-invasive imaging tests, and a variety of more sensitive invasive tests are used to localise the tumour preoperatively. Endoscopic ultrasonography (EUS) is safe and highly effective when performed by experienced users and may replace the routine use of other preoperative localisation studies.[31–33] An endoscope is passed into the duodenum and a balloon is inflated against the intestinal wall with saline. A 5–10 MHz transducer is used to generate an image of the pancreas through the intestinal and stomach walls. Tumours as small as 2–3 mm in diameter can be identified in the pancreatic head by moving the transducer through the duodenum at the junction of the pancreas. The endoscope must be passed well into the third portion of the duodenum to adequately visualise the uncinate process. Insulinomas in the pancreatic body and tail are imaged by positioning the transducer in the stomach and scanning the posterior wall. Sensitivity for EUS ranges from 70–90% and specificity is near 100% (Table 5.3).[32,34–36] It more accurately detects tumours in the head of the pancreas (as compared with tumours in the body and tail) because the head can be viewed through three angles (from the third portion of the duodenum, through the bulb and through the stomach) whereas the body and tail can only be viewed through the stomach. A case–control study evaluating the cost effectiveness of EUS on preoperative localisation of pancreatic endocrine tumours showed a greater than $2000 cost saving per patient for preoperative localisation studies, mainly because of the reduced need for angiograms and venous sampling procedures.[37] Total surgical and anaesthesia times were also reduced in the EUS group. EUS is cost effective when used early in the preoperative localisation strategy and may avoid unnecessary morbidity associated with more invasive tests.[37]

In patients with negative results after non-invasive imaging studies or EUS, a regional localisation study—either calcium arteriography or portal venous sampling (PVS)—may be obtained. These two studies rely on the functional activity of the insulinoma (i.e. excessive insulin production) and not on the capability to image the tumour (i.e. tumour size). The calcium arteriogram seems to be the most informative preoperative test for localising insulinomas. It is replacing PVS as the invasive localising study of choice.[22] Calcium provocation may identify the region of the pancreas containing the tumour (head, body or tail). Arteries that perfuse the pancreatic head (gastroduodenal artery and superior mesenteric artery) and the body/tail (splenic artery) are selectively catheterised sequentially, and a small amount of calcium gluconate (0.025 mEq Ca^{2+} kg^{-1} body weight) is injected into each artery during different runs. A catheter positioned in the right hepatic vein is used to collect blood for measurement of insulin concentrations 30–60 seconds after the calcium injection. Calcium stimulates a marked increase in insulin secretion from the insulinoma. A greater than two-fold increase in the hepatic vein insulin concentration indicates localisation of the tumour to the area of the pancreas being perfused by the injected artery (**Fig. 5.3**). Additionally, injection of contrast may reveal a tumour blush, confirming the location of the insulinoma by imaging the tumour. It may be necessary to obtain multiple views (including oblique images) to evaluate lesions obscured by vessels and bones. This test therefore combines the functionality advantage of PVS with the more exact localisation capability of an arteriogram. These combined features are especially useful in patients with MEN-1 who may have multiple functional islet cell tumours. The reported sensitivity of calcium stimulation is between 88 and 94% and few false positive results occur (**Table 5.3**).[22,38,39] The calcium arteriogram may also aid in the diagnosis because calcium does not stimulate normal pancreatic β cells to secrete insulin, and indirectly it may help exclude other causes of hypoglycaemia.

Figure 5.3
Calcium angiogram in a patient with an insulinoma localised to the pancreatic tail. Intra-arterial calcium was selectively injected into splenic, superior mesenteric, hepatic and gastroduodenal arteries in four different runs. Blood samples were taken serially from hepatic vein and insulin concentrations measured at 0, 1 and 2 minutes before and after calcium injection. After injection into the splenic artery, there was a rapid marked increase in hepatic vein insulin concentrations at 1 and 2 minutes. This finding localised the insulinoma to the pancreatic tail.

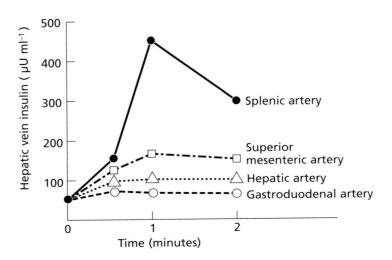

PVS is performed by measuring insulin concentrations in the portal vein and its tributaries.[32] A catheter is passed through the liver into the portal vein. It may be associated with complications, including haemobilia and haemorrhage.[40] It is more costly because approximately 20 blood samples are assayed for insulin concentration. Sensitivity ranges from 67–80% (**Table 5.3**) and there are few false positives.[3,22–25] Because the calcium angiogram provides similar information, can image the tumour and is less costly and invasive, it should replace PVS for invasive localisation.

A small proportion of insulinomas remain unlocalised even after all localisation studies are obtained and are therefore considered occult. When the diagnosis is certain on the basis of the results of the fast, surgical exploration with careful inspection, palpation and intraoperative ultrasonography (IOUS) of the pancreas is still indicated. Most of these patients (>90%) will still have an insulinoma identified and removed by experienced surgeons.[1,41] Recent retrospective reviews have shown that the combination of surgical exploration with IOUS will identify almost all insulinomas.[42–46]

Operative management

The only curative treatment for patients with insulinoma is surgical resection, and surgery should accurately identify and remove all islet cell tumours. Blind pancreatic resection with the hope of including an unidentified insulinoma in the specimen is no longer indicated, and IOUS should be used to identify clearly the tumour to preserve as much normal pancreatic tissue as possible. Accurate preoperative localisation correlates with a high probability of identifying the tumour in the same location at surgery, and eventual cure. However, even with successful preoperative localisation, a careful pancreatic exploration should be performed at the time of surgery, including palpation and IOUS. The possibility of multiple insulinomas or a false positive result with a preoperative localisation test may result in surgical failure. IOUS also helps to define the relationship of the tumour to the common bile duct, pancreatic duct, portal vein and adjacent blood vessels. When preoperative localisation studies are inconclusive, adequate mobilisation of the pancreas with the use of IOUS results in successful identification and resection of the insulinoma in nearly all cases.

Operative approach

A mechanical bowel preparation is advised. Pneumococcal vaccination is used preoperatively because distal pancreatectomy with splenectomy may be necessary. The prophylactic use of octreotide preoperatively to reduce complications of pancreatic surgery such as fistulae and pseudocysts has not been proven to be beneficial.[47] A standard midline laparotomy or bilateral subcostal incision is recommended to give adequate exposure to the abdomen, which is facilitated by a fixed upper abdominal retractor. The entire abdomen, including regional lymph nodes, is initially inspected for potential metastases, which occur in 10% of sporadic cases. Metastatic insulinoma deposits on the surface of the liver typically appear as firm nodules. IOUS with a 5 MHz transducer may be helpful in identifying deep hepatic metastases.

Suspicious hepatic lesions that are small and peripheral should be excised by wedge resection, and larger or deeper lesions should be biopsied. Samples are sent for immediate frozen-section analysis to exclude tumour. In general, resection of localised tumour metastases is indicated to decrease symptoms associated with hyperinsulinaemia, which may be poorly controlled long term by medical means. To expose adequately the pancreas, the hepatic and splenic flexures of the colon are mobilised out of the upper abdomen, and the gastrocolic ligament is divided to open the lesser sac.

Pancreatic mobilisation

In contradistinction to gastrinomas, virtually all insulinomas are located within the pancreas and are uniformly distributed throughout the entire gland.[3] Therefore, the head, body and tail of the pancreas must be sufficiently mobilised to permit evaluation of the entire organ. This requires an extended Kocher manoeuvre to lift adequately the head of the pancreas out of the retroperitoneum and division of attachments at the inferior and posterior border of the pancreas, to permit evaluation of the posterior body and tail (**Fig. 5.4**). Because the head of the pancreas is thick, small tumours that are centrally located may not be easily palpated. The entire pancreatic head must be sufficiently mobilised so that the posterior surface can be adequately examined visually and palpated

Figure 5.4
Operative manoeuvres to identify insulinoma. (a) Kocher manoeuvre with careful palpation of head of pancreas. (b) Opening gastrocolic ligament, superior retraction of stomach, inferior retraction of transverse colon and careful palpation of body and tail of pancreas after incision along inferior border.

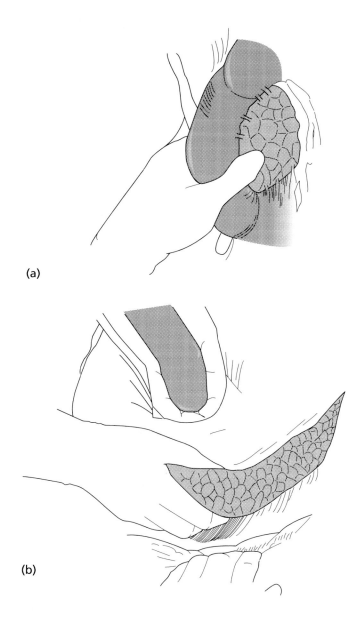

(a)

(b)

between the thumb and forefinger. The splenic ligaments may be divided to completely mobilise the spleen out of the retroperitoneum for complete examination and palpation of the pancreatic tail.

Intraoperative manoeuvres to find insulinoma

Direct inspection of the entire pancreatic surface is carried out first because an insulinoma may appear as a brownish-red purple mass, like a cherry. Most insulinomas are encompassed by pancreatic parenchyma and may not be directly visible, but careful palpation of the pancreas between the thumb and forefinger may identify some of these. The tumour feels like a firm, nodular and discrete mass. Approximately 65% of insulinomas may be identified by the traditional operative manoeuvres of inspection and palpation.[3] Tumours are more difficult to identify when the pancreas is scarred from previous surgery or alcoholism and when tumours arise centrally within the thick pancreatic head.

IOUS is the best intraoperative method to find and remove insulinoma. It is performed by placing the transducer on the surface of the pancreas, which is covered in a pool of saline to maximise image quality. A 10 MHz or 7.5 MHz real-time probe is used, which has a short focal length and high resolution. An insulinoma appears as a sonolucent mass with margins distinct from the uniform more echodense pancreas parenchyma (**Fig. 5.5**).

IOUS can localise an occult insulinoma that has not been identified preoperatively[48] and can identify tumours that are not visible or palpable (Fig. 5.5).[3,41] It is particularly helpful in evaluation of the pancreatic head. In conjunction with simultaneous palpation, ultrasonography further clarifies lesions.[41] The sensitivity for detecting insulinomas using IOUS is greater than 75%[24,26] and approaches 100% (**Table 5.3**).[3,22]

Figure 5.5
Intraoperative ultrasonography of insulinoma (arrow). The insulinoma appears sonolucent compared with more echodense pancreas. This tumour measures 1 cm in diameter and was not palpable within the pancreatic head.

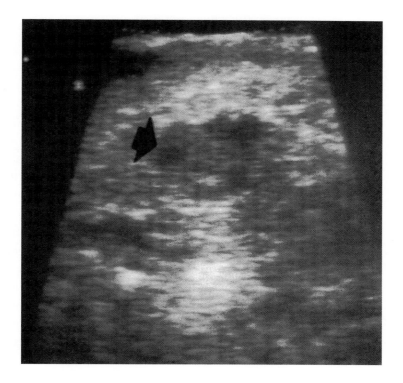

Insulinoma resection

Enucleation means to excise only the adenoma with minimal normal pancreatic tissue. It is currently the operation of choice for benign insulinomas. With the use of preoperative localisation and IOUS, blind distal pancreatectomy is no longer advocated. Tumour size, location and surrounding anatomy determine whether enucleation or pancreatic resection is performed. It is important to consider the relationship of the tumour to the pancreatic duct by imaging both structures with IOUS prior to tumour excision. Small tumours that are separated from the pancreatic duct and major vessels by normal pancreas can be safely enucleated (Fig. 5.5). IOUS allows a precise, safe tumour enucleation and helps plan the shortest, most direct route to the tumour while avoiding the pancreatic duct. If a clear margin of normal pancreatic tissue does not exist between the insulinoma and other structures, then a distal or subtotal pancreatectomy and splenectomy is advised.[3,48] Ductal injury in an attempt to resect a tumour in close proximity to the pancreatic duct results in most postoperative morbidity. Evidence of malignancy, such as involvement of peripancreatic lymph nodes or tumour invasion, mandates pancreatic resection and not enucleation.[41] Large tumour size may also be an indication for pancreatic resection. Rarely, pancreaticoduodenectomy is indicated if enucleation cannot be performed safely. A study reviewing 50 patients treated by pancreaticoduodenectomy for periampullary neuroendocrine tumours showed a postoperative mortality rate of 2%, with no postoperative deaths occurring after 1967.[49] The most common complications were wound infection (24%), pancreatic fistula (24%) and delayed gastric emptying (15%). Patients with benign tumours had a significantly higher 5-year survival rate (94%) compared with those with malignant tumours (61%).[49]

Insulinoma and MEN-1

Approximately 10% of insulinomas occur in the setting of MEN-1 syndrome, and 20% of patients with MEN-1 develop insulinomas. Insulinomas in MEN-1 syndrome may be multiple and may occur simultaneously and diffusely throughout the pancreas.[50] The goal of treatment is to ameliorate the hypoglycaemia by eliminating the source of insulin hypersecretion. Difficulty arises in identifying which tumour or tumours produce the excessive insulin, but there is usually a dominant large tumour (>3 cm) that is readily identified on abdominal CT.[51] An invasive regional localisation test such as the calcium angiogram or PVS is indicated to determine if the imaged tumour is responsible for the excessive secretion of insulin. Other small islet cell tumours may also be identified, but these tumours are most likely clinically insignificant. If the insulinoma(s) arises within the body or tail of the pancreas, then a subtotal or distal pancreatectomy is indicated because multiple other islet cell tumours are virtually always present.[52] A tumour that arises in the head of the pancreas is enucleated, if possible, or alternatively resected by pancreaticoduodenectomy. The use of PVS or calcium angiogram can determine the region of the pancreas that contains the insulinoma. Intraoperative measurements of insulin concentration can accurately predict the completeness of surgery.[53] Medical management for this condition is reserved for those occasional patients who have failed surgical therapy, those who are poor surgical risks or those in whom a single source of hyperinsulinism cannot be found.[54]

Laparoscopic surgery

Laparoscopic surgery offers many advantages to patients, including decreased hospital stay, reduced pain, smaller incisions and a shorter recovery period. There is an ever-widening array of procedures that can now be safely performed laparoscopically with very successful results. Because insulinomas are usually small, benign and almost always located within the pancreas, laparoscopic surgery with laparoscopic IOUS is a logical approach to treat these patients. There are several successful case reports of laparoscopic enucleation of pancreatic insulinomas and laparoscopic distal pancreatectomies.[55–58] Operative times ranged from 180–360 minutes for those operations that were successfully completed laparoscopically. Complications included pancreatic fistula and some procedures required conversion to open surgery. Minimally invasive surgery for pancreatic insulinomas is feasible in the hands of the experienced surgeon but requires further development and study.

Outcome

Most patients with insulinoma are cured of hypoglycaemia and return to a normal, fully functional lifestyle. Appropriate localisation of sporadic insulinoma and surgical resection of all adenomatous tissue results in a cure rate of greater than 95%.[3,26] Virtually all patients with benign, sporadic insulinomas are cured of their disease and have a normal long-term survival (**Table 5.4**).[59] Symptoms resolve postoperatively and the fasting serum concentration of glucose normalises.[3] Although successful resection of the tumour(s) responsible for hyperinsulinism renders most MEN-1 patients asymptomatic postoperatively,[51] persistent or recurrent hypoglycaemia owing to a missed insulinoma or metastatic disease from the original tumour may develop.[1]

In general, pancreatic surgery for insulinoma should have an associated morbidity rate less than 20% and a mortality rate approaching 0%.[1] Potential complications specifically associated with pancreatic surgery include fistula, pseudocyst, pancreatitis and abscess. Octreotide reduces the amount of pancreatic drainage[18] and may reduce complications when give both preoperatively and postoperatively.[47,60] The use of IOUS decreases complications from ductal injury.

Series	No	Tumour found (%)	Initial remission (%)
Insulinoma			
Brown et al.[38]	36	100	100
Huai et al.[43]	28	100	100
Hashimoto and Walsh[44]	21	95	94
Lo et al.[46]	27	100	96
Pasieka et al.[124]	45	100	100
Doherty et al.[3]	25	96	96
Grant et al.[26]	36	100	97
Gastrinoma			
Norton et al.[107]	123	86/100[a]	51[b]
Mignon et al.[125]	125	81	26
Norton et al.[63]	73	77	58[c]
Howard et al.[91]	11	91	82
Thompson et al.[89]	5	100	100

[a] Gastrinomas were found in 86% of initial surgical explorations and 100% of subsequent explorations.
[b] 5-year disease-free survival was maintained at 49%.
[c] 5-year survival was decreased to 30%.

Table 5.4   *Results of recent series for insulinoma and localised gastrinoma*

Gastrinoma

Each year, approximately 0.1–3 people per million population develop gastrinoma, the second most common pancreatic endocrine tumour (**Table 5.1**).[61] The clinical features of this tumour were first described by Zollinger and Ellison in 1955.[62] Because of an increased awareness of Zollinger–Ellison syndrome (ZES) and the widespread availability of accurate immunoassays to measure serum concentrations of gastrin, gastrinoma is increasingly diagnosed and treated at an early stage of disease.

Patient presentation

Gastrinomas secrete excessive amounts of the hormone gastrin, which may cause epigastric abdominal pain, diarrhoea and oesophagitis. The most common sign is peptic ulcer disease. Diarrhoea, caused by gastrin-induced hypersecretion and increased bowel motility, is the second most common symptom and may be the only manifestation of ZES in 20% of patients. Oesophagitis with or without stricture occurs with more severe forms of the syndrome. Approximately 20% of patients with ZES will have it as part of MEN-I,[1] and this syndrome must always be excluded. A significant family history of ulcers, peptic ulceration occurring at a young age and peptic ulcers in association with hyperparathyroidism and/or nephrolithiasis all may be indicative of MEN-1. These patients may have multiple subcutaneous lipomas.

As a result of increased serum gastrin concentrations, the gastric chief cells are under constant stimulation to produce acid, which causes peptic ulceration and epigastric abdominal pain in 80% of patients with ZES. Approximately 0.1–1% of patients who present with peptic ulcer disease have ZES.[61]

Patients with ZES usually have a solitary ulcer in the proximal duodenum, similar to patients with peptic ulcer disease unrelated to gastrinoma, and 'typical' ulceration does not exclude ZES. All patients with peptic ulcer disease severe enough to require surgery should be screened preoperatively for gastrinoma by obtaining a fasting serum gastrin concentration. Recurrent ulceration after appropriate medical treatment or after acid-reducing surgical procedures, or peptic ulceration in multiple locations or unusual locations such as distal duodenum or jejunum, are all suspicious of the ZES. Patients with ZES may present with a perforated ulcer, which may occur in the jejunum. Not all patients with ZES have peptic ulcer disease, and 20% of patients with ZES have no evidence of peptic ulceration at the time of presentation.[63]

Diagnosis

The evaluation of a patient suspicious for having ZES begins by obtaining a fasting serum concentration of gastrin (**Fig. 5.6**). Hypergastrinaemia occurs in almost all patients with ZES and is defined as a serum gastrin concentration greater than 100 pg ml^{-1}.[64] Therefore, a normal fasting serum gastrin concentration effectively excludes ZES. Antacid medications may cause a false positive increase in serum gastrin concentration, and those medicines should be withheld for 3 days before measurement of the serum gastrin concentration.

Achlorhydria is a common cause of hypergastrinaemia, and gastric acid secretion is measured to exclude this condition (Fig. 5.6). A basal acid output (BAO) greater than 15 mEq/h (greater than 5 mEq/h in patients who have undergone previous acid-reducing operations) is abnormal and occurs in 98% of patients with ZES. Measurement of gastric pH is a simpler but less accurate indicator of gastric acid hypersecretion. A gastric pH greater than 3 essentially excludes ZES, whereas a pH less than or equal to 2 is consistent with ZES.

An extremely increased fasting serum gastrin concentration (greater than 1000 pg ml^{-1}) and abnormally elevated BAO establish the diagnosis of ZES. Many patients with ZES have gastric acid hypersecretion and minimally increased fasting serum gastrin concentrations (100–1000 pg ml^{-1}). For these patients, the secretin stimulation test is the provocative test of choice.[1] The secretin test is carried out after an overnight fast; secretin 2 U kg^{-1} by intravenous injection is administered, and blood samples are collected immediately before

Figure 5.6
Flow diagram for diagnosis and evaluation of patients with suspected Zollinger–Ellison syndrome (gastrinoma).

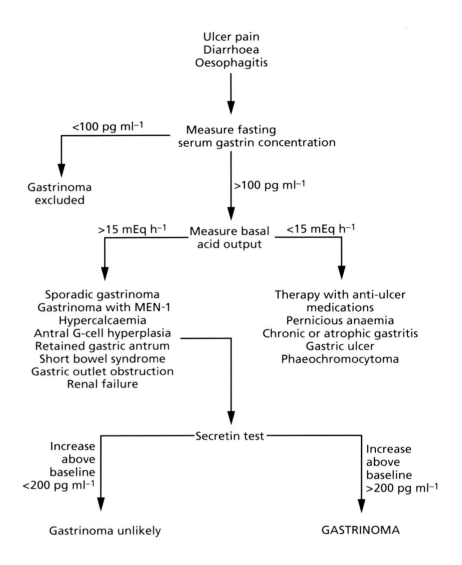

and at 2, 5, 10 and 15 minutes after giving the secretin. A 200 pg ml^{-1} increase of gastrin concentration above baseline is diagnostic of ZES. The test sensitivity is not 100%, and approximately 15% of patients with gastrinoma may have a negative secretin test.

Medical control of gastric acid hypersecretion

The management of patients with gastrinoma consists of two phases: to control the symptoms associated with acid hypersecretion and to remove the tumour, which is potentially malignant and life threatening. The development of H$_2$-receptor antagonists and Na$^+$-K$^+$-ATPase inhibitors has made medical control of gastric acid hypersecretion possible in all patients. Patients with ZES typically require 2–5 times the usual dose of anti-ulcer medications to keep the BAO <15 mEqh^{-1}. Omeprazole at 20–40 mg p.o. twice a day will usually control acid hypersecretion. Patients who have reflux oesophagitis or who have had prior operations to reduce acid secretion, such as subtotal gastrectomy, should have the acid output maintained at <5 mEqh^{-1}. If acid hypersecretion is controlled, epigastric discomfort resolves and ulcers heal in virtually all patients.[62,65,66] Because of the recent advances in the medical treatment of peptic ulcer disease, total gastrectomy is not indicated in patients with gastrinoma.

Adequate medical control of gastric acid hypersecretion with resolution of symptoms and decreased ulcerogenic complications has resulted in increased concern about the potential malignancy of the primary tumour. The most important determinant of long-term survival in patients with ZES is the growth of the primary tumour and its metastatic spread.[66] Tumour progression accounted for most deaths when patients were followed long term.[66] Development of liver metastases is associated with subsequent death from tumour, and surgical resection of the primary can reduce the incidence of liver metastases. In a recent study, hepatic metastases developed in only 3% of patients with gastrinoma treated by surgical excision of the primary compared with 23% managed without surgery.[67] Therefore, the current goal of surgery for ZES has shifted away from controlling gastric-acid hypersecretion to aggressive resection of the primary tumour as well as localised metastatic disease. Surgical intervention can obviate the need for long-term medical therapy, which is important since experimental rodent studies suggest that the long-term use of omeprazole is associated with the development of gastric carcinoid tumours.[68] The authors have recently diagnosed diffuse malignant gastric carcinoids in two patients with ZES and MEN-1 who have been taking omeprazole for several years. It is imperative that such patients are monitored with periodic endoscopy to screen for the development of carcinoid tumours.

The natural history of longstanding ZES in patients in whom the excessive acid secretion is controlled is largely unclear, primarily because effective medical therapy is relatively new. A longitudinal study of 212 patients with ZES and well controlled acid secretion showed that none of these patients died of acid-related complications.[69] This study evaluated the long-term clinical course of patients with gastrinoma. Pancreatic location of tumour and a tumour diameter greater than 3 cm were found to be associated with an increased risk of death from gastrinoma, and higher serum gastrin concentrations correlated with more malignant disease and a shortened survival time.[69] Extensive liver metastases had increased negative effects on survival, as did the development of bone metastases or ectopic Cushing's syndrome. These results lend further support to early surgical intervention (as surgery decreases the rate of development of liver metastases), as well as aggressive surgical therapy of limited hepatic metastases.[69,70]

Preoperative tumour localisation

In contradistinction to insulinoma, gastrinoma is malignant in 60–90% of patients.[2] Duodenal gastrinomas as small as 2 mm in diameter may have associated regional lymph node metastases.[71] At the time of diagnosis, approximately 25–40% of patients have liver metastases.[72,73] Imaging studies must carefully assess the liver, and all patients with ZES should undergo preoperative testing to localise the tumour and to define the extent of disease so that appropriate surgical treatment can be undertaken.

Non-invasive tumour localising studies

Initial tumour localisation studies should be non-invasive, should attempt to image the primary tumour and should adequately assess the liver for metastases. As with localising insulinoma, abdominal ultrasonography has a low sensitivity of only 20–30% for gastrinoma (Table 5.3). Abdominal CT detects approximately 50% of gastrinomas overall, but sensitivity depends greatly on tumour size, tumour location and the presence of metastases.[74] Gastrinomas that are greater than 3 cm in diameter are reliably detected by CT, whereas tumours less than 1 cm in diameter are rarely detected (Fig. 5.7).

Primary gastrinomas that arise within the pancreas are identified much more reliably than those in extrapancreatic, extrahepatic locations (80% vs. 35%). CT scanning identifies 50% of liver metastases. Abdominal MRI has a low sensitivity (25%) in localising primary gastrinomas but is the study of choice to show hepatic metastases (Table 5.3). Gastrinoma metastases in the liver appear bright on dynamic T2 weighted images and show a distinct ring with gadolinium enhancement.[75] MRI is especially useful to differentiate gastrinoma metastases within the liver from haemangiomas.

Recent studies indicate that somatostatin receptor scintigraphy (SRS) may significantly improve the preoperative localisation of gastrinomas.[76] SRS images gastrinomas on the basis of the density of somatostatin type 2 receptors. Because a high proportion of gastrinomas have these type 2 receptors, approximately 80% of primary tumours can be identified, and the true extent of metastatic disease is delineated more accurately than by CT or MRI.[77] SRS is now the non-invasive imaging modality of choice for gastrinomas (**Fig. 5.7**).

Several prospective studies have evaluated the utility of SRS compared with conventional studies. In a prospective study of 35 patients, SRS had a greater sensitivity than all other conventional studies combined (angiography, MRI, CT, ultrasonography).[78] The rate of detection correlated closely with tumour size detecting 30% of gastrinomas less than 1.1 cm in diameter and 96% of those greater than 2 cm. A positive SRS study strongly predicts the presence of tumour, but the high negative predictive value (33–100%) cautions against excluding a

Figure 5.7
(a) Computed tomography scan and (b) somatostatin receptor scintigraphy preoperatively identified large gastrinomas in this patient.

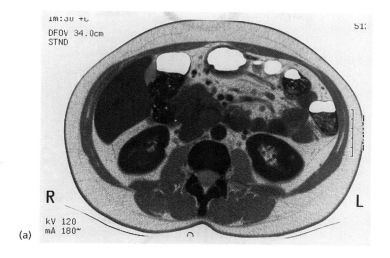

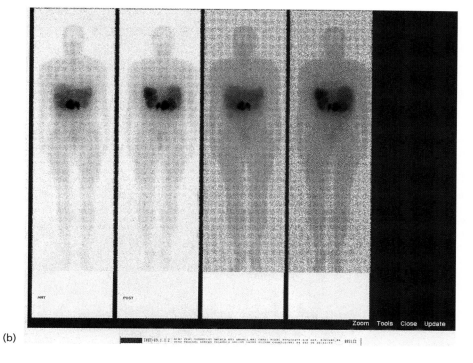

tumour on the basis of a negative study.[79] Another recent prospective study in 146 patients found a sensitivity of 71%, specificity of 86%, positive predictive value of 85% and a negative predictive value of 52%. These 146 patients underwent 480 SRS studies, with a false positive localisation rate of 12%. Extra–abdominal false positive localisation studies were more common than intra-abdominal false positive scans and were attributed to thyroid, breast or granulomatous lung disease.[80]

The most common causes of false positive intra-abdominal SRS scans were accessory spleens, localisation to prior operative sites and renal parapelvic cysts. Only 2.7% of these false positive studies actually altered management, suggesting the importance of a high awareness of other potential causes for a positive SRS scan in the clinical setting.

Invasive tumour localising modalities

Although non-invasive imaging studies are important as initial tests to exclude gross hepatic metastases and unresectable disease, these studies may fail to image the primary gastrinoma. Invasive modalities may be useful to localise accurately the primary tumour prior to surgery. EUS has a reported sensitivity of 85% for detecting gastrinomas and a specificity of 95% (**Table 5.3**).[32,35,36] Tumours in the pancreas as small as 2–3 mm may be imaged. Duodenal gastrinomas can be visualised as a submucosal mass with EUS (**Fig. 5.8**). The ability to detect duodenal wall gastrinomas directly has been disappointing, and liver metastases are not reliably imaged. The combination of EUS and SRS for gastrinomas has been found to be 93% in a small series of patients.[81]

Previously the best imaging modality to localise a primary gastrinoma was selective angiography. Angiograms are obtained by selectively catheterising gastroduodenal, hepatic, superior mesenteric and splenic arteries. A hypervascular tumour 'blush' is characteristically observed in the location of the gastrinoma (**Fig. 5.9**). Sensitivity is 68% overall for extrahepatic gastrinomas and 86% for hepatic metastases, but only 34% for duodenal gastrinomas (**Table 5.3**).[82,83]

Figure 5.8
View of duodenal wall gastrinoma through endoscope. The tumour appears as a small submucosal mass, which was biopsied and confirmed as a gastrinoma.

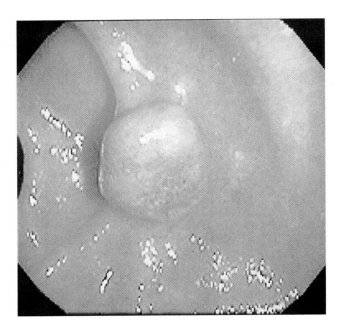

Figure 5.9
Secretin angiogram in patient with Zollinger–Ellison syndrome and gastrinoma localised to duodenum. (a) Results of secretion injection of selective arteries that perfuse the pancreas and duodenum (gastroduodenal artery, hepatic artery, superior mesenteric artery, splenic artery). Gastrin concentrations were measured in the hepatic vein before secretin injection and at intervals after secretin injection. (b) When secretin was injected into the gastroduodenal artery gastrinoma was visualised in the wall of the duodenum as a 'blush' (arrow), and the hepatic vein gastrin concentrations were most increased (a).

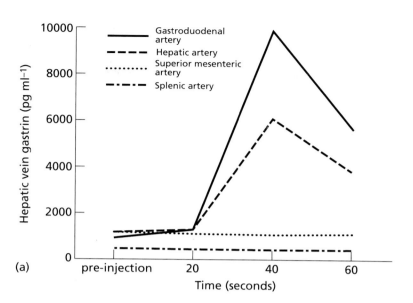

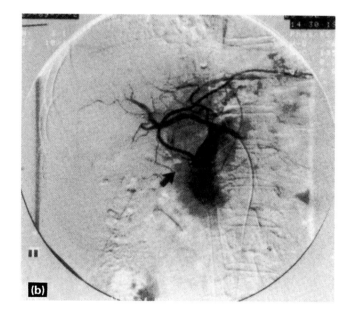

Tumours less than 1–2 cm in size are less reliably detected. Selective arterial secretin injection (SASI) during angiography, and collection of blood samples from a hepatic vein as well as a peripheral vein for measurement of the gastrin concentration, increases the sensitivity for localising the primary tumour to 90–100%, with a specificity of virtually 100% (**Fig. 5.9**).[84] Injection of secretin into the artery supplying the gastrinoma causes an increase in the hepatic vein gastrin concentration by more than 80 pg ml^{-1} in 40 seconds. In this way the gastrinoma can be localised to either the pancreatic head, body/tail of the pancreas or the liver. Gastrinomas are usually only found in the gastroduodenal artery territory and occult tumours are usually in the gastrinoma triangle. PVS for gastrin is similar and provides regional localisation, with similar sensitivity to the SASI test. Neither study is particularly useful in patients with ZES because gradients are nearly always found in the gastrinoma triangle.

Surgery for tumour eradication

If preoperative imaging studies reveal no evidence of unresectable metastatic disease, then patients with sporadic gastrinoma and acceptable risks should undergo abdominal exploration for tumour resection.

Operative approach

Mechanical bowel preparation and pneumococcal vaccination are required preoperatively. The prophylactic use of octreotide may reduce complications from pancreatic surgery.[47] The surgeon should be prepared for hepatic resection if unsuspected liver metastases are identified intraoperatively. An upper abdominal incision that provides adequate exposure for exploration of the entire pancreas, regional lymph nodes and liver is necessary. The abdomen is initially inspected for metastases, with particular attention to possible ectopic sites of tumour such as the ovaries, jejunum and omentum. The entire surface of the liver is then palpated for metastatic lesions. Metastases typically appear tan in colour and feel firm. Deep hepatic metastases may be identified by using IOUS with a 5 MHz transducer. All suspicious hepatic lesions must be either excised or biopsied to exclude malignant gastrinoma. In general, liver metastases that are not identified preoperatively by abdominal MRI or SRS are small and potentially resectable at the time of operation. Similarly, hilar and peripancreatic regional lymph nodes are carefully evaluated for metastatic disease.

Intraoperative manoeuvres to find the primary gastrinoma

Successful intraoperative localisation and resection of tumours may be extremely challenging because tumours only 2 mm in size may be in the wall of the duodenum. There is also a high rate of associated lymph node metastases and a possible occurrence of primary gastrinomas within lymph nodes with no other identifiable primary tumour.[85] The initial finding of a single involved lymph node may, therefore, represent a primary tumour or metastatic disease from a very small, unlocalised primary tumour. Preoperative studies, such as SRS, accurately localise the primary gastrinoma and metastases and greatly facilitate the operative management, allowing a surgical approach directed to the area containing the tumour. Intraoperative localisation is still necessary because 20–40% of patients in whom the tumour is not apparent with preoperative studies will still have tumour identified at surgery. A potentially useful new tool is the measurement of intraoperative gastrin concentrations. In a series of 20 patients, this test had an accuracy of 94% in predicting the successful removal of all gastrin-secreting tumours.[86] Both the positive predictive value and specificity were 100%, and the negative predictive value 88%, with a sensitivity of 91%. Although a small series of patients, the study showed that intraoperative measurements of gastrin concentration may provide an additional tool to help guide complete resection.

Successful tumour identification requires knowledge of where primary gastrinomas arise. The so-called 'gastrinoma triangle,' bounded by the neck and body of the pancreas medially, the junction of the cystic and common bile ducts superiorly and the second and third portions of the duodenum inferiorly, contains more than 80% of primary gastrinomas.[87] In this region, most gastrinomas arise within the duodenum. The head of the pancreas and duodenum are first exposed by mobilising the hepatic flexure of the colon out of the upper abdomen and dividing the gastrocolic ligament to open the lesser sac. A Kocher manoeuvre is performed to lift the head of the pancreas out of the retroperitoneum. The entire pancreatic surface is carefully examined visually and palpated between the thumb and forefinger (Fig. 5.4). IOUS is very useful for localising intrapancreatic gastrinomas (Table 5.3). The body and tail of the pancreas may be mobilised and similarly examined after dividing the inferior and posterior pancreatic attachments to find the few gastrinomas that may arise in the distal pancreas.

Primary gastrinomas have increasingly been recognised as occurring in extrapancreatic locations.[87–89] IOUS is poor at detecting gastrinomas within the duodenum (**Table 5.3**), and the surgeon must rely more on inspection, palpation and duodenotomy to find these tumours.[41] In 30–40% of patients, the gastrinoma is located in the submucosa of the duodenum. Duodenal gastrinomas are usually very small—less than 6 mm in size—and are difficult to palpate. Endoscopic transillumination of the duodenum may allow small duodenal tumours to be seen and guide precise tumour resection.[90] The gastrinoma appears as a dark, opaque shadow surrounded by the semitransparent red glow of the duodenal wall. If the tumour is not localised by endoscopic transillumination, then duodenotomy is recommended to allow direct inspection and exploration of the duodenal mucosa. Duodenal wall gastrinomas occur in greatest density more proximally in the duodenum (**Fig. 5.10**). Tumours are detected most usually by duodenotomy, followed by intraoperative endoscopy with transillumination and least often by palpation (**Fig. 5.10**). Regional lymph nodes should be systematically sampled, as lymph node metastases may be inapparent at exploration and will be found in 55% of patients with duodenal tumours. Gastrinomas can be found by an experienced surgeon in 80–90% of patients (**Table 5.4**).[89,91]

Figure 5.10
Density of duodenal gastrinomas found at surgery and method of operative identification. Gastrinomas within the wall of the duodenum are most common in the first portion (D1) and decrease in density move distally (D3). Duodenotomy identified the most tumours, followed by intraoperative endoscopy and then palpation.

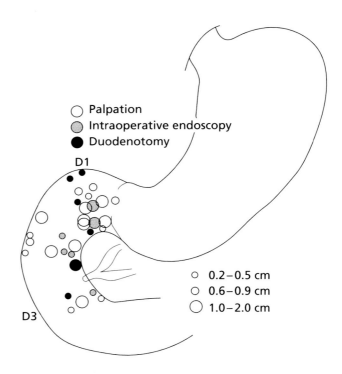

○ Palpation
◍ Intraoperative endoscopy
● Duodenotomy

D1

○ 0.2–0.5 cm
○ 0.6–0.9 cm
◯ 1.0–2.0 cm

D3

Approximately 5–24% of gastrinomas are found in extrapancreatic, extra-intestinal lymph nodes only, with no apparent primary pancreatic or duodenal tumour.[92–95] Whether these represent primary tumours or metastases from occult pancreatic or intestinal primary tumours is controversial. Primary tumours as small as 2 mm may have associated lymph node metastases[71] and are easily missed intraoperatively without meticulous exploration. There are at least six reported patients without previous gastric or pancreatic resections who seem to be bio-chemically cured after the excision of only lymph nodes containing gastri-noma.[94–96] Peripancreatic lymph nodes from patients undergoing Whipple resection for non-endocrine tumour may contain cells that stain positive for neuroendocrine markers, giving a plausible explanation for lymph node primary gastrinoma.[85] A prospective study of 215 patients with ZES found eight patients to have extrapancreatic, extraduodenal, extralymphatic primary gastrinomas. These tumours were located in the liver (three patients), common bile duct (one), jejunum (one), omentum (one), pylorus (one) and ovary (one).[97] Seven of these patients were cured biochemically after resection.

It is reasonable to conclude the operation if careful exploration, including examination of the duodenum with duodenotomy, does not reveal a primary tumour, all involved lymph nodes have been resected and other ectopic sites have been examined carefully.

Tumour resection

As described for insulinoma, tumour enucleation remains the procedure of choice for resecting sporadic gastrinomas. Tumours that arise within the pancreas and that are not near the pancreatic duct or major vessels are safely enucleated. Large pancreatic tumours with vital structures in close proximity must be removed by pancreatic resection. Duodenal gastrinomas may be precisely resected using endoscopic transillumination of the duodenum.[90] Some normal duodenal wall around the tumour is removed, but as much of the duodenal wall as possible is preserved to allow a non-constricting closure. Special attention is paid to avoid the ampulla of Vater. Involved regional lymph nodes should be excised. Although most gastrinomas are malignant, performing a more radical pancreatic resection that includes regional lymph nodes (e.g. pancreaticoduo-denectomy) is currently not indicated. Small tumours can be easily enucleated and because of the slow progression of disease, symptomatic relief with medical treatment is easily achieved. Pancreaticoduodenectomy can be performed with acceptable morbidity and mortality and may be indicated for patients with larger, locally aggressive tumours.[49]

The presence of lymph node metastases at the time of operation should not discourage an aggressive surgical approach to remove all gross tumour. Gastrinoma is associated with lymph node involvement in 50–80% of patients and, unlike many other types of cancer, lymph node involvement alone without hepatic or distant metastases does not seem to decrease survival.[2,98,99] Resection of all apparent tumour to eradicate disease increases disease-free survival and may extend overall survival. The development of hepatic and distant metastatic disease occurs in 25–90% of patients and is the most common cause of morbidity and mortality associated with tumour.[63,83,99,100] Patients should be carefully followed by screening for recurrent disease because if a patient develops an increased serum gastrin concentration in conjunction with a tumour that has been imaged, reoperation should be considered. Approximately one third of these patients can be rendered free of disease.[101]

Gastrinoma and MEN-1

Parathyroidectomy should be performed first in patients with MEN-1 who have hyperparathyroidism and ZES because normalisation of the serum calcium concentration usually results in a marked decrease in serum gastrin, allowing better medical control of the symptoms of ZES.[102] Whether patients should undergo abdominal exploration is controversial. Earlier surgical series suggest that resecting gastrinoma does not cure these patients of ZES. More recent studies show that aggressive surgical approaches may result in normalisation of serum gastrin concentrations.[103] Most gastrinomas in patients with MEN-1 are currently thought to be malignant.[51] Only 3% of patients without hepatic metastases who undergo resection of the gastrinoma eventually develop liver metastases compared with 23% of similar patients who are managed medically over a similar period.[67] Hepatic metastases are associated with decreased survival from ZES.[99] All patients with MEN-1 and ZES should undergo SASI to determine the pancreatic region of the tumour secreting gastrin and then undergo surgery to resect the primary tumour and metastases. Tumours that are at least 3 cm in size usually have lymph node metastases.[104] Preoperative abdominal CT is necessary to identify hepatic metastases and plan surgical resection. SRS is also useful in determining the true extent of disease. In patients with MEN-1, 70% of gastrinomas are found within the duodenum, and approximately 50% of patients may have multiple duodenal tumours.[104] Some advocate performing routine duodenotomy and peripancreatic lymph node sampling whenever a duodenal gastrinoma is found in a patient with MEN-1, as well as enucleation of palpable tumours in the pancreas.[103] Others report discouraging results despite similar procedures.[51]

The appropriate extent of surgical resection in patients with ZES and MEN-1 is controversial because these tumours are uncommon and only a few studies have enough patients to allow for an analysis of surgical outcome. Thompson argues for an aggressive surgical approach.[105,106] In a series of 34 patients with ZES and MEN-1 who had undergone surgery, 68% remained eugastrinaemic, with a 15-year survival rate of 94%. He recommends performing a distal pancreatectomy (because of the concomitant neuroendocrine tumours in the neck, body and tail of the pancreas in these patients), enucleation of any tumours in the pancreatic head or uncinate process, duodenotomy and exision of any tumours from the first to fourth portions of the duodenum, and a peripancreatic lymph node dissection in those patients with a duodenal tumour or a pancreatic tumour greater than 3 cm in diameter.[105,106] Norton et al., however, found that patients with MEN-1 and ZES rarely became free of disease despite extensive duodenal exploration, with only 16% of patients free of disease immediately after surgery and only 6% at 5 years.[107] This is in contrast to a surgical cure of approximately 50% of patients with sporadic gastrinomas.[107]

Outcome

The overall survival for patients with sporadic gastrinoma not metastatic to the liver is greater than 90% at 5 years and greater than 85% at 10 years (**Table 5.4**). An immediate postoperative cure rate of 60% can be obtained if all tumour is identified and resected, and over 50% of these patients remain free of disease at 5 years follow-up.[63] Patients with liver metastases at presentation have an overall survival of only 20–38%.[99]

Other rare endocrine tumours of the pancreas

Other pancreatic endocrine tumours include vasoactive intestinal peptide (VIP)-oma, glucagonoma, somatostatinoma, growth hormone-releasing factor (GRF)-oma, adrenocorticotrophic hormone (ACTH)-oma, parathyroid hormone (PTH)-like-oma, neurotensinoma and non-functional islet cell tumour or pancreatic peptide (PP)-oma (Table 5.1).[108] These neoplasms occur in less than 0.2 people per million per year. In general, these tumours resemble gastrinoma in that all are associated with a high incidence of malignancy. Each of these tumours can also arise in association with MEN-1, including GRFoma (30%) and PPoma (80–100%). The hormones, symptoms and signs, diagnostic tests, sites of occurrence, proportions malignant and frequency of associated MEN-1 for each tumour are given in Table 5.1.

PPomas produce pancreatic polypeptide and neurone-specific enolase, which have no clinically appreciable biologically active function, and therefore patients do not present with a typical hormonal syndrome. Symptoms arise because of mass effect and include abdominal pain, gastrointestinal bleeding and obstruction. Diagnosis may only be made after palpation of an abdominal mass or incidental identification of a pancreatic mass on imaging studies. Malignant spread to lymph nodes or liver is common and related to tumour size (more than 50% for tumours >3 cm).

For all of these tumours, preoperative abdominal CT is necessary in attempting to localise the primary tumour and to exclude liver metastases.[104] The goals of surgical treatment are to control symptoms caused by excessive hormone production and to potentially cure or decrease disease bulk. The only potentially curative treatment for malignant endocrine tumours is surgical resection.[109–113] Patients with extensive bilobar hepatic metastases are typically not candidates for surgery, and symptoms may respond to chemotherapy, interferon-α or octreotide.[109]

Occult pancreatic endocrine tumours

An 'occult' islet cell tumour is an unlocalised tumour by non-operative tests that occurs in a patient with a definitively diagnosed clinical hormonal syndrome, such as fasting hyperinsulinaemic hypoglycaemia or ZES. The tumour is biochemically proven, but its anatomical site remains unclear. Approximately 10–20% of insulinomas and 15% of gastrinomas are occult. Patients with insulinoma should undergo a regional localisation study such as the calcium angiogram preoperatively in an attempt to localise the tumour to a specific anatomical area (**Fig. 5.3**).

Patients with occult gastrinomas need not undergo a regional localisation study as these tumours are nearly always in the duodenum within the gastrinoma triangle. Exploratory laparotomy is then the last resort to identify the location of the tumour and to resect it. Surgery should not be performed in patients with insulinoma unless IOUS is available, given its advantages in finding small tumours within the pancreas (**Fig. 5.5**).[1] Surgery in patients with occult gastrinoma should focus on the duodenum, including transillumination and duodenotomy (**Fig. 5.10**).

Abdominal exploration by an experienced pancreatic endocrine surgeon, knowledge of the sites of occurrence of specific tumours and the use of IOUS results in identification and removal of the tumour in all but a few patients. In the rare instance that a tumour remains unlocalised and unresected after thorough exploration, the decision whether to perform a pancreatectomy depends on the particular patient's response to medical management and the results of the preoperative regional localisation study. Pancreatic resection is not indicated if the patient's hormonal syndrome can be well controlled by medical management. When medical management is unsatisfactory, the only alternative is to perform a pancreatectomy on the basis of the regional localisation data. Blind pancreatectomy is never indicated.

Malignant pancreatic endocrine tumours

With improvements in the medical management of syndromes of hormonal excess, growth and metastatic spread of primary islet cell tumours has increasingly become more problematic. Except for insulinomas, which are malignant in only 5–10% of cases, more than 60% of pancreatic endocrine tumours overall are malignant.[109,112,113] Data concerning the management of these patients are mainly derived from experience with malignant gastrinomas, which occur more commonly than other more obscure pancreatic neuroendocrine tumours.

No diagnostic histological criteria from examination of tumour biopsy samples or resected primary tumours exist to define malignancy for pancreatic endocrine tumours. Malignancy is definitively established with surgical exploration and histological evidence of tumour remote from the primary lesion, usually in peripancreatic lymph nodes or the liver. Recurrence of tumour at a location distant from a resected primary tumour site also definitively indicates malignancy. Gross invasion of blood vessels, surrounding tissues or adjacent organs usually suggests a malignant tumour.[110] IOUS showing a pancreatic tumour with indistinct margins may imply local invasion and malignancy.[48] Very large tumours (>5 cm) have an increased risk of being malignant.[2] Tumour DNA ploidy and tumoral growth fraction determined by flow cytometry may provide an indication of biological behaviour of some of these tumours. Because islet cell tumours generally grow slowly, metastases may not become evident until years after the initial primary tumour resection.

Evaluation of metastatic disease

Evaluation of a patient with a malignant neuroendocrine tumour begins by assessing the extent of disease using radiological imaging studies. SRS seems to be the single best imaging study to select patients for aggressive surgery to remove metastatic disease.[1] If the tumour binds this isotope, then disease anywhere in the body can be identified. Miliary or extensive bilobar hepatic disease and distant metastases are considered inoperable and, if identified preoperatively, can prevent unnecessary surgery. CT or MRI may identify disease in the chest and abdomen. Specific complaints of bone pain are elicited and, if present, evaluated with bone scan and radiography.

Malignant primary insulinomas are relatively large—approximately 6 cm— and can usually be readily detected by non-invasive imaging studies.[41] Gastrinomas may metastasise to regional lymph nodes when only millimetres in size. In one study, duodenal primary gastrinomas have been found to have a higher incidence of lymph node metastases (55%) than pancreatic gastrinomas (22%).[1] Some suggest that rare gastrinomas to the left of the superior mesenteric artery in the pancreatic tail are always malignant and more commonly produce liver metastases. Metastatic tumour must be distinguished from multiple tumours, which occur simultaneously. If multiple insulinomas or gastrinomas are found in a patient, then MEN-1 should be suspected.

Surgical management

Pancreatic neuroendocrine carcinomas have a better prognosis than adenocarcinoma of the exocrine pancreas and are often managed with aggressive surgical resection.[76] Surgery is undertaken to decrease tumour bulk so that hormonal syndromes are more effectively controlled by medical management, relieve symptoms of mass effect, and/or eliminate cancerous tissue and improve disease-free or overall survival. Preoperative staging studies are important to exclude patients from surgery who would not benefit from resection.

Limited metastases as well as the primary tumour should be resected to adequately debulk tumour and to eliminate the hormonal syndrome.[114] Incomplete tumour resection may not improve the ability to control the hormonal syndrome medically. For medically fit patients with metastatic insulinoma in whom hypoglycaemia is poorly controlled by medical management, tumour debulking may control symptoms for prolonged time periods, even in the setting of distant metastases.[63] Approximately 50% of patients with metastatic insulinoma undergoing resection have complete biochemical remission.[115]

Although treatment is generally palliative and not curative for patients with locally advanced tumours and limited metastatic disease, surgery may be the only therapy that effectively ameliorates life-threatening symptoms. It may increase survival because these tumours are generally indolent, slow-growing neoplasms.[115,116] Limited regional metastatic disease can often be successfully resected and may be curative if no liver metastases are present.[114] Complete resection of localised or regional nodal metastases with negative margins at the initial surgery provides the highest probability of cure.[1] Although disease-free survival is prolonged in most patients, most eventually develop recurrent tumour.

Approximately 30% of patients with metastatic insulinoma can undergo complete resection of tumour.[115,116] Median survival is increased from 11 months in patients with metastatic insulinoma who cannot undergo resection to 4 years in those in whom tumour debulking is possible.[99] Palliative re-resection of recurrent tumour extends median survival from 11–19 months to 4 years.[117] Surgery may also be the most effective treatment for patients with metastatic gastrinoma if most or all of the tumour can be resected.[1] Aggressive resection of liver metastases of gastrinoma, considered resectable by preoperative radiological imaging studies, improves 5-year survival from 28% in patients with inoperable metastases to 79–85%.[114,118]

Patients with solitary, localised metastatic disease benefit most. Recurrence of disease in more than one lobe of the liver may be treated by hepatic arterial embolisation or orthotopic liver transplant. Laparoscopic thermal ablation is a novel, minimally invasive method of providing effective cytoreduction of neuroendocrine tumours metastatic to the liver.[119] Patients may also have symptoms such as obstruction secondary to mass effect from the size or location of the tumour or gastrointestinal bleeding from direct tumour invasion into adjacent bowel, which are effectively eliminated by resection of the tumour.[114] Pain secondary to neural invasion may be effectively palliated by percutaneous coeliac axis nerve block.

Non-surgical management

Symptoms from extensive metastases may respond to chemotherapy or octreotide, but these treatments are not curative.[1] Combination chemotherapy with streptozocin and 5-fluorouracil is the most effective regimen for metastatic insulinoma, producing at least a partial response in 60% of patients. Doxorubicin may also be used. Patients with metastatic gastrinoma are treated with streptozocin, doxorubicin and/or 5-fluorouracil. Treatment with octreotide results in unpredictable responses, causing decreased tumour growth in some patients and having no effect in others.[100,108,120] The addition of interferon-α to octreotide therapy may benefit a subgroup of patients with advanced metastatic disease that is unresponsive to octreotide monotherapy.[121] Dacarbazine may be effective in controlling the clinical and biochemical manifestations of gastrinoma.[122] Cryosurgery may be a useful adjuvant in patients with refractory hepatic neuro-endocrine metastases. Cryosurgery can relieve symptoms and causes a reduction in tumour markers, which may allow a better response to subsequent systemic therapy.[123] Octreotide may ameliorate symptoms, especially in patients with malignant VIPoma (**Fig. 5.11**), and when symptoms are adequately controlled, patients can live comfortably and productively for many years with metastatic disease.

Figure 5.11
Use of octreotide in patient with metastatic VIPoma. The patient had voluminous diarrhoea (5–6 kg d⁻¹) and hypokalaemia (serum K⁺= 3 mmol l⁻¹) and required large potassium supplements. After octreotide 100 μg b.i.d. was started, the diarrhoea stopped, the patient gained weight and the serum concentrations of bicarbonate and potassium normalised.

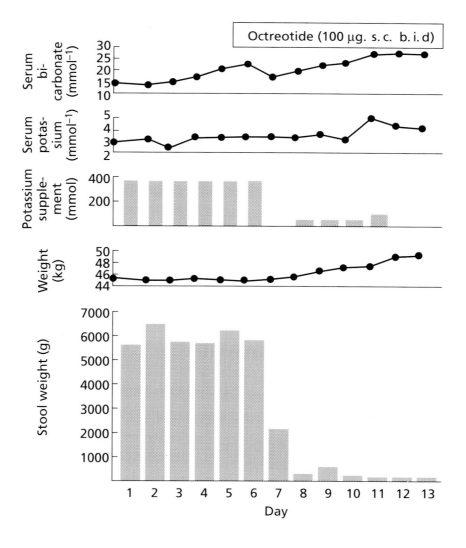

References

1. Norton JA. Neuroendocrine tumors of the pancreas and duodenum. Curr Probl Surg 1994; 31: 77–164.

2. Peplinski GR, Norton JA. Gastrointestinal endocrine cancers and nodal metastases: biological significance and therapeutic implications. Surg Oncol Clin North Am 1996; 5: 159–71.

3. Doherty GM, Doppman JL, Shawker TH *et al*. Results of a prospective strategy to diagnose, localize and resect insulinomas. Surgery 1991; 110: 989–97.

4. Dizon AM, Kowalyk S, Hoogwerf BJ. Neuroglycopenic and other symptoms in patients with insulinomas. Am J Med 1999; 106: 307–10.

5. Thompson NW, Lloyd RV, Nishiyama RH *et al*. MEN I pancreas: a histological and immunohistochemical study. World J Surg 1984; 8: 561–74.

6. Chandrasekharappa SC, Guru SC, Manickam P *et al*. Positional cloning of the gene for multiple endocrine neoplasia-type 1. Science 1997; 276: 404–7.

7. Lemmens I, Van de Ven WJM, Kas K *et al*. Identification of the multiple endocrine neoplasia type 1 (MEN1) gene. Hum Mol Genet 1997; 6: 1169–75.

8. Marx SJ, Agarwal SK, Heppner C *et al*. The gene for multiple endocrine neoplasia type 1—recent findings. Bone 1999; 25: 119–22.

9. Bartsch D, Kopp I, Bergenfelz A *et al*. MEN1 gene mutations in 12 MEN1 families and their associated tumors. Eur J Endocrinol 1998; 139: 416–20.

10. Burgess JR, Greenaway TM, Parameswaran V *et al*. Enteropancreatic malignancy associated with multiple endocrine neoplasia type 1. Cancer 1998; 83: 428–34.

11. Grunberger G, Weiner JL, Silverman R *et al*. Factitious hypoglycemia due to surreptitious administration of insulin: diagnosis, treatment and long-term follow-up. Ann Intern Med 1988; 108: 252–7.

12. Gorden P, Skarulis MC, Roach P *et al*. Plasma proinsulin-like component in insulinoma: a 25-year experience. J Clin Endocrinol Metab 1995; 80: 2884–7.

13. Farley DR, van Heerden JA, Myers JL. Adult pancreatic nesidioblastosis: unusual presentations of a rare entity. Arch Surg 1994; 129: 329–32.

14. Goudswaard WB, Houthoff HJ, Koudstaal J *et al*. Nesidioblastosis and endocrine hyperplasia of the pancreas: a secondary phenomenon. Hum Pathol 1986; 17: 46–54.

15. Grant CS. Insulinoma. Surg Oncol Clin North Am 1998; 7: 819–44.

16. Thornton PS, Alter CA, Katz LE *et al*. Short- and long-term use of octreotide in the treatment of congenital hyperinsulinism. J Pediatr 1993; 123: 637–43.

17. Glaser B, Hirsch HJ, Landau H. Persistent hyperinsulinemic hypoglycemia of infancy: long-term octreotide treatment without pancreatectomy. J Pediatr 1993; 123: 644–50.

18. Gorden P, Comi RJ, Maton PN *et al*. Somatostatin and somatostatin analogue (SMS 201-995) in treatment of hormone-secreting tumors of the pituitary and gastrointestinal tract and non-neoplastic diseases of the gut. Ann Intern Med 1989; 110: 35–50.

19. Arnold R, Frank M, Kajdan U. Management of gastroenteropancreatic endocrine tumors: the place of somatostatin analogues. Digestion 1994; 55 (Suppl 3): 107–13.

20. von Eyben FE, Grodum E, Gjessing HJ *et al*. Metabolic remission with octreotide in patients with insulinoma. J Intern Med 1994; 235: 245–8.

21. Arnold R, Neuhaus C, Benning R *et al*. Somatostatin analog sandostatin and inhibition of tumor growth in patients with metastatic endocrine gastroenteropancreatic tumors. World J Surg 1993; 17: 511–9.

22. Doppman JL, Chang R, Fraker DL *et al*. Localization of insulinomas to regions of the pancreas by intra-arterial stimulation with calcium. Ann Intern Med 1995; 123: 269–73.

23. Vinik AI, Delbridge L, Moattari R *et al*. Transhepatic portal vein catheterization for localization of insulinomas: a ten-year experience. Surgery 1991; 109: 1–11.

24. Gianello P, Gigot JF, Berthet F *et al*. Pre- and intraoperative localization of insulinomas: report of 22 observations. World J Surg 1988; 12: 389–97.

25. Fraker DL, Norton JA. Localization and resection of insulinomas and gastrinomas. JAMA 1988; 259: 3601–5.

26. Grant CS, van Heerden J, Charboneau JW *et al*. Insulinoma: the value of intraoperative ultrasonography. Arch Surg 1988; 123: 843–8.

27. Boukhman MP, Karam JM, Shaver J *et al*. Localization of insulinomas. Arch Surg 1999; 134: 818–23.

28. Lamberts SW, Bakker WH, Reubi JC *et al*. Somatostatin receptor imaging in the localization of endocrine tumors. N Engl J Med 1990; 323: 1246–9.

29. Lamberts SW, Hofland LJ, van Koetsveld PM *et al.* Parallel in vivo and in vitro detection of functional somatostatin receptors in human endocrine pancreatic tumors: consequences with regard to diagnosis, localization and therapy. J Clin Endocrinol Metab 1990; 71: 566–74.

30. Virgolini I, Raderer M, Kurtaran A *et al.* Vasoactive intestinal peptide-receptor imaging for the localization of intestinal adenocarcinomas and endocrine tumors. N Engl J Med 1994; 331: 1116–21.

31. Owens LV, Huth JF, Cance WG. Insulinoma: pitfalls in preoperative localization. Eur J Surg Oncol 1995; 21: 326–8.

32. Thompson NW, Czako PF, Fritts LL *et al.* Role of endoscopic ultrasonography in the localization of insulinomas and gastrinomas. Surgery 1994; 116: 1131–8.

33. Bottger TC, Junginger T. Is preoperative radiographic localization of islet cell tumors in patients with insulinoma necessary? World J Surg 1993; 17: 427–32.

34. Heyder N. Localization of an insulinoma by ultrasonic endoscopy. N Engl J Med 1985; 312: 860–1.

35. Glover JR, Shorvon PJ, Lees WR. Endoscopic ultrasound for localization of islet cell tumors. Gut 1992; 33: 108–10.

36. Rosch T, Lightdale CJ, Botet JF *et al.* Localization of pancreatic endocrine tumors by endoscopic ultrasonography. N Engl J Med 1992; 326: 1721–6.

 37. Bansal R, Tierney W, Carpenter S *et al.* Cost effectiveness of EUS for preoperative localization of pancreatic endocrine tumors. Gastrointest Endosc 1999; 49: 19–25.

 38. Brown CK, Barlett DL, Doppman JL *et al.* Intraarterial calcium stimulation and intraoperative ultrasonography in the localization and resection of insulinomas. Surgery 1997; 122: 1189–94.

39. Cohen MS, Picus D, Lairmore TC *et al.* Prospective study of provocative angiograms to localize functional islet cell tumors of the pancreas. Surgery 1997; 122: 1091–100.

40. Miller DL, Doppman JL, Metz DC *et al.* Zollinger-Ellison syndrome: technique, results, and complications of portal venous sampling. Radiology 1992; 182: 235–41.

41. Norton JA, Cromack DT, Shawker TH *et al.* Intraoperative ultrasonographic localization of islet cell tumors. Ann Surg 1988; 207: 160–8.

42. Boukhman MP, Karam JH, Shaver J *et al.* Insulinoma—experience from 1950 to 1995. West J Med 1998; 169: 98–104.

43. Huai J, Zhang W, Niu H *et al.* Localization and surgical treatment of pancreatic insulinomas guided by intraoperative ultrasound. Am J Surg 1998; 175: 18–21.

44. Hashimoto LA, Walsh RM. Preoperative localization of insulinomas is not necessary. J Am Coll Surg 1999; 189: 368–73.

 45. Norton JA. Intraoperative methods to stage and localize pancreatic and duodenal tumors. Ann Oncol 1999; 10(Suppl 4): 182–4S.

46. Lo C, Lam K, Kung AWC *et al.* Pancreatic insulinomas—a 15-year experience. Arch Surg 1997; 132: 926–30.

47. Buchler M, Friess H, Klempa I *et al.* Role of octreotide in the prevention of postoperative complications following pancreatic resection. Am J Surg 1992; 163: 125–31.

48. Norton JA, Sigel B, Baker AR *et al.* Localization of an occult insulinoma by intraoperative ultrasonography. Surgery 1985; 97: 381–4.

49. Phan GQ, Yeo CJ, Cameron JL *et al.* Pancreaticoduodenectomy for selected periampullary neuroendocrine tumors: fifty patients. Surgery 1997; 122: 989–97.

 50. Demeure MJ, Klonoff DC, Karam JH *et al.* Insulinomas associated with multiple endocrine neoplasia type 1: the need for a different surgical approach. Surgery 1991; 110: 998–1004.

51. Sheppard BC, Norton JA, Doppman JL *et al.* Management of islet cell tumors in patients with multiple endocrine neoplasia: a prospective study. Surgery 1989; 106: 1108–18.

52. O'Riordain DS, O'Brien T, van Heerden JA *et al.* Surgical management of insulinoma associated with multiple endocrine neoplasia type I. World J Surg 1994; 18: 488–93.

 53. Prove C, Pattou F, Carnaille B *et al.* Intraoperative insulin measurement during surgical management of insulinomas. World J Surg 1998; 22: 1218–24.

54. Veldhuis JD, Norton JA, Wells SA *et al.* Therapeutic controversy: surgical versus medical management of multiple endocrine neoplasia (MEN) type 1. J Clin Endocrinol Metab 1997; 82: 357–64.

55. Dexter SPL, Martin IG, Leindler L *et al.* Laparoscopic enucleation of a solitary pancreatic insulinoma. Surg Endosc 1999; 13: 406–8.

56. Yoshida T, Bandoh T, Ninomiya K *et al.* Laparoscopic enucleation of a pancreatic insulinoma: report of a case. Surg Today 1998; 28: 1188–91.

57. Vezakis A, Davides D, Larvin M *et al.* Laparoscopic surgery combined with preservation of the spleen for distal pancreatic tumors. Surg Endosc 1999; 13: 26–9.

58. Gagner M, Pomp A, Herrera MF. Early experience with laparoscopic resections of islet cell tumors. Surgery 1996; 120: 1051–4.

59. Service FJ, McMahon MM, O'Brien PC et al. Functioning insulinoma—incidence, recurrence, and long-term survival of patients: a 60-year study. Mayo Clin Proc 1991; 66: 711–9.

60. Lange JR, Steinberg S, Doherty GM et al. A randomized prospective trial of postoperative somatostatin analogue in patients with neuroendocrine tumors of the pancreas. Surgery 1992; 112: 1033–8.

61. Eriksson B, Oberg K, Skogseid B. Neuroendocrine pancreatic tumors: clinical findings in a prospective study of 84 patients. Acta Oncol 1989; 28: 373–7.

62. Zollinger RM, Ellison EH. Primary peptic ulceration of the jejunum associated with islet cell tumors of the pancreas. Ann Surg 1955; 142: 709–28.

63. Norton JA, Doppman JL, Jensen RT. Curative resection in Zollinger–Ellison syndrome: results of a 10 year prospective study. Ann Surg 1992; 215: 8–18.

64. Wolfe MM, Jensen RT. Zollinger–Ellison syndrome, current concepts in diagnosis and management. N Engl J Med 1987; 317: 1200–9.

65. Fox PS, Hofmann JW, DeCosse JJ et al. The influence of total gastrectomy on survival in malignant Zollinger–Ellison tumors. Ann Surg 1974; 180: 558–66.

66. Zollinger RM, Ellison EC, O'Dorsio TM et al. Thirty years' experience with gastrinoma. World J Surg 1984; 8: 427–35.

67. Fraker DL, Norton JA, Alexander HR et al. Surgery in Zollinger–Ellison syndrome alters the natural history of gastrinoma. Ann Surg 1994; 220: 320–30.

68. Larsson H, Carlsson E, Matsson H. Plasma gastrin and gastric enterochromaffin cell activation and proliferation—studies with omeprazole and ranitidine in intact and adrenalectomized rats. Gastroenterology 1986; 90: 391–9.

69. Yu F, Venzon DJ, Serrano J et al. Prospective study of the clinical course, prognostic factors, causes of death, and survival in patients with long-standing Zollinger–Ellison syndrome. J Clin Oncol 1999; 17: 615–30.

70. Norton JA. Gastrinoma—advances in localization and treatment. Surg Oncol Clin North Am 1998; 7: 845–61.

71. Thompson NW, Pasieka J, Fukuuchi A. Duodenal gastrinomas, duodenotomy, and duodenal exploration in the surgical management of Zollinger–Ellison syndrome. World J Surg 1993; 17: 455–62.

72. Sutliff VE, Doppman JL, Gibril F et al. Growth of newly diagnosed, untreated metastatic gastrinomas and predictors of growth patterns. J Clin Oncol 1997; 15: 2420–31.

73. vonSchrenck T, Howard JM, Doppman JL et al. Prospective study of chemotherapy in patients with metastatic gastrinoma. Gastroenterology 1988; 94: 1326–34.

74. Wank SA, Doppman HL, Miller DL et al. Prospective study of the ability of computerized axial tomography to localize gastrinomas in patients with Zollinger–Ellison syndrome. Gastroenterology 1987; 92: 905–12.

75. Semelka RC, Cumming MJ, Shoenut JP et al. Islet cell tumors: comparison of dynamic contrast-enhanced CT and MR imaging with dynamic gadolinium enhancement and fat suppression. Radiology 1993; 186: 799–802.

76. Schirmer WJ, Melvin WS, Rush RM et al. ^{111}In-Pentetreotide scanning versus conventional imaging techniques for the localization of gastrinoma. Surgery 1995; 118: 1105–13.

77. Gibril F, Reynolds JC, Doppman JL et al. Somatostatin receptor scintigraphy: its sensitivity compared with that of other imaging methods in detecting primary and metastatic gastrinomas. Ann Intern Med 1996; 125: 26–34.

78. Alexander HR, Fraker DL, Norton JA et al. Prospective study of somatostatin receptor scintigraphy and its effect on operative outcome in patients with Zollinger–Ellison syndrome. Ann Surg 1998; 228: 228–38.

79. Meko JB, Doherty GM, Siegel BA et al. Evaluation of somatostatin-receptor scintigraphy for detecting neuroendocrine tumors. Surgery 1996; 120: 975–84.

80. Gibril F, Reynolds JC, Chen CC et al. Specificity of somatostatin receptor scintigraphy: a prospective study and effects of false-positive localizations on management in patients with gastrinomas. J Nucl Med 1999; 40: 539–53.

81. Proye C, Malvaux P, Pattou F et al. Noninvasive imaging of insulinomas and gastrinomas with endoscopic ultrasonography and somatostatin receptor scintigraphy. Surgery 1998; 124: 1134–44.

82. Maton PN, Miller DL, Doppman HL et al. Role of selective angiography in the management of Zollinger–Ellison syndrome. Gastroenterology 1987; 92: 913–9.

83. Thom AK, Norton JA, Axiotis CA et al. Location, incidence and malignant potential of duodenal gastrinomas. Surgery 1991; 110: 1086–93.

84. Imamura M, Takahashi K. Use of selective arterial secretin injection test to guide surgery in patients with Zollinger–Ellison syndrome. World J Surg 1993; 17: 433–8.

85. Perrier ND, Batts KP, Thompson GB et al. An immunohistochemical survey for neuroendocrine

cells in regional pancreatic lymph nodes—a plausible explanation for primary nodal gastrinomas. Surgery 1995; 118: 957–65.

86. Proye C, Pattou F, Carnaille B *et al.* Intraoperative gastrin measurements during surgical management of patients with gastrinomas: experience with 20 cases. World J Surg 1998; 22: 643–50.

87. Stabile BE, Morrow DJ, Passaro E. The gastrinoma triangle: operative implications. Am J Surg 1984; 147: 25–31.

88. Pipeleers-Marichal M, Donow C, Heitz PU *et al.* Pathologic aspects of gastrinomas in patients with Zollinger–Ellison syndrome with and without multiple endocrine neoplasia type I. World J Surg 1993; 17: 481–8.

89. Thompson NW, Vinik AI, Eckhauser FE. Microgastrinomas of the duodenum. Ann Surg 1989; 209: 396–404.

90. Frucht H, Norton JA, London JF *et al.* Detection of duodenal gastrinomas by operative endoscopic transillumination, a prospective study. Gastroenterology 1990; 99: 1622–7.

91. Howard TJ, Zinner MJ, Stabile BE *et al.* Gastrinoma excision for cure. Ann Surg 1990; 211: 9–14.

92. Norton JA. Advances in the management of Zollinger–Ellison syndrome. Adv Surg 1994; 27: 129–59.

93. Wolfe MM, Alexander RW, McGuigan JE. Extrapancreatic, extraintestinal gastrinoma: effective treatment by surgery. N Engl J Med 1982; 306: 1533–6.

94. Norton JA, Doppman JL, Collen MJ *et al.* Prospective study of gastrinoma localization and resection in patients with Zollinger–Ellison syndrome. Ann Surg 1986; 204: 468–79.

95. Bornman PC, Marks IN, Mee AS *et al.* Favourable response to conservative surgery for extra-pancreatic gastrinoma with lymph node metastases. Br J Surg 1987; 74: 198–201.

96. Richardson CT, Peters MN, Feldman M. Treatment of Zollinger–Ellison syndrome with exploratory laparotomy, proximal gastric vagotomy, and H₂-receptor antagonists. Gastroenterology 1985; 89: 357–67.

97. Wu PC, Alexander HR, Bartlett DL *et al.* A prospective analysis of the frequency, location, and curability of ectopic (nonpancreaticoduodenal, nonnodal) gastrinoma. Surgery 1997; 122: 1176–82.

98. Kisker O, Bastian D, Bartsch D *et al.* Localization, malignant potential, and surgical management of gastrinomas. World J Surg 1998; 22: 651–8.

99. Ellison EC. Forty year appraisal of gastrinoma: back to the future. Ann Surg 1995; 222: 511–21.

100. Norton JA, Sugarbaker PH, Doppman JL *et al.* Aggressive resection of metastatic disease in selected patients with malignant gastrinoma. Ann Surg 1986; 203: 352–9.

101. Jaskowiak NT, Fraker DL, Alexander R *et al.* Is reoperation for gastrinoma excision indicated in Zollinger–Ellison syndrome? Surgery 1996; 120: 1055–63.

102. Norton JA, Cornelius MJ, Doppman JL *et al.* Effect of parathyroidectomy in patients with hyperparathyroidism, Zollinger–Ellison syndrome, and multiple endocrine neoplasia type 1: a prospective study. Surgery 1987; 102: 958–66.

103. Thompson NW. Surgical treatment of the endocrine pancreas and Zollinger–Ellison syndrome in the MEN I syndrome. Henry Ford Hosp Med J 1992; 40: 195–8.

104. Macfarlane MP, Fraker DL, Alexander HR *et al.* A prospective study of surgical resection of duodenal and pancreatic gastrinomas in MEN-1. Surgery 1995; 118: 973–9.

105. Thompson NW. Current concepts in the surgical management of multiple endocrine neoplasia type 1 pancreatic-duodenal disease. Results in the treatment of 40 patients with Zollinger–Ellison syndrome, hypoglycaemia or both. J Intern Med 1998; 243: 495–500.

106. Thompson NW. Management of pancreatic endocrine tumors in patients with multiple endocrine neoplasia type I. Surg Oncol Clin North Am 1998; 7: 881–91.

107. Norton JA, Fraker DL, Alexander HR *et al.* Surgery to cure the Zollinger–Ellison syndrome. N Engl J Med 1999; 341: 635–44.

108. Carty S, Jensen RT, Norton JA. Prospective study of aggressive resection of metastatic pancreatic endocrine tumors. Surgery 1992; 112: 1024–32.

109. Vinik AI, Strodel WE, Eckhauser FE *et al.* Somatostatinomas, PPomas, neurotensinomas. Semin Oncol 1987; 14: 263.

110. Verner JV, Morrison AB. Endocrine pancreatic islet disease with diarrhea: report of a case due to diffuse hyperplasia of no beta islet tissue with a review of 54 additional cases. Arch Intern Med 1974; 133:492–9.

111. Capella C, Polak JM, Butta R *et al.* Morphologic patterns and diagnostic criteria of VIP-producing endocrine tumors. A histologic, histochemical, ultrastructural and biochemical study of 32 cases. Cancer 1983; 52: 1860.

112. Caplan PH, Koob L, Abellera RM *et al.* Cure of acromegaly by operative removal of an islet cell tumor of the pancreas. Am J Med 1978; 64: 874.

113. Bresler L, Boissel P, Conroy T *et al.* Pancreatic islet cell carcinoma with hypercalcemia: complete remission 5 years after surgical excision and chemotherapy. Am J Gastroenterol 1991; 86: 635.

114. Danforth DN, Gorden P, Brennan MF. Metastatic insulin secreting carcinoma of the pancreas. Clinical course and the role of surgery. Surgery 1984; 96: 1027–36.

115. Rothmund M, Stinner B, Arnold R. Endocrine pancreatic carcinoma. Eur J Surg Oncol 1991; 17: 191–9.

116. Modlin IM, Lewis JJ, Ahlman H *et al.* Management of unresectable malignant endocrine tumors of the pancreas. Surg Gynecol Obstet 1993; 176: 507–18.

117. Zogakis TG, Norton JA. Palliative operations for patients with unresectable endocrine neoplasia. Surg Clin North Am 1995; 75: 525–38.

118. Norton JA, Doherty GM, Fraker DL *et al.* Surgical treatment of localized gastrinoma within the liver: a prospective study. Surgery 1998; 124: 1145–52.

119. Siperstein AE, Rogers SJ, Hansen PD *et al.* Laparoscopic thermal ablation of hepatic neuroendocrine tumor metastases. Surgery 1997; 122: 1147–55.

120. Mozell E, Woltering EA, O'Dorisio TM *et al.* Effect of somatostatin analog on peptide release and tumor growth in the Zollinger–Ellison syndrome. Surg Gynecol Obstet 1990; 170: 476–84.

121. Frank M, Klose KJ, Wied M *et al.* Combination therapy with octreotide and alpha-interferon: effect on tumor growth in metastatic endocrine gastroenteropancreatic tumors. Am J Gastroenterol 1999; 94: 1381–7.

122. Ohshio G, Hosotani R, Imamura M *et al.* Gastrinoma with multiple liver metastases: effectiveness of dacarbazine (DTIC) therapy. J Hepatobiliary Pancreat Surg 1998; 5: 339–43.

123. Bilchik AJ, Sarantou T, Foshag LJ *et al.* Cryosurgical palliation of metastatic neuroendocrine tumors resistant to conventional therapy. Surgery 1997; 122: 1040–8.

124. Pasieka JH, McLeod MK, Thompson NW *et al.* Surgical approach to insulinomas assessing the need for localization. Arch Surg 1992; 127: 442–7.

125. Mignon M, Ruszniewski R, Haffan S *et al.* Current approach to the management of tumoural process in patients with gastrinoma. World J Surg 1986; 10: 702–9.

6 Carcinoid syndrome

Nigel D.S. Bax
H. Frank Woods

Incidence of carcinoid tumours

The symptoms of the carcinoid syndrome are well known, but it is extremely unusual for physicians or surgeons to make a diagnosis prior to an appropriate biopsy sample being examined or a laparotomy being performed. In a series of 52 patients with abdominal carcinoid tumours in Northern Ireland the diagnosis was not made preoperatively on any occasion[1] and in over 140 patients seen in Sheffield over the past 14 years the clinical or biochemical diagnosis has not been made before histological diagnosis.

Carcinoid tumours are apparently rare. Ten years ago, reports from Sweden and Northern Ireland put the incidence of metastatic carcinoid tumours at between 0.3 and 0.7 patients per 100 000 of the population per year.[1,2] Similar figures were found in the Trent Region in the UK.[3] A large UK series examined approximately 4000 registrations of carcinoid tumours of all types and found the incidence per 100 000 for males and females in England to be 0.71 and 0.87 and in Scotland 1.17 and 1.36, respectively.[4]

The largest and most recent epidemiological report combines data from 5468 patients registered with the Surveillance, Epidemiology and End-Results (SEER) programme of the National Cancer Institute in the USA[5] with those from a previously reported group of 2837 patients.[6] The period of study was from 1951 to 1991. Despite the reporting methods changing during data collection, the overall picture that the surveys give is invaluable, covering an estimated 9.5% of the American population over about 40 years. The all-sites age-adjusted incidence of carcinoid tumours per 100 000 of the population was between 1.2 and 2.16.[5] As with the large UK survey,[6] there was a slightly higher incidence in white females but there was an almost two fold increase in the chance of a black American male developing a carcinoid tumour compared with a white American male. It seems that there may have been a particular increase in the incidence of gastric carcinoids in black Americans over the past 20–30 years.[5]

These rates may be underestimates as postmortem studies suggest an incidence two to three times higher, but it is not known whether such patients were symptomatic in life.[7,8] Between 1958 and 1969, 63% of the population of Malmo who died underwent postmortem examination by one department of pathology.[7] Of the 16 294 patients examined, 199 (1.22%) were found to have carcinoid tumours, with the overwhelming majority of these being found in the gastrointestinal tract. These figures give an annual incidence of 8.4 per 100 000 population per year.

Just over 100 of the patients seen in Sheffield over the past 12 years have come from within 20 miles of the hospital, an area with a population of about 1.6 million. This gives a crude incidence figure of about 0.5 cases per 100 000 population per year. These data imply that there may be an underdiagnosis of carcinoid tumours. If the postmortem data of the incidence are correct, then it might be that there are about 1000 new patients in the UK each year, and a general practitioner will be likely to see one new patient every 30 years. It is not surprising, therefore, that even when a patient presents with flushing and diarrhoea, the diagnosis of a carcinoid tumour does not come instantly to mind.

Diagnosis

Clinical history

The presenting features of the commonest carcinoid tumours are shown in **Table 6.1**. The classification is based on the site of the primary—namely, the foregut, midgut and hindgut.[9]

Almost all primary carcinoid tumours occur either in the gastrointestinal tract (74%) or the lungs (25%).[5] The ovary was the site of approximately 0.5% of primary tumours in the SEER programme. Lung carcinoid tumours often cause symptoms at a relatively early stage in their natural history and thus present in a younger group of patients.[5] Many of the appendiceal tumours are discovered incidentally during abdominal operations.

An abdominal carcinoid tumour is difficult to diagnose because of the intermittent nature of the symptoms, especially in the early stages of the condition. The natural history of such tumours has been well described,[11] with special emphasis being placed on the vague abdominal symptoms that often result in a patient being diagnosed as having the irritable bowel syndrome (**Table 6.2**). These symptoms may persist for some years before the diagnosis of a carcinoid tumour is made. Patients may experience symptoms intermittently for up to 4–5

Site (% of all carcinoid tumours)	Usual age of presentation (years)	Symptoms	Carcinoid syndrome present
Foregut (25%)			
Lung (2% of all lung tumours)	40–50	Haemoptysis Cough Infection Chest pain	Very rare
Gastric (1% of all gastric tumours)	50–70 (75% cases with chronic atrophic gastritis and 5–10% with Zollinger–Ellison syndrome. About 15–25% are 'sporadic' cases)	Anaemia Abdominal pain	No, but may see bright red facial flushing thought to be due to histamine release
Midgut			
Terminal ileum (15–25%)	50–70	Abdominal pains Intermittent obstruction Diarrhoea Flushing	Yes after spread to the liver
Appendix (19%)	30–50	Many found incidentally About 10% cause pain	No, unless spread to the liver
Caecum (4%)	55–70	Abdominal pains Intermittent obstruction Weight loss	Yes, after spread to the liver
Hindgut			
Colon (Transverse, descending and sigmoid: 2%)	60–70	Abdominal pains Weight loss	Rare
Rectal (12%)	50–60	Rectal bleeding Rectal pain Constipation Many asymptomatic	Very rare

Data from references 5, 6, 9, 10, 11 and 22

Table 6.1 *Clinical details of the more common carcinoid tumours*

years before carcinoid tumour is diagnosed.[2,12] Typical antecedent diagnoses include the irritable bowel syndrome, peptic ulcer disease, gastritis and Crohn's disease. Barium radiography studies may show what are thought to be typical appearances of Crohn's disease in the terminal ileum, with ulcerated mucosa. This imitation has been described previously[13] and in a series of 176 consecutive patients with ileal carcinoid tumours four (2%) were initially diagnosed on the basis of radiographic appearances of Crohn's disease.[14]

Flushing and diarrhoea are the two symptoms ubiquitously reported in the syndrome (**Table 6.2**). Aggregating data from five studies totalling about 500

Symptom	Character	Differential diagnoses
Abdominal pains	Intermittent Right upper quadrant and right iliac fossa May be a long history Often previous negative investigations	Inflammatory bowel disease Peptic ulcer disease Gallstones Irritable bowel syndrome Neoplasm
Diarrhoea	Intermittent At first occurs in episodes lasting a few days Mainly first thing in the morning May be associated with flushing May occur immediately after eating	Inflammatory bowel disease Irritable bowel syndrome Neoplasm (including endocrine)
Flushing	From barely perceptible to florid Typically affects face and neck May be provoked by chocolate, alcohol and food Palpitations and hypotension may occur Telangiectases on cheeks and nose Patient may not notice all flushes Mild lachrymation and rhinorrhoea	The menopause Emotion Alcohol Medullary carcinoma of thyroid Mastocytosis

Table 6.2 *History of abdominal carcinoid tumour*

patients showed that at the time of presentation to a tertiary referral centre, a mean of 75% (range 30–94%) had flushing and 73% (range 38–86%) diarrhoea.[2,11,12,15,16] Four of these studies reported asthma as a presenting feature in a mean of 15% (range 2–23%) of patients. Three studies reported abdominal pains in a mean of 49% (range 25–73%) of patients, peripheral oedema in a mean of 29% (range 3–66%) and pellagra in a mean of 4% (range 0–6%). The large ranges may reflect differences in the times at which patients presented to the referral centres and highlight the difficulties in comparing data between centres.

Abdominal pain, diarrhoea and flushing

In 122 consecutive patients with abdominal carcinoid tumours presenting in Sheffield, 69% had abdominal pain at the time of diagnosis, 36% had diarrhoea and 29% were flushing (**Fig. 6.1**). Thirty (36%) of the 84 patients with abdominal pain experienced it solely in the epigastrium or right upper quadrant area, with 19 (23%) experiencing it solely in the right lower quadrant. Twenty one patients (25%) had generalised abdominal pains, but only five (6%) had pain solely on the left side of the abdomen.

In some patients the symptoms had been present for many years before the condition was diagnosed, and it would be difficult to attribute the symptoms in all patients to the presence of a carcinoid tumour. Nevertheless, at the time of diagnosis abdominal pain was both the commonest and most persistent symptom. A common pattern of symptoms was for patients to have initially a few episodes of abdominal pains, sometimes localised, sometimes colicky in nature,

Figure 6.1
The length of history of (a) abdominal pains, (b) diarrhoea and (c) flushing in 122 patients with abdominal carcinoid tumours.

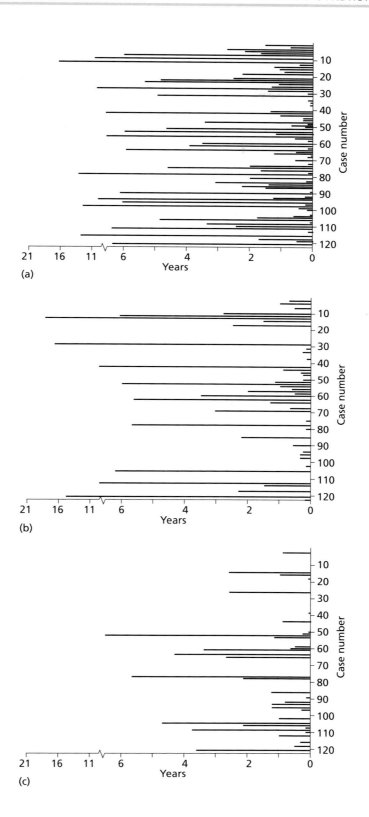

each separated by weeks or even months. The pains became more frequent and by the time of diagnosis most patients had either diarrhoea or flushing or both. A few patients seemed to have none of these symptoms and were usually diagnosed after an enlarged liver or other abdominal mass had been found.

Patients with abdominal pain alone had often been investigated with a barium enema, upper alimentary endoscopy, abdominal ultrasonography and blood tests without finding an abnormality. In one series, 45% of patients with an abdominal carcinoid tumour presented with intestinal obstruction,[1] and data from the 103 patients in the series from Uppsala showed that the patients with intestinal obstruction were diagnosed more quickly than those with diarrhoea or flushing.[2]

Many other clinical features occur, including palpitations, bronchial asthma, heart failure, pellagra, other endocrine conditions such as Cushing's syndrome or hyperparathyroidism in association with multiple endocrine neoplasia type 1 (MEN-1), weight loss and depression. Echocardiographic abnormalities are found in 45% of patients presenting with the carcinoid syndrome,[17] although not all these patients will have heart failure requiring drug therapy at this time. However, the progression of the heart valve disorders (tricuspid and pulmonary) may be rapid over the ensuing year or so to the extent that valve replacement is indicated. Heart failure secondary to valvular fibrosis was considered to be the cause of death in 26 of 63 patients with midgut carcinoids.[18] The urinary excretion of 5-hydroxyindole acetic acid and the plasma 5-hydroxytryptamine concentration are higher in patients with carcinoid heart disease than in those not so affected,[19] but the precise cause of the valvular fibrosis remains unknown. MEN occurred in 0.5% of patients from Northern Ireland with carcinoid tumours,[20] although in a series of 191 Italian patients with gastric carcinoids, 12 were found to have this association.[21]

Although any of the above clinical features may be associated with the syndrome, their presence in isolation in the absence of either abdominal pain, diarrhoea, wheezing or an abdominal mass should not cause suspicion of a carcinoid tumour.

There is no particular pattern to the diarrhoea except that it tends to occur most commonly immediately on rising in the morning and diminishes as the day progresses. It is unusual to see patients with nocturnal diarrhoea.

The flushing attacks are usually confined to the face and upper chest. They occur spontaneously or sometimes may be triggered by drinking alcohol, eating chocolate, occasionally eating hot food or opening the bowels. A flush may be nothing more than a feeling of warmth or mild sweating across the forehead for 10–20 seconds. At the other extreme the whole body may flush for 5–10 minutes or occasionally longer. The latter type of flush is extremely rare but seen most commonly at the time of induction of anaesthesia and may be associated with rapid changes in the systemic blood pressure and with bronchospasm. The most common flushing attacks last for between 30 seconds and 2–3 minutes and affect only the face, the front of the neck and sometimes the upper chest, accompanied in some by running of the nose and eyes. Patients occasionally report concurrent palpitations.

Flushing attacks do not occur until the carcinoid tumour has metastasised to the liver. Occasionally, ultrasonography and computed tomography do not reveal any abnormality of the liver in patients who are flushing, and the situation may be further confused by the excretion of urinary 5-hydroxyindole acetic acid within the reference range. Diagnosis in such extremely rare patients is difficult.

After a few years of flushing episodes, there may be a permanent flush across the cheeks and nose. This may vary from mild telangiectasis to a deep ruby or a very dark purple discoloration and, rarely, a blackening of the skin. The flushing attacks in patients with a gastric primary are reported as being bright red and patchy[22] and possibly due to the release and effect of histamine. The distinction of colours of flushing is not easy to characterise clinically. The presence of a flush of any hue is the important physical sign. Despite flushing that is obvious to others, some patients do not notice that they are flushing or only notice a few of their attacks. This makes the number of flushes per day a potentially unreliable way of measuring the response to therapy.

Site of the primary tumour

Gastric carcinoid tumours

The main sites of primary tumours in the gastrointestinal (GI) tract are the jejuno-ileum, rectum and colon.[11] Gastric primaries occur in between 2 and 3.8% of patients with carcinoid tumours,[5,6] and some reports suggest that the stomach may be a far more common primary site—accounting for 10–30% of patients.[22,23] Such apparent anomalies emphasise the value of large scale studies and the need for collaborative work in this rare condition.

About 80% of gastric carcinoid tumours are associated with chronic atrophic gastritis and hypergastrinaemia. They may be multifocal, and in up to 50% of affected patients are linked with pernicious anaemia.[21,25,26] About 6% are seen as part of the MEN-1 syndrome,[20,21] and a further 14% of gastric carcinoid tumours often showing highly malignant features, occur sporadically and have no apparent association with other conditions. There has probably been an increase in the incidence of gastric carcinoid tumours over the past few decades, which is most evident in black American males.[27] The cause is unknown.

Lung carcinoid tumours

Patients with lung carcinoid tumours, which account for about 2% of all pulmonary tumours and about 25% of all carcinoid tumours, usually present with haemoptysis or pneumonia. Such a clear clinical presentation often results in patients being diagnosed at an earlier stage, and the survival figures in this group are better than in those with bowel carcinoid tumours.[5] Between 50 and 85% of lung primaries are to found in the main stem or lobar bronchi, with the remainder in the lung periphery.[5,28] Patients with lung carcinoids may present with Cushing's syndrome and have been reported to account overall for about 3% of patients with this condition.[29]

Appendiceal carcinoid tumours

Of the 8305 patients included in the End Results Group, the Third National Cancer Survey and the SEER programs 1570 (19%) had appendiceal carcinoid tumours.[30] They were 1.7 times more common in women and showed evidence of metastasis in 35% of patients. These data show that appendiceal carcinoid tumours are not as indolent as had been previously assumed and that affected patients may require long-term follow-up. The chance of an appendiceal carcinoid tumour producing metastases at the time of presentation is 30–60% for primary tumours greater than 2 cm in diameter, 0–11% for tumours between 1 and 2 cm in diameter and nil for tumour less than 1 cm in diameter.[31]

Rectal carcinoid tumours

Secondary spread from rectal carcinoid tumours is found in less than 2% of patients with rectal primaries less than 1 cm in diameter, up to 15% with primaries between 1 and 1.9 cm in diameter and up to 80% with primaries equal to or greater than 2 cm diameter.[31] Patients with carcinoid tumours of the rectum or appendix, as with lung carcinoid tumours, have better 5-year survival figures than those with tumours in other primary sites, probably because they present and are diagnosed at an earlier stage (**Table 6.1**).[5]

A precise site of the primary tumour was not reported for almost 11% of patients in the End Results Group, the Third National Cancer Survey and the SEER programmes.[5] In a series of 434 patients with GI primaries or primaries of unknown origin, the clinical and biochemical behaviour of the latter group resembled that found in patients with midgut carcinoid primaries with distant metastases.[33]

Associated cancers

A recent large population-based study, which included just over 1000 patients with carcinoid tumours, showed no overall increased risk of a patient having a second tumour.[34] A postmortem study found a prevalence of second, non-carcinoid, malignancies in 41%, a value which was almost the same as the prevalence of malignant tumours in all patients, including those without carcinoid tumours.[6] The finding by others, including the SEER programme, of prevalence rates of second, non-carcinoid, malignant tumours of 13–25%, in the absence of control data, does not confirm that carcinoid tumours are associated with the development of non-related tumours. This makes it difficult to justify the advice given that patients should be investigated and followed-up for other malignancies.[5]

Clinical examination (Table 6.3)

There may be no abnormalities on physical examination. Facial telangiectasia may be present as may peripheral oedema and pellagra.[14] The percentage of patients affected by these conditions varies between studies and probably reflects the stage of the disease. Pellagra-like rash may be found in up to 6% of patients.[14] The patient may flush intermittently while at rest, after eating, on abdominal palpation or as a result of emotional stress.

There may be a mass in the right iliac fossa, which is often tender. The mass is usually larger than the primary tumour itself and contains fibrous tissue, which may involve the bowel wall and the mesentery. The liver may be enlarged, sometimes with discrete masses palpable on the surface, which may be tender. Central abdominal masses may be due to enlargement of lymph nodes. Ascites is rarely

General
May be normal
Flushing—face and neck, sometimes chest, rarely trunk and arms
Weight loss
Peripheral oedema
Telangiectasia
Bright eyes and sometimes lachrymation during a flush

Abdomen
Mass in right iliac fossa/para-aortic region
Hepatomegaly
Ascites
Rectal mass

Cardiovascular
Raised jugular venous pressure
Tricuspid regurgitation/stenosis
Pulmonary stenosis

Skin
Pellagra (rare)
Peripheral oedema (rare initially)

Bones
Tender with secondaries

Respiratory
Wheezing (rare)

Table 6.3 *Clinical examination*

detected except in very advanced disease, and jaundice is uncommon, even in the period shortly before death.

Examination of bones for tenderness on percussion or 'springing' may result in pain where secondary deposits are present.

A raised jugular venous pressure increases the possibility of tricuspid or pulmonary valve disease.

Metastases to the eye are rare, but fundoscopy and slit-lamp examination should be performed if suspected. In a series of 410 patients with such metastases, carcinoid was responsible in 2.2%.[35] Decreased vision is the commonest symptom of a choroidal secondary tumour, with proptosis and diminished eye movements the commonest symptoms of orbital secondaries. Choroidal carcinoid secondaries are orange on fundoscopy.

Investigations (Table 6.4)

Urine and blood

The carcinoid syndrome is diagnosed by the presence of diarrhoea and flushing, either singly or together, combined with an increase in the excretion of urinary 5-hydroxyindole acetic acid (5-HIAA) over 24 hours. To diagnose the syndrome there needs to be both clinical and biochemical evidence of hormone excess. The excess of urinary 5-HIAA excretion is a marker of the syndrome rather than it or its precursors necessarily being the cause.

5-HIAA is formed from tryptophan, which is metabolised to 5-hydroxytryptophan (5-HTP) and thence rapidly to 5-hydroxytryptamine (5-HT). The 5-HT, which is carried mainly in the platelets, is subsequently metabolised through an intermediate step to 5-HIAA. Neither the blood concentration of 5-HT nor the urine excretion of 5-HTP are reliable indicators of the carcinoid syndrome. Patients with tumours of the foregut (lung, stomach, duodenum, jejunum and pancreas) often excrete less 5-HIAA than patients with tumours of the midgut.[24,36] In a series of 301 patients with carcinoid tumours, an increased excretion of 5-HIAA was found in 76% of those with carcinoid tumours of the midgut, 31% of those with tumours of the foregut and in none with tumours of the hindgut.[37] Over 75% of patients within each group had hepatic metastases.

The clinical utility of estimating plasma concentrations of the various hormones from the gut and elsewhere as well as the numerous markers that may be produced in patients with carcinoid tumours is still in the process of being established. The potential value of estimating plasma chromogranin A concentration as a marker of the presence and activity of carcinoid tumours has been described recently.[37] Chromogranin A is found in the vesicles of neuroendocrine cells and may be broken down into about eight smaller glycoprotein components.

Urine	Minimum of two 24-hour urines for 5-HIAA estimation Use quantitative not qualitative assay If borderline result, repeat urine collection with diet control 5-HIAA excretion relates to tumour mass and activity 5-HIAA excretion >300 μmol 24 h⁻¹: median survival of 45 months 5-HIAA excretion <300 μmol 24 h⁻¹: median survival of 72 months[37] Some patients produce little or no 5-HIAA excess Ensure laboratory has acid in urine collection bottle (otherwise 5-HIAA degrades)
Blood	Basic tests may be normal ↑ alkaline phosphatase and γ-glutamyl transferase ↓ prognosis Alkaline phosphatase and γ-glutamyl transferase may increase quickly in 3–6 months before death Plasma chromogranin A concentration ↑ with neuroendocrine tumours Plasma chromogranin A concentration over 5 mg l⁻¹ may indicate relapse Estimation of plasma concentration of many gut peptides of unknown value Estimation of plasma serotonin concentration of unknown value Measure other hormones as indicated (e.g. ACTH, PTH, gastrin)
Radiography	Barium follow-through may show terminal ileal distortion/stricture Chest X-ray film may show consolidation/mass/be normal Bone secondaries may be sclerotic (typically seen in vertebrae)
Ultrasonography	Mass lesions in liver Occasionally see primary Rectal tumours and local spread seen with transrectal views May be used to measure tumour size change with therapy
CT scan	Mass lesions in liver See mesenteric lesions with 'star-burst' appearance May see primary tumour Use spiral CT with at least dual-phase imaging
¹¹¹In-octreotide scintigraphy	Shows 80–85% of tumours (20% may not have relevant somatostatin receptors) Binds to receptors on cell surface Shows unsuspected lesions Shows sites of tumours Perform whole body single photon emission CT scanning Not specific for carcinoid tumours Possible false negative result
¹²³I-MIBG scintigraphy	Shows about 60% of tumours Binds to intracellular granules Use to determine if ¹³¹I-MIBG therapy is suitable
Bone scan	Symptomless patients may have positive scan results Perform if any bone tenderness or pain
Angiography	Not a routine investigation Mesenteric angiography prior to bowel surgery Hepatic angiography prior to embolisation/chemoembolisation
Cardiac echocardiography	Perform in all Cardiac changes rarely seen until syndrome present for over 3 years

Table 6.4 *Investigations*

Plasma chromogranin A concentrations have been found to be increased in 87, 78 and 100% of patients with carcinoid tumours of the midgut, foregut and hindgut, respectively.[37] It has been suggested that chromogranin A plasma concentrations above a certain threshold identify patients in whom the condition is about to relapse,[37] with a high degree of sensitivity (92%) and specificity (97%).[38] The finding of a more precise marker for the presence and behaviour of carcinoid tumours may be of considerable clinical importance, and further studies will determine the role of plasma chromogranin A estimations with greater precision. Some patients with the irritable bowel syndrome may have an increased plasma chromogranin A concentration,[39] and because this condition causes similar symptoms to those experienced by patients with carcinoid tumours, distinguishing the two may be difficult.

Neuropeptide K, substance P, urinary histamine, serum gastrin, serum pancreatic polypeptide, calcitonin and chromogranin B may be increased in patients with carcinoid tumours but, with the exception of histamine and gastrin, their clinical utility remains unclear.

The estimation of 5-HIAA concentrations in the urine may be qualitative or quantitative. A recent quality control exercise of several clinical chemistry laboratories showed that when a qualitative method was used 10 of 25 (40%) of the results were incorrect. When a quantitative method was used only 2 of 40 (5%) of the results were incorrect (Forrest, personal communication). The use of qualitative methods of 5-HIAA analysis should cease.

Urinary excretion of 5-HIAA is variable, and reliance should not be placed on results from a single 24-hour urine collection. Many protocols for diagnosis and follow-up rely on two 24-hour urine collections. Food that contains large amounts of 5-HT, such as aubergines, avocado pears, bananas and many nuts may cause a slight increase of the urinary 5-HIAA, but this is not thought to be of relevance in most patients.[8]

There are no basic blood tests that are of any diagnostic assistance. Often, the serum albumin concentration is normal and the serum alkaline phosphatase and γ-glutamyl transferase are only slightly increased—even in the presence of considerable metastatic disease in the liver. Increased concentrations of these enzymes have been found to be inversely related to survival.[49] Within the 3–6 months prior to death, the activities of these enzymes increase to as much as 10 times the upper limit of the reference range.

Imaging

The diagnosis of a carcinoid tumour is not infrequently made as a result of abdominal ultrasonography, the identification of hepatic secondary tumours and a positive biopsy result in patients in whom the diagnosis had not been suspected. In the Sheffield series of patients this has become the commonest route of establishing the diagnosis.

A consensus plan of imaging to determine the site of the primary tumour and the extent of the metastases has been proposed by the European Neuroendocrine Tumour Network (ENET) (**Fig. 6.2**).[40]

Performing both an octreoscan and a CT scan makes it likely that carcinoid tumour will be seen in about 95% of cases. The typical CT appearances of carcinoid tumour deposits within the mesentery are of a discrete mass with radiating spokes (**Fig. 6.3**). About 40% of abdominal carcinoid tumours contain calcification.[41] Evidence of intestinal obstruction, thickening of the bowel wall and lymphadenopathy may also be seen on CT scans. Carcinoid liver metastases are heterogeneous in their vascularity and therefore to optimise detection, arterial and portal venous phase spiral CT should be performed.[42]

The scintigraphic localisation of a carcinoid tumour was first described in 1989[43] and since then the Dutch group who initially developed this technique have reported their experience in over 1000 patients.[44] The technique relies on attaching a radioligand to a somatostatin analogue, which in turn attaches itself to somatostatin receptors that are abundant on the surface of carcinoid tumour cells. Previously unsuspected carcinoid deposits have been found in over 50% of patients studied using ^{111}In-octreotide (Pentetreotide; also known as an Octreoscan). A ^{111}In-octreotide scan showing abnormal uptake in the right iliac fossa region and in hepatic secondaries is shown in **Fig. 6.4(a)** (a terminal ileal tumour was removed at operation **Fig. 6.4(b)**). An octreoscan, with whole-body single photon emission CT, ideally should be performed in all patients in whom surgical or medical treatment is being considered as this will allow optimal planning of treatment.

Postoperative studies in patients in whom it had been thought there had been complete removal of tumour showed probable residual tumour in about 30%. It may be possible to improve the outcome of tumour debulking by intraoperative scintigraphic scanning. Up to about 15% of carcinoid tumours are octreoscan negative,[45] and this may be a result of such tumours not having the specific somatostatin receptors that bind to the radiolabelled octreotide.

Radiolabelled metaiodobenzylguanidine (MIBG) has been used to localise phaeochromocytomas and neuroblastomas. Scintigrams with ^{131}I-MIBG were positive in 51 of 70 patients with metastatic carcinoid disease.[46] MIBG scanning is not as sensitive as scanning with CT or ^{111}In-octreotide.[47] In 28 patients with carcinoid tumours of the midgut ^{111}In-octreotide, CT and MIBG scans identified tumours in 92, 76 and 66% of patients, respectively. MIBG is taken up into the secretory granules of neuroendocrine cells, unlike radiolabelled octreotide, which binds to cell membrane receptors. Patients who do not respond to somatostatin analogues might, therefore, benefit from radiolabelled MIBG therapy, and a positive MIBG scan would indicate those patients suitable for such treatment.[48]

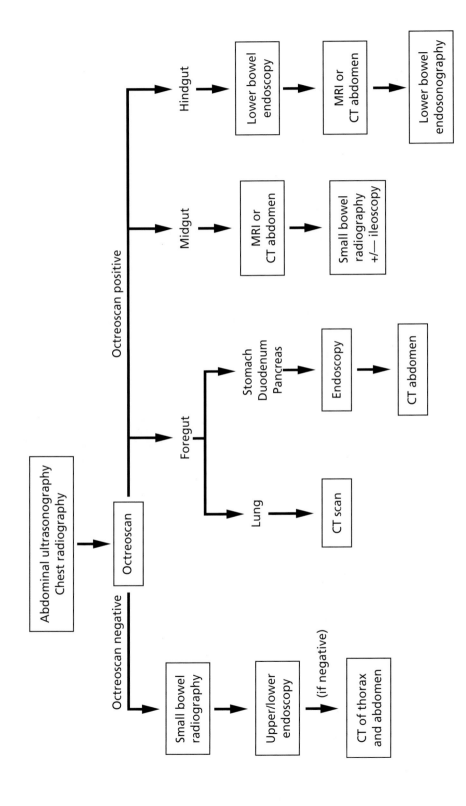

Figure 6.2
European Neuroendocrine Tumour Network recommendations for imaging neuroendocrine tumours.

Figure 6.3
A mesenteric secondary carcinoid tumour showing radiating spokes.

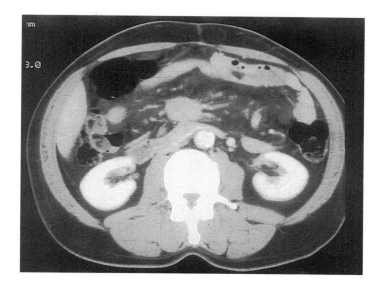

Figure 6.4
An ^{111}In-octreotide scan (a) showing increased uptake in the region of the terminal ileum and within the liver, and the operative finding (b) showing the terminal carcinoid. At operation it was possible to remove all hepatic secondary deposits. (b) Courtesy of Professor A. Johnson.

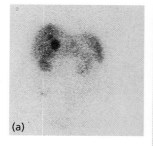

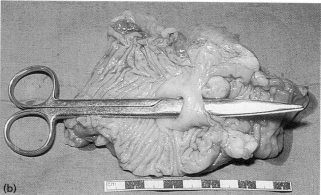

(a)

(b)

Mesenteric angiography gives valuable information when planning for a resection of a bowel carcinoid mass. The bowel may be tethered into a mass of fibrous tissue, making resection difficult, and a knowledge of the vascular supply is useful. Hepatic angiography need not be performed routinely but only in those undergoing embolisation and chemoembolisation therapy.

Histopathology

Expert histopathology is essential in establishing the diagnosis, which should not be made solely on the basis of whether the cells are argyrophil or argentaffin positive. Carcinoid tumours of the foregut are argyrophil positive. The enterochromaffin-like cells that from the major cell type in gastric carcinoid tumours are argentaffin negative.[50] Carcinoid tumours of the midgut are predominately argentaffin positive and those of the hindgut typically non-reactive. Carcinoid tumours can look like adenocarcinomas and may be diagnosed as such unless the tissue is examined for neurone-specific enolase and chromogranin.[11]

The term 'carcinoid' was introduced to describe a tumour that looked like a cancer but had more benign behaviour. The diversity of these tumours is so great, however, that a new classification is required. It has been suggested that the term 'carcinoid' be replaced by 'neuroendocrine' and tumours described on the basis of their site, size, symptoms, histopathology, hormone secretion and exhibition of tumour markers.[51,52]

The degree of cellular differentiation may be determined by assessing the expression of the proliferating antigen Ki-67, and this is related to the length of survival of the patient[53,54] and may assist in determining which patients might benefit from chemotherapy. The so-called atypical carcinoids, usually of foregut origin, have a high expression of Ki-67 antigen and are the carcinoid tumours most likely to respond to chemotherapy.

Antibodies raised to the various subtypes of chromogranin have been used for immunohistochemical staining of a range of neuroendocrine tumours, but the clinical relevance of knowing which subtypes of chromogranin are present in a tumour is not known.[55]

Treatment

The aim of treatment in patients with the carcinoid syndrome is to relieve the local and distant effects caused by the tumour and its secretions. Optimal control of the carcinoid syndrome results from removal of tumour, and surgery affords the only method of cure. If surgery is not possible or leaves, as is usual, residual tumour, then the biological activity of this tissue may be diminished by a variety of therapies, virtually none of which have been studied in randomised controlled clinical trials. Uncontrolled trials, often with less than 100 patients, provide the basis of the therapeutic approach to carcinoid tumours. The current treatment options are summarised in **Table 6.5**.

Surgery

If a patient is fit for surgery then debulking the patient of tumour or as much of the tumour as possible provides the best outcome of all available therapies.[56–58] Surgical debulking may greatly diminish the symptoms of the syndrome,[59,60] decreases the urinary 5-HIAA excretion[61] and should be attempted whenever possible.

Many patients still present with an acute intestinal problem, requiring urgent surgery. Typically, the findings at operation are of a mass, often in the right iliac

Surgery	Attempt to remove as much tumour as possible
	Cover operation with octreotide
	Gives the best long-term results—the only therapy that may result in cure (rare)
	Hepatic resection diminishes symptoms—effect on survival not known
Biotherapy	Octreotide for patients with the carcinoid syndrome
	Increasing the dosage of octreotide (up to 500 μg t.d.s.) increases the clinical effect
	Clinical effect of somatostatin analogues may decrease with time
	Interferon-α probably not as effective as octreotide in controlling symptoms
	Interferon-α may have a flat dose–response curve >3–5 mega units three times a week
	Adverse effects of interferon may limit its use
	Slow-release somatostatin analogues (lanreotide and octreotide-LAR) may give same degree of symptom control as octreotide
	Place of interferon-α unclear but consider using in patients unresponsive to somatostatin analogues
	Somatostatin analogues and interferon are expensive
Tumour-targeted treatment	^{111}In-octreotide decreases symptoms of syndrome—ideal time to administer unknown
	^{131}I-MIBG may be of value in patients with carcinoid syndrome not responding to biotherapy or surgery and with a life expectation of over 6–12 months
	No trials comparing ^{131}I-MIBG with octreotide or ^{111}In-octreotide therapy
	^{90}Y-DOTA-octreotide therapy at present of unknown benefit
Embolisation of hepatic secondaries	Indicated when surgical removal of tumour not possible and liver function normal
Chemoembolisation	Unknown whether the intrahepatic artery administration of cytotoxics gives additional benefit than embolisation to patients with midgut carcinoid tumours and hepatic secondaries
Drugs	Simple therapy such as codeine phosphate or loperamide may control diarrhoea
Radiotherapy	Decreases pain from bone secondaries
	Possible value in shrinking tumours

Table 6.5 *Treatment*

fossa, which consists of loops of small bowel adherent to each other and the ascending colon. The tumour, which may be no more than 1–2 cm in diameter forms the nidus of the mass. There may be mesenteric deposits, together with seedlings in the peritoneum. In addition, secondary deposits are usually seen on the surface of the liver. Faced with such a situation, it is not surprising that a diagnosis of inoperable disseminated malignancy is made, a defunctioning bowel procedure performed and biopsies taken. A few days later the histopathology report raises the possibility of carcinoid tumour. Nearly half the patients in a series from Belfast presented in this manner.[1]

The survival of patients with operable carcinoid disease is longer than that of patients with inoperable disease.[56] In a series of 48 patients all with hepatic metastases, 11 who had had surgery alone were alive and apparently free of tumour 3 months later, 6 of the 27 who had been treated with embolisation and octreotide had died and 8 of the 10 treated with octreotide alone had died.[57] This study highlights the difficulties in conducting trials of therapy in patients with carcinoid tumours. The numbers in each treatment group were small, and the groups seemed not well matched for stage of disease.

The Gothenburg group has shown a 70% 5-year survival in 64 patients with carcinoid tumours of the midgut and bilobar hepatic secondary spread.[58] These patients had undergone removal of the primary tumour and local spread as well as repeated hepatic embolisation. The same group has proposed a treatment protocol for the management of gastric carcinoid tumours, with endoscopic removal of small lesions, antrectomy for larger lesions and gastrectomy for invasive tumours that have metastasised to local lymph nodes.[62] Patients should be monitored with regular upper alimentary endoscopy.

Secondary tumours on the surface of the liver have long been removed but hepatic resection is now being used by some as a method of debulking. In 74 patients—50 with carcinoid tumours and 23 with islet cell tumours—treated with hepatic resection, 60% were of symptoms 1 year after the operation and 40% after 2 years.[60]

No prospective trials have been conducted to determine whether patients live longer after the resection of liver metastases in carcinoid syndrome. Current practice is not to undertake this form of treatment unless it is possible to resect at least 90% of the liver metastases[63] and to remove the primary tumour and any local spread.

Some patients have undergone liver transplantation for hepatic carcinoid secondaries,[64,65] but as yet the nature of the studies and the numbers of patients included is such that the role of this treatment remains unclear.

At any time during the course of the operation, but particularly at the time of induction of anaesthesia, patients may have sudden and marked changes in blood pressure. Hypotension or hypertension can occur at various times, with prolonged and extensive flushing and bronchospasm, and these latter features are those of a carcinoid crisis. There are no indicators as to which patients might react adversely to anaesthesia or surgery, except that there is evidence to suggest that hypotension may provoke a carcinoid crisis.[66] Patients with a greatly increased urinary 5-HIAA excretion and a presumed large tumour load seem to be no more likely to have a carcinoid crisis than do patients with only a minimal increase. Octreotide therapy has prevented these complications.[60] In patients not already receiving octreotide, treatment is started the day before surgery using the following protocol: A first dose of 50 μg is followed 8 hours later by 100 μg and continued eight hourly thereafter so that by the time a patient is anaesthetised four or five doses have been given. The octreotide is given subcutaneously at this stage. The final preoperative dose is given an hour before induction. Further doses of 10–20 μg may be given intravenously during the operation as the clinical state dictates. Episodes of hypotension caused by the tumour releasing vasoactive peptides respond well to such treatment. Patients who are already receiving octreotide prior to operation continue the therapy but are given their regular dose 1 hour before induction.

Somatostatin analogues

A chance observation led to the use of somatostatin analogues in the treatment of the carcinoid syndrome. Two patients with MCT flushed when they received pentagastrin, and it was thus postulated that gastrin might be the cause of the carcinoid flush. Somatostatin was known to inhibit gastrin release and when given to patients with carcinoid disease it abolished pentagastrin-induced flushing.[68] Gastrin is now known not to be responsible for carcinoid flushing, but the serendipity of these early experiments resulted in the production of several somatostatin analogues that have a beneficial effect in the carcinoid syndrome.

A single dose of somatostatin has a very short duration of effect owing to its rapid metabolism, which makes it of no practical value in controlling carcinoid symptoms. The somatostatin molecule was modified to make it longer acting and by 1986 a study of the effects of this new drug, octreotide, was reported.[69]

 A review of over 60 published studies showed that diarrhoea and flushing may be controlled in about 80% of patients. As many as 90% of patients may benefit with appropriate dose titration but few obtain complete relief from their symptoms.[70]

The initial dosage of octreotide should be 100 µg t.d.s. subcutaneously, increasing by 50–100 µg every 8 hours until symptoms are controlled.

Octreotide does not seem to cause regression of carcinoid tumours. There are frequent references in the literature to octreotide 'stablising' the disease process, with tumour growth rate being slowed but there are no agreed criteria to determine the precise rate of tumour growth, and 'stabilisation' may suggest a degree of precision that is unwarranted. Regrettably, the only control data in studies quoting survival figures is historical and there is uncertainty as to whether octreotide prolongs life.

There is nevertheless circumstantial evidence that the range of therapies now available to treat carcinoid tumours may have a beneficial effect on survival. An overview of several reports indicates that currently one would anticipate a group of patients with midgut primaries and hepatic metastases to have a median survival of about 7 years, whereas in the era prior to biotherapy, embolisation and radical surgery, the 5-year survival rate was about 20%.[18] One difficulty in interpreting survival data is that the length of time patients had the tumour prior to treatment varied between studies.

A disadvantage of octreotide is that it has to be given several times each day by repeated subcutaneous injections. Two 'long-acting', or perhaps better entitled, 'slow-release,' somatostatin analogues, lanreotide and octreotide-LAR help to circumvent this problem. They are administered intramuscularly once every 2 or 4 weeks, respectively and seem to control the symptoms of carcinoid syndrome as well as octreotide.[71,72,73] The two studies of lanreotide[71,72] lasted 6 months and were without control arms. Symptoms remained suppressed in 38–56% of patients 6 months after starting treatment. About 60% of patients taking either octreotide or octreotide-LAR had continuing symptomatic relief 24 weeks after starting treatment.[73]

There may be a reappearance of symptoms towards the end of a dosing interval, necessitating an increased frequency of drug administration or increased dosage. It is unknown whether lanreotide or octreotide-LAR have any effect on tumour growth. Their effect on longevity is unknown. There are no trials directly comparing lanreotide with octreotide-LAR.

The response to octreotide may diminish with time,[69] but the cause for this is not known. Octreotide therapy is well tolerated, although its injection may cause a slight and transient stinging sensation. Many patients complain of smelly motions. This is due to the increase in the fat content of the stools secondary to the inhibition of cholecystokinin release caused by octreotide. Occasionally a patient may notice worsening of diarrhoea, and in some, gallstones and biliary sludge may be caused by octreotide therapy. In a retrospective review of a group of 44 patients taking octreotide for between 18 and 84 months, gallstones or gallbladder sludge developed in 4 and 23 patients, respectively.[74] Gallstones did not develop in patients receiving octreotide 150 µg t.d.s., but only in those receiving higher dosages. Overall, six patients required surgery for symptomatic gallbladder disease. Stopping octreotide therapy has been associated with biliary colic and pancreatitis.

It is often recommended that when octreotide therapy by itself is not controlling the symptoms of the carcinoid syndrome interferon-α should be added. The administration of interferon-α 5 mega units three times a week to patients already receiving octreotide 200 µg t.d.s. resulted in improved symptom control,[75] but this dosage of octreotide is below the recommended maximum.

Interferon-α

Oberg et al. gave human leucocyte interferon to a small group of patients with metastatic carcinoid tumour[76] and symptoms were improved in two thirds. A larger study provided evidence of clinical benefit and a decrease in urinary excretion of 5-HIAA in about half the patients for a median of 34 months.[77] Further studies have shown that, overall, the beneficial effects of interferon-α are probably less marked than those of octreotide and that, similar to octreotide, there are no data other than circumstantial to support it having an effect on tumour size. The dosages commonly used vary between 3 and 6 mega units three times weekly. Far higher dosages have been given but it is uncertain if they produce any therapeutic advantage.

Side effects with interferon are more troublesome than with octreotide. The commonest is a feeling of an influenza-like illness a few hours after the injection. Paracetamol 1 g taken at the time of the injection may lessen this problem. Many patients (about 70%) experience fatigue, which may be severe and the reason they stop taking the drug. There may be disturbances of liver enzymes and serum lipids as well as the appearance of thyroid antibodies and the development of hypothyroidism.[78]

An area of clinical uncertainty and considerable debate is whether somatostatin analogues or interferon should be given to patients who have metastatic disease in the liver but not the syndrome. There are no published data relating to this situation. One view is that patients without the syndrome who have progressive disease should start taking a somatostatin analogue. This view is based on the belief that patients who have received such drugs, and other treatments, have a slower rate of progression of tumour mass and an increased length of survival compared with historical controls. An alternative view is that a trial should be mounted to answer the question as to whether this therapeutic strategy is appropriate.

If a patient fails to respond to octreotide with the dosage having been titrated up to 500 μg t.d.s. then it is appropriate to give interferon-α in addition. The reason for a patient not responding to octreotide therapy might be that the tumour is relatively deplete of receptors to which octreotide binds. If diarrhoea is the sole problem then codeine phosphate may help and at considerably less expense than octreotide, which costs approximately £6000 a year at a dosage of 100 μg t.d.s. Three mega units of interferon-α three times a week for a year costs about £2600, and the slow release somatostatin analogues would cost between £9000 and 11 000 per patient per year.

Targeted radiotherapy

There are recent reports of the use of radiolabelled formulations of octreotide and of MIBG to treat patients with metastatic carcinoid disease.[48,79,80] The treatment with the octreotide compounds has been with [111]Indium and [90]Yttrium preparations, although the latter is not at present available for use in treating neuroendocrine tumours. The indications for their use have not been established.

Cytotoxic therapy and the use of other drugs

There is no evidence to support the use of cytotoxic therapy in patients with well differentiated metastatic carcinoid tumours of the midgut. The initial studies using drugs such as streptozotocin and 5-fluorouracil were conducted about 15–25 years ago and both they and subsequent studies with compounds such as dacarbazine, adriamycin, cisplatin and etoposide have shown only a weak effect in modifying symptoms and biochemical markers. The effect of chemotherapy is quite different in patients with an undifferentiated neuroendocrine tumour of the foregut such as might be found in the pancreas. A combination of etoposide and cisplatin resulted in a tumour regression rate of 67% in 18 patients with anaplastic neuroendocrine tumours whereas there was no response in patients with well differentiated carcinoid tumours.[81] Pancreatic neuroendocrine tumours also show a response rate of about 60% to a combination of streptozotocin and 5–fluorouracil.[82,83]

Several other drugs, including ketanserin, cyproheptadine, calcitonin, codeine phosphate and, in the past, methysergide and parachlorophenylalanine, have been used in an attempt to control the symptoms of the disease. None have been compared directly with octreotide or interferon.

Hepatic embolisation and chemoembolisation

The treatment of obliterating the arterial supply to hepatic secondary carcinoid tumours was first reported in 1977.[84] It is now an established treatment in controlling the symptoms of the carcinoid syndrome and is probably effective because it causes necrosis of the tumour. Embolisation of hepatic tumours through the hepatic artery is possible because they receive their blood supply from the hepatic artery whereas about 75% of the blood supply to the rest of the liver is from the portal vein.

Embolisation alone, without additional hepatic artery chemotherapy, resulted in a decrease in hepatic tumour volume of greater than 50% in 13 of 27 patients with hepatic metastases from carcinoid tumours of the midgut.[85] A retrospective review of 29 patients, also with metastatic carcinoid tumours of the midgut, treated with intrahepatic artery gel foam powder showed an objective response in 15, which lasted for a median of 12 months and gave a 5–year survival of 60%.[86] Similar clinical benefit and survival figures have been found after embolisation with polyvinyl alcohol particles.[87]

Patients considered for embolisation therapy will be those for whom surgery would not be possible, and typically they will have a large hepatic tumour load. It is usually not possible to treat all the metastases in one session of embolisation, and the procedure may be repeated at intervals of between 1 and 3 months.

Before embolisation, hepatic arteriography should be performed to assess the position and number of metastases as well as to ensure that the portal vein is patent. The patient must be adequately hydrated prior to the procedure and be receiving octreotide, antimicrobial cover and treatment to prevent pain and nausea. The procedure should not be performed if there is obstruction to the portal vein of if there is impairment of liver function.[88]

Cytotoxic drugs such as doxorubicin,[88] 5–fluorouracil[89] and streptozotocin[90] have been administered prior to treatment with embolising agents. The objective responses are similar to those seen with embolisation alone but have not been compared directly. The numbers of patients studied have been few and there have been no controlled trials and thus it is not known whether this combination therapy gives any advantage over embolisation alone. There were more survivors at 5 years and a greater degree of biochemical response in patients who received embolisation plus interferon compared with a group who received interferon alone, but embolisation was not found to have a statistically significant effect on survival.[91]

Patients may experience pain over the right upper abdomen and lower right chest for 3 or 4 days after embolisation. The pain may be pleuritic, which raises the possibility of a pulmonary embolus. There may be an intermittent pyrexia, probably related to tissue necrosis, which raises concern about a hepatic abscess or septicaemia. The pain usually lasts only a day or two, but the pyrexia may persist for a week or slightly longer. An example of vaso-obliterative therapy using absolute alcohol injected into the hepatic artery branch going to a carcinoid hepatic secondary from the midgut is shown in **Figure 6.5**.

Embolisation and vaso-obliterative therapy causes symptomatic benefit, but it is unclear at what stage of the disease such therapy should be given. Some have used it in patients unsuitable for surgical debulking and when symptoms have not been controlled by biotherapy. Others recommend its use after surgical debulking,[58] or instead of it if this is not possible, as well as starting a patient on biotherapy. There are currently no data to suggest that after embolisation treatment, either with or without accompanying intrahepatic artery chemotherapy, patients live longer, but symptoms that have escaped from control with biotherapy may be lessened in about 50% of patients.

Radiotherapy

Carcinoid tumours are thought to be radio-resistant, but radiotherapy is excellent in relieving the pain from bone secondaries. A few recent reports have raised the possibility that secondary deposits in the liver and elsewhere shrink in response to radiotherapy,[92] but there are no trials that determine whether radiotherapy has more than a palliative role.

Monitoring the response to therapy

A reasonable aim is an 80% or greater decrease in the frequency of flushing and diarrhoea. Relief of pain should also be achieved. A decrease in the urinary excretion of 5-HIAA should be seen. Such a decrease is associated with a decrease in the frequency and severity of symptoms but does not seem to be related to changes in tumour growth. Plasma chromogranin concentrations may be as helpful a marker of disease status as the urinary excretion of 5-HIAA and give equal warning of deterioration. Any lessening of the response to therapy is not of predictive value as regards survival. Tumour size may be evaluated by routine scanning techniques, but as the tumour is typically slow growing, scans usually do not need to be performed more than six monthly.

Figure 6.5
Hepatic angiogram showing a carcinoid tumour (a) before and (b) after injection of absolute alcohol into the artery supplying the tumour. Photo courtesy of Dr P. Gaines.

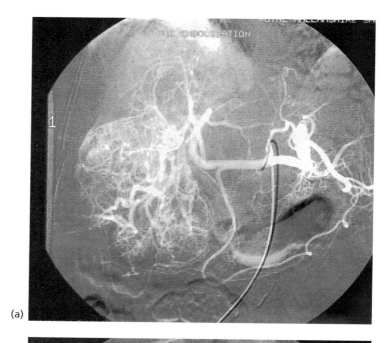

(a)

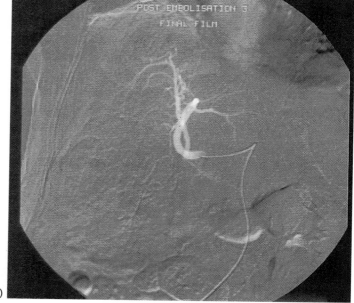

(b)

Survival data in relation to carcinoid disease are difficult to interpret because they are based on survival from the time of diagnosis rather than from the time of onset of the disease. With this reservation one might expect 60% of patients with operable disease to be alive 10 years after abdominal carcinoid tumour was

Figure 6.6
Percentage of patients surviving 5 years with carcinoid tumours of various primary sites and with varying extents of metastases. Data from the Surveillance, Epidemiology and End Results (SEER) programme in the USA as reported by Modlin and Sandor in 1997.[5] Overall numbers of patients within each group and percentages of patients with localised (L), regional (R) and distant (D) metastases were: appendix, n=410 (L62, R27, D9); lung, n=1756 (L67, R20, D7); rectum, n=545 (L72, R7, D7); small intestine, n=1770 (L25, R39, D31); stomach, n=204 (L53, R10, D21).

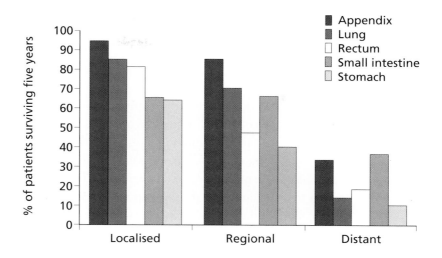

diagnosed, compared with 40% and 20% of patients with inoperable disease or hepatic metastases, respectively.[56]

The SEER programme[5] gives the most recent and cohesive data on survival, and a summary is given in **Figure 6.6**.

The survival of patients with gastric carcinoid tumours depends on the nature of the tumour. Survival is best in patients with tumours secondary to chronic atrophic gastritis and those related to the MEN-1 syndrome.[21] There were no deaths in a group of 152 with chronic atrophic gastritis and one death in 12 patients with MEN-1 over a follow-up period of about 4 years, whereas 7 of 27 patients with sporadic gastric carcinoid tumours had died in 2 years.

Conclusion

The symptoms occurring in patients with metastatic carcinoid tumour were first recognised to conform to a pattern in the 1950s and were labelled as the carcinoid syndrome.[14,93] A feature of the disease that had been described over 100 years ago[94] and often mentioned in the literature until about 1950, was that of abdominal pain. A recent report has re-emphasised the predominance of pain in the presentation of patients with carcinoid tumours.[95] Abdominal pain occurred in 60 of 150 (40%) patients of whom 27 had metastatic disease, 13 the syndrome, all with diarrhoea and 9 had flushing.

There is an important distinction to make between carcinoid disease and the carcinoid syndrome. If the development of the syndrome occurs before diagnosis then the opportunity to cure the disease will almost certainly have been lost, and this is usually the case. The challenge is to diagnose the condition in a patient who presents with intermittent abdominal pain. Even in the absence of the syndrome, any patient with a long history of small bowel obstruction should be suspected of having a carcinoid tumour.[96]

The significant drug development over the past few years has been the new formulations of somatostatin analogues necessitating injection every 2–4 weeks compared with the two or three injections a day with octreotide. Targeted therapy with radiolabelled octreotide and MIBG remains to be fully evaluated.

Current treatment of carcinoid tumours would be to remove the primary tumour and as much secondary tumour as possible and to administer a somatostatin analogue concurrently and thereafter. The methods of reducing hepatic tumour mass include resection and embolisation, but the optimal approach is not known. Chemotherapy is of no proven value for carcinoid tumours of the midgut.

The recent developments that may be of clinical value in the future are the cloning of the *MEN-1* gene[97] and a better understanding of the biology of neuroendocrine cells and the functions of the five somatostatin receptors currently identified. Different receptors seem to control hormone release and apoptosis, and receptor-specific agonists may offer therapeutic opportunities in the future.[98–101]

Carcinoid tumours are diverse and would more appropriately be called neuroendocrine tumours and categorised on the basis of their site of origin and biological, chemical and clinical behaviour.

The evidence base from which therapeutic decisions might be made is small and incomplete—a reflection in part of the design of past clinical studies and the small numbers of patients participating. The recognition of the need to collaborate in basic research, clinical trials and in the formulation of clinical guidelines as regards neuroendocrine tumours has led to the formation of groups focusing on these tumours—in the UK, the UK Network Group and in Europe, the European Neuroendocrine Tumour Network (ENET).

Acknowledgements

The management of carcinoid tumours requires close liaison between pathologists, clinical chemists, radiologists, surgeons, anaesthetists and clinical oncologists and physicians, and we thank our colleagues Alan Johnson, Bill Thomas, Ali Majeed, John Smith, Tony Blakeborough, Peter Gaines, Tim Stephenson, Robert Forrest, Gary Mills, Charles Reilly, John Peacock, David Radford, Wilf Yeo and Thelma Broadhead for their help and guidance. We thank too, all those other colleagues who have referred patients to us.

References

1. Buchanan KD, Johnston CF, O'Hare MMT *et al.* Neuroendocrine tumours. A European view. Am J Med 1986; 81 (suppl 6B): 14–22.

2. Norheim I, Oberg K, Theodorsson-Norheim E *et al.* Malignant carcinoid tumours. Ann Surg 1987; 206: 115–25.

3. Woods HF, Bax NDS, Ainsworth I. Abdominal carcinoid tumours in Sheffield. Digestion 1990; 45 (suppl): 17–22.

4. Newton JN, Swerdlow AJ, dos Santos Sliva IM *et al.* The epidemiology of carcinoid tumours in England and Scotland. Br J Cancer 1994; 70: 939–42.

 5. Modlin IM, Sandor A. An analysis of 8305 cases of carcinoid tumors. Cancer 1997; 79: 813–34.

6. Godwin DJ. Carcinoid tumours: an analysis of 2,837 cases. Cancer 1975; 36: 560–9.

7. Berge T, Linell F. Carcinoid tumours. Acta Pathol Microbiol Scand 1976; 84: 322–30.

8. Weil C. Gastroenterohepatic endocrine tumours. Klin Wochenschr 1985; 63: 433–59.

9. Williams ED, Sandler M. The classification of carcinoid tumours. Lancet 1963; i: 1084–90.

10. Ballantyne GH, Savoca PE, Flannery JT *et al.* Incidence and mortality of carcinoids of the colon. Data from the Connecticut Tumor Registry. Cancer 1992; 69: 2400–5.

11. Vinik AI, Thompson N, Eckhauser F *et al.* Clinical features of carcinoid syndrome and the use of somatostatin analogue in its management. Acta Oncol 1989; 28: 389–402.

12. Bax NDS, Woods HF, Batchelor A *et al.* The clinical manifestations of carcinoid disease. World J Surg 1996; 20: 142–6.

13. Stark S, Bluth I, Rubenstein S. Carcinoid tumour of the ileum resembling regional ileitis clinically and roentgenologically. Gastroenterology 1961; 40: 813–7.

14. Hsu EY, Feldman JM, Lichtenstein GR. Ileal carcinoid tumours simulating Crohn's disease: incidence among 176 consecutive cases of ileal carcinoid. Am J Gastroenterol 1997; 92: 2062–5.

15. Thorson AH. Studies on carcinoid disease. Acta Med Scand 1958; 161, suppl 334.

16. Kahler HJ, Heilmeyer L. Klinik and Pathophysiologie des Karzinoids und Karzinoid syndroms unter Berucksichtigung der Pharmacologie des 5-Hydroxytryptamins. Ergeb Inn Med Kinderheilk 1961; 16: 292–5.

 17. Moyssakis IE, Rallidas LS, Guida GF *et al.* Incidence and evolution of carcinoid syndrome in the heart. J Heart Valve Dis 1997; 6: 625–30.

18. Makridis C, Ekbom A, Bring J *et al.* Survival and daily physical activity in patients treated for advanced midgut carcinoid tumours. Surgery 1997; 122: 1075–82.

19. Robiolio PA, Rigolin VH, Wilson JS *et al.* Carcinoid heart disease. Correlation of high serotonin levels with abnormalities detected by cardiac catheterisation and echocardiography. Circulation 1995; 92: 790–5.

20. Watson RG, Johnston CF, O'Hare MM *et al.* The frequency of gastrointestinal endocrine tumours in a well-defined population—Northern Ireland 1970–1985. Q J Med 1989; 72: 647–57.

21. Rindi G, Bordi C, Rappel S *et al.* Gastric carcinoids and neuroendocrine carcinomas: pathogenesis, pathology and behaviour. World J Surg 1996; 20: 168–72.

22. Grahame-Smith DG. The carcinoid syndrome. London: W Heinemann, 1972.

23. Hauser H, Wolf G, Uranus S *et al.* Neuroendocrine tumours in various organ systems in a ten-year period. Eur J Surg Oncol 1995; 21: 297–300.

24. Gilligan CJ, Lawton GP, Tang LH *et al.* Gastric carcinoid tumours: the biology and therapy of an enigmatic and controversial lesion. Am J Gastroenterol 1995; 90: 338–52.

25. Sjoblom SM, Sipponen P, Miettinen M *et al.* Gastroscopic screening for gastric carcinoids and carcinoma in pernicious anaemia. Endoscopy 1988; 20: 52–6.

26. Granberg D, Wilander E, Strinsberg M *et al.* Clinical symptoms, hormone profiles, treatment, and prognosis in patients with gastric carcinoids. Gut 1998; 43: 223–8.

27. Modlin IM, Sandor A, Tang LH *et al.* A 40-year analysis of 265 gastric carcinoids. Am J Gastroenterol 1997; 92: 633–8.

28. Okike N, Bernatz PE Woolner LB. Carcinoid tumors of the lung. Ann Thorac Surg 1976; 22: 270–7.

29. Limper AH, Carpenter PC, Scheithauer B *et al.* The Cushing syndrome induced by bronchial carcinoid tumours. Ann Intern Med 1992; 117: 209–14.

30. Sandor A, Modlin IM. A retrospective analysis of 1570 appendiceal carcinoids. Am J Gastroenterol 1998; 93: 422–8.

31. Memon MA, Nelson H. Gastrointestinal carcinoid tumours. Dis Colon Rectum 1997; 40: 1101–18.

32. Mani S, Modlin IM, Ballantyne GH et al. Carcinoids of the rectum. J Am Coll Surg 1994; 179: 231–48.

33. Kirshbom PM, Kherani AR, Onaitis MW et al. Carcinoids of unknown origin: comparative analysis with foregut, midgut and hindgut carcinoids. Surgery 1998; 1063–70.

34. Westergaard T, Frisch M, Melbye M. Carcinoid tumours in Denmark 1978–1989 and the risk of subsequent cancers. A population-based study. Cancer 1995; 76: 106–9.

35. Harbour JW, Potter PD, Shields CL et al. Uveal metastases from carcinoid tumour. Ophthalmology 1993; 101: 1084–90.

36. Creutzfeldt W, Stockman F. Carcinoids and carcinoid syndrome. Am J Med 1987; 82: (suppl 5B): 5–16.

37. Janson ET, Holmberg L, Stridsberg M et al. Carcinoid tumours: analysis of prognostic factors and survival in 301 patients from a referral center. Ann Oncol 1997; 8: 685–90.

38. Pirker RA, Pont J, Pohnl R et al. Usefulness of chromogranin A as a marker for the detection of relapses of carcinoid tumours. Clin Chem Lab Med 1998; 36: 837–40.

39. Eriksson B. Tumour markers. Presentation at the European Neuroendocrine Tumour Network Conference. Innsbruck, Feb 2000.

40. Klose K-J. E.N.E.T. Guidelines for CT-MR-UL. Presentation at the European Neuroendocrine Tumour Network Conference. Innsbruck, Feb 2000.

41. Woodard PK, Feldman JM, Paine SS et al. Midgut carcinoid tumours: CT findings and biochemical profiles. J Comput Assis Tomograph 1995; 19: 400–5.

42. Paulson EK, McDermott VG, Keogan MT et al. Carcinoid metastases to the liver: role of triple-phase helical CT. Radiology 1998; 206: 143–50.

43. Krenning EP, Bakker WH, Breeman WAP et al. Localization of endocrine related tumours with radioiodinated analogue of somatostatin. Lancet 1989; i: 242–5.

44. Krenning EP, Kwekkeboom DJ, Bakker WH et al. Somatostatin receptor scintigraphy with [111In-DPTA-d Phe1]- and [123I-Tyr3]- octreotide: the Rotterdam experience with more than 1000 patients. Eur J Nucl Med 1993; 20: 716–31.

45. Kalkner K-M, Janson ET, Nilsson S et al. Somatostatin receptor scintigraphy in patients with carcinoid tumours: comparison between radioligand uptake and tumour markers. Cancer Res 1995; (suppl) 55: 5801–4s.

46. Hoefnagel CA, Taal BG, Valdes Olmos RA. Role of 131I-metaiodobenzylguanidine therapy in carcinoids. J Nucl Biol Med 1991; 35: 346–8.

47. Dresel S, Tatsch K, Zachoval R et al. 111In-octreotide and 123I-MIBG scintigraphy in the diagnosis of small intestinal carcinoid tumours—results of a comparative investigation. (Paper in German-title translated) Nuklearmedizin 1996; 35: 53–8.

48. Zuetenhorst H, Taal BG, Boot H et al. Long-term palliation in metastatic carcinoid tumours with various applications of meta-iodobenzylguanidine (MIBG): pharmacological MIBG, 131I-labelled MIBG and the combination. Eur J Gastroenterol Hepatol 1999; 11: 1157–64.

49. Neijt JP, Lacave AJ, Splinter TA et al. Mitoxantrone in metastatic apudomas: a phase II study of the EORTC Gastro-Intestinal Cancer Cooperative Group. Br J Cancer 1995; 71: 106–8.

50. Sundler F, Hakanson R. Gastric endocrine cell typing at the light microscopic level. In: Hakanson R, Sundler F (eds) The stomach as an endocrine organ. Amsterdam: Elsevier Science Publishers, 1991, pp. 9–26.

51. Capella C, Heitz PU, Hofler H et al. Revised classification of neuroendocrine tumours of the lung, pancreas and gut. Digestion 1994; 55 (suppl 3): 11–23.

52. Solacia E, Rindi G, Paolotti D et al. Clinicopathological profile as a basis for classification of the endocrine tumours of the gastroenteropancreatic tract. Ann Oncol 1999; 10 (suppl 2): 9–15S.

53. Chaudhry A, Oberg K, Wilander E. A study of biological behavior based on the expression of a proliferating antigen in neuroendocrine tumours of the digestive system. Tumor Biol 1992; 13: 27–35.

54. Costes V, Marty-Ane C, Piccot MC et al. Typical and atypical bronchopulmonary carcinoid tumours: a clinicopathologic and KI-67-labelling study. Hum Pathol 1995; 26: 740–5.

55. Stridsberg M, Oberg K, Li Q et al. Measurements of chromogranin A, chromogranin B (secretogranin I), chromogranin C (secretogranin II) and pancreastatin in plasma and urine from patients with carcinoid tumours and endocrine pancreatic tumours. J Endocrinol 1995; 144: 49–59.

56. Moertel CG. Karnofsky memorial lecture. An odyssey in a land of small tumours. J Clin Oncol 1987; 5: 1502–22.

57. Wangberg B, Getered K, Nilsson O et al. Embolisation therapy in the midgut carcinoid syndrome: just tumour ischaemia? Acta Oncol 1993; 32: 251–6.

58. Ahlman H, Westberg G, Wangberg B et al. Treatment of liver metastases of carcinoid tumours. World J Surg 1996; 20: 196–202.

59. Ahlman H, Schersten T, Tisell LE. Surgical treatment of patients with carcinoid syndrome. Acta Oncol 1989; 28: 403–7.

60. Que FG, Nagorney DM, Batts KP *et al*. Hepatic resection for metastatic neuroendocrine carcinomas. Am J Surg 1995; 169: 36–42.

61. Woods HF, Bax NDS, Smith JARS. Small bowel carcinoid tumours. World J Surg 1985; 9: 921–9.

62. Ahlman H, Kolby L, Lundell L *et al*. Clinical management of gastric carcinoid tumours. Digestion 1994; 55 (suppl 3): 77–85.

63. Ahlman H. Surgery including liver transplantation. Presentation at the European Neuroendocrine Tumour Network Conference. Innsbruck, Feb 2000.

64. Dousset B. Saint-Marc O, Pitre J *et al*. Metastatic endocrine tumours: medical treatment, surgical resection, or liver transplantation. World J Surg 1996; 20: 908–14.

65. Curtiss SI, Mor E, Schwartz ME *et al*. A rational approach to the use of hepatic transplantation in the treatment of metastatic neuroendocrine tumors. J Am Coll Surg 1995; 180: 184–7.

66. Ahlman H, Nilsson O, Wangberg B *et al*. Neuroendocrine insights from the laboratory to the clinic. Am J Surg 1996; 172: 61–7.

67. Veall GRQ, Peacock JE, Bax NDS *et al*. Review of the anaesthetic management of 21 patients undergoing laparotomy for carcinoid syndrome. Br J Anaes 1994; 72: 335–41.

68. Frolich JC, Bloomgarten ZT, Oates JA *et al*. The carcinoid flush: provocation by pentagastrin and inhibition by somatostatin. N Engl J Med 1978; 299: 1055–7.

69. Kvols LK, Moertel CG, O'Connell MJ *et al*. Treatment of the malignant carcinoid syndrome. Evaluation of a long-acting somatostatin analogue. N Engl J Med 1986; 315: 663–6.

70. Harris AG, Redfern JS. Octreotide treatment of carcinoid syndrome: analysis of dose titration data. Aliment Pharm Ther 1995; 9: 387–94.

71. Wymenga ANM, Eriksson B, Salmela PI *et al*. Efficacy and safety of prolonged-release lanreotide in patients with gastrointestinal neuroendocrine tumours and hormone related symptoms. J Clin Oncol 1999; 4: 1111–7.

72. Ruszniewski P, Ducreux M, Chayvialle J-A *et al*. Treatment of the carcinoid syndrome with the longacting somatostatin analogue lanreotide: a prospective study in 39 patients. Gut 1996; 39: 279–83.

73. Rubin J, Ajani J, Schirmer W *et al*. Octreotide acetate long-acting formulation versus open-label subcutaneous octreotide acetate in malignant carcinoid syndrome. J Clin Oncol 1999; 17: 600–6.

74. Trendle MC, Moertel CG, Kvols LK. Incidence and morbidity of cholelithiasis in patients receiving chronic octreotide for metastatic carcinoid and malignant islet cell tumours. Cancer 1997; 79: 830–4.

75. Frank F, Klose KJ, Weid M *et al*. Combination therapy with octreotide and alpha interferon: effect on tumour growth in metastatic endocrine gastroenteropancreatic tumours. Am J Gastroenterol 1999; 94: 1381–7.

76. Oberg K, Funa K, Alm G. Effects of leucocyte interferon on clinical symptoms and hormone levels in patients with mid-gut carcinoid tumours and carcinoid syndrome. Lancet 1983; 309: 129–33.

77. Oberg K, Norheim I, Lind E *et al*. Treatment of malignant carcinoid tumours with human leucocyte interferon—long term results. Cancer Treat Rep 1986; 70: 1297–1304.

78. Oberg K. Interferon review. Presentation at the European Neuroendocrine Tumour Network Conference. Innsbruck, Feb 2000.

79. Otte A, Mueller-Brand J, Dellas S *et al*. Yttrium-90-labelled somatostatin-analogue for cancer treatment. Lancet 1998; 351: 417–8.

80. McCarthy KE, Woltering EA, Espenan GD *et al*. In situ radiotherapy with ^{111}In-pentetreotide: initial observations and future directions. Can J Sci American 1998; 4: 94–102.

81. Moertel CG, Kvols LK, O'Connell MJ *et al*. Treatment of neuroendocrine carcinomas with combined etoposide and cisplatin. Evidence of major therapeutic activity in the anaplastic variants of these neoplasms. Cancer 1991; 68: 227–32.

82. Moertel CG, Hanley JA, Johnson LA. Streptozocin compared with streptozocin plus fluorouracil in the treatment of advanced islet-cell carcinoma. N Engl J Med 1980; 303: 1189–94.

83. Moertel CG, Lefkopoulo M, Lipsitz S *et al*. Streptozocin doxorubicin, streptozocin–fluorouracil or chlorozotocin in the treatment of advanced islet-cell carcinoma. N Engl J Med 1992; 326: 563–5.

84. Allison DJ, Modlin IM, Jenkins WJ. Treatment of carcinoid liver metastases by hepatic artery embolisation. Lancet 1977; ii: 1323–5.

85. Wangberg B, Geterud K, Nilsson O *et al*. Embolisation therapy in the midgut carcinoid syndrome: just tumour ischaemia? Acta Oncol 1993; 32: 251–6.

86. Eriksson BK, Larsson EG, Skogseid BM *et al*. Liver embolizations of patients with malignant neuroendocrine gastrointestinal tumors. Cancer 1998; 83: 2293–301.

87. Brown KT, Koh BY, Brody LA *et al*. Particle embolisation of hepatic neuroendocrine metastases for control of pain and hormonal symptoms. J Vasc Interv Radiol 1999; 10: 397–403.

88. Ruszniewski P, Rougier P, Roche A *et al.* Hepatic arterial chemoembolization in patients with liver metastases of endocrine tumours. Cancer 1993; 71: 2624–30.

89. Diaco DS, Hajarizadeh H, Mueller CR *et al.* Treatment of metastatic carcinoid tumours using multimodality therapy of octreotide acetate, intra-arterial chemotherapy, and hepatic arterial chemoembolization. Am J Surg 1995; 169: 523–8.

90. Tommasseti P, Del Vecchio E, Faccioli P *et al.* Treatment of liver metastases of an endocrine pancreatic tumour by hepatic artery chemoembolisation. J Clin Gastroenterol 1994; 18: 170–2.

91. Jacobsen MB, Hanssen LE, Kolmannskog F *et al.* Interferon-alpha 2b, with or without prior hepatic artery embolization: clinical response and survival in mid-gut carcinoid patients. The Norwegian carcinoid study. Scand J Gastroenterol 1995; 30: 789–96.

92. Chakravarth A, Abrams RA. Radiation therapy in the management of patients with malignant carcinoid tumours. Cancer 1994; 75: 1386–90.

93. Sjoerdsma A, Weissbach H, Udenfriend S. A clinical, physiologic and biochemical study of patients with malignant carcinoid (argentaffinoma). Am J Med 1956; 20: 520–32.

94. Ransom WB. A case of primary carcinoma of the ileum. Lancet 1890; ii: 1020–3.

95. Shebani KO, Souba WW, Finkelstein DM *et al.* Prognosis and survival in patients with gastrointestinal tract carcinoid tumours. Ann Surg 1999; 229: 815–21.

96. Stewart WH, Bartlett RM, Bishop HM *et al.* Carcinoid tumours presenting with acute abdominal signs. Ann Surg 1961; 154: 112–20.

97. Chandrasekharappa SC, Guru SC, Manickam U *et al.* Positioning cloning of the gene for multiple endocrine neoplasia-type 1. Science 1997; 276: 404–7.

98. Sharma K, Patel YC, Srikant CB. Subtype-selective induction of wild-type p53 apoptosis, but not cell cycle arrest, by human somatostatin receptor 3. Mol Endocrinol 1996; 10: 1688–96.

99. Cordelier P, Esteve JP, Bousquet C *et al.* Characterisation of the antiproliferative signal mediated by the somatostatin receptor subtype sst5. Proc Natl Acad Sci 1997; 94: 9343–8.

100. Caron P, Buscail L, Beckers A *et al.* Expression of somatostatin receptor SST4 in human placenta and absence of octreotide effect on human placental growth hormone concentration during pregnancy. J Clin Endocrinol Metab 1997; 82: 3771–6.

101. Pages P, Benali N, Saint-Laurent N *et al.* sst2 somatostatin receptor mediates cell cycle arrest and induction of p27 (Kip1). Evidence for the role of SHP-1. J Biol Chem 1999; 274: 15186–93.

7 Clinical governance and quality in endocrine surgery

B. J. Harrison

Clinical governance

'Expert knowledge is often incomplete and influenced by strongly held beliefs and personal interest'

The measurement and regulation of clinical activity is here to stay. Most surgeons would agree that unacceptable variations in standards of care and outcomes must be reduced. Yet, despite best intentions, therapeutic activity that is ineffective or unsubstantiated may take many years to disappear from clinical practice. In addition, our individual practice and the interventions that we use inevitably reflect the current fashion, albeit inappropriate in terms of any evidence base. We should not, however, lose sight of the fact that the 'evidence base' and systematic reviews may be adversely affected by subjective analysis, interpretations of variations in the results from previous studies, publication bias and missing data. Changes in clinical practice can be exciting, but surgeons should be wary of advancing through errors. From an idea and hypothesis through technical development there should be systematic progression, which ends in appropriate outcome measure development and assessment.[1] This certainly applies to the development of minimally invasive surgery of the thyroid and parathyroid glands.[2] Are mortality and readmission rates, complications and duration of hospital stay sufficient to compare the new with what has gone before? Insisting that all studies are randomised and that all studies should use historical controls shares one thing in common. Both are equally wrong.

The key points of clinical governance are to avoid risk, to detect adverse events rapidly and to improve clinical care. We can effect these by continued professional development, quality improvement, risk management and clinical effectiveness. Guidelines should help us make decisions about what is appropriate, leading to change and improvement in patient care. Guidelines that are of use will identify the key decisions and consequences in association with review of the relevent evidence required to inform such decisions. We should not succumb to the reactionary view that the development and use of guidelines for endocrine surgery can be avoided. A dogmatic approach to what are 'appropriate' treatments is inappropriate. Examination of new and old controversies in endocrine surgery as shown below tells us that there is currently little evidence to support a rigid approach in how we advise our patients.

Thyroid disease

- Do all patients with retrosternal goitre require surgery?
- Radioiodine or surgery for patients with retrosternal goitre?
- The extent of surgery for differentiated thyroid cancer?
- The extent of lymph node surgery in differentiated and medullary thyroid cancer?
- When to complete primary surgery/reoperate in patients with medullary thyroid cancer?

Parathyroid

- The indications for surgery in those with mild hypercalcaemia
- What are the indications for reoperative parathyroid surgery?
- Which, if any, imaging studies are appropriate prior to first time surgery?
- Which imaging studies are appropriate prior to reoperative surgery?
- Unilateral or bilateral neck exploration?
- Minimally invasive surgery?

Adrenal

- Transperitoneal or retroperitoneal laparoscopic surgery?
- What size of incidentaloma should be removed?
- Partial adrenalectomy in familial disease?

Pancreas

- Which preoperative localisation/regionalisation studies are required in patients with insulinoma/gastrinoma?
- When to operate on the pancreas in patients with multiple endocrine neoplasia type I syndrome?

Clinical governance and quality are synonomous with achieving and maintaining good practice. These in turn require that the appropriate surgeon (and trainee) is available to appropriately treat the patient with appropriate outcome and morbidity against appropriate standards. The endocrine surgeon must be part of a team that includes endocrine physicians, oncologists, radiologists, cytopathologists, histopathologists, chemical pathologists and clinical/molecular geneticists.

What is good practice?

There are few if any emergencies in endocrine surgery, thus endocrine surgeons have ample time before any elective intervention to ask:

- Which biochemical/cytological tests and imaging studies are necessary prior to surgery, and will their results alter the management of the patient?
- Should we operate? How will this benefit the patient? What is the purpose and aim of the procedure?
- Which operation is appropriate in this specific case?
- Does the patient understand the indications, implications and risks of surgery in order to give informed consent?
- Are there alternative therapies other than surgery?

Critical review of our current practice with these questions in mind will benefit our patients prior to, during and after surgery.

Who should perform surgery on the endocrine glands and the 'turf' war?

In the USA, thyroid operations comprise fewer than 5% of an average general surgeon's practice. This figure justifies the 1996 consensus statement on thyroid disease by the Royal College of Physicians of London and the Society of Endocrinology,[3] which stated that 'each district general hospital should have access to an experienced thyroid surgeon.' Although the domain of surgery of the endocrine glands is currently debated between general surgeons—endocrine/upper gastrointestinal tract/hepatobiliary, head and neck, oromaxillo-facial, ENT and urologists—no individual group has an unassailable right to care for and treat the patients. The needs of the patient must come first. The introduction to the British Association of Endocrine Surgeons (BAES) guidelines states

'...[*the guidelines do*] not define an endocrine surgeon or specify who should practice endocrine surgery ... Elective endocrine surgery will not be in the portfolio of every district general hospital, but where it is, based on experience and caseload, it should be in the hands of a nominated surgeon with an endocrine interest. Those patients requiring more complex investigation and care as detailed in the guidelines should be referred to an appropriate centre. These rare and complex diseases will only be managed effectively by multidisciplinary teams in units familiar with these disorders ... this category includes patients with endocrine pancreatic tumours, adrenal tumours, thyroid malignancy especially medullary thyroid carcinoma, familial syndromes and those requiring reoperative thyroid and parathyroid surgery...'

Subspecialisation

The advantages of subspecialisation to the patient are better outcome and fewer complications.

It is all too easy to lose sight of the important issues:

1.   The experienced surgeon should be part of an experienced multidisciplinary team.

There is evidence from the UK to support a continued need for subspecialisation in endocrine surgery i.e. to further good practice. This is exemplified both by the use of fine needle aspiration cytology (FNAC) in patients with thyroid disease and by morbidity from surgery. FNAC, in addition to clinical examination, is the most sensitive and specific test for the diagnosis of thyroid nodules and will reduce the need for surgery by at least 25%. Isotope scanning and ultrasonography contribute little to the diagnostic investigation of a euthyroid patient with nodular thyroid disease. Although more than 25 years have passed since FNAC of the thyroid was introduced, in a retrospective study from the South West Thames region, only 8% of the patients who underwent surgery had undergone preoperative needle aspiration of the thyroid;[4] 34% of 186 operations were deemed avoidable. In the same region 50 surgeons undertook a caseload of less than 500 thyroidectomies per year. In a retrospective study from a single district hospital, only 42% of patients with thyroid cancer presenting with a thyroid nodule had preoperative FNAC.[5] The BAES audit in 1995 demonstrated that FNAC use related to the number of thyroid operations performed.[6] Surgeons who performed less than 25 thyroidectomies per year used preoperative fine needle aspiration in only 42% of cases overall and in 50% of the cases in which the final diagnosis was cancer. Among 107 non-specialist surgeons interviewed by postal questionnaire in the North West/Mersey regions,[7] a median of 10 thyroidectomies were performed per year, and 20% of district general hospital surgeons never used FNAC. In the same study, 40% of surgeons replied that they would perform nodule excision alone or subtotal lobectomy for a solitary nodule, an operation that is to be condemned in the management of this condition.

Complication rates of thyroid and parathyroid procedures will vary according to the experience of the surgeon, being higher in patients treated by non-specialists, as shown in Europe[8] and the USA.[9] In the UK, a retrospective study from North Trent identified that over a 10-year period, 32 surgeons operated on 148 patients with thyroid cancer subsequently referred to a thyroid cancer clinic. Recurrent laryngeal nerve palsy and hypoparathyroidism were more common after surgery by non-specialists, and more than 50% of the surgeons had treated only a single patient with thyroid cancer in 10 years. A further 101 patients over the same period were never referred to a multidisciplinary thyroid cancer clinic for consideration of adjuvant therapy.[10]

2. As the quality of the care received by the patient is paramount, it should be subjected to assessment by audit and benchmarking against agreed standards.

It is clear from the above studies that there is a need to collect prospective information on endocrine surgical activity in the UK, not only for issues of surgical subspecialisation, but for education and training. The BAES have initiated a long-term prospective audit that will provide much needed information on activity and outcome. Membership of the association will be conditional on providing information. The following standards and outcome measures are suggested as being applicable to current endocrine surgical practice.

Thyroid

Standards

- The indications for operation, risks and complications should be discussed with patients prior to surgery.
- FNAC should be performed routinely in the investigation of solitary thyroid nodules.
- The recurrent laryngeal nerve should be routinely identified in patients undergoing thyroid surgery.
- All patients scheduled for reoperative thyroid surgery should undergo preoperative examination of their vocal cords by an appropriately skilled independent doctor (e.g. an ENT surgeon). All patients reporting voice change after thyroid surgery should undergo examination of their vocal cords. Permanent vocal cord palsy should not occur in more than 1% of patients.
- A return to theatre to control postoperative haemorrhage should occur in less than 5% of patients.
- All patients with thyroid cancer should be reviewed by the cancer center designated specialist multidisciplinary team.

Outcome measures

There should be documented evidence to support that:

- The patient was informed of the indications for surgery and its risks and complications.
- FNAC was performed in at least 90% of patients prior to operation for solitary/dominant nodules.
- The recurrent laryngeal nerve/s were identified during a surgical procedure.
- The permanent postoperative vocal cord palsy rate is not more than 1%.
- All patients scheduled for reoperative thyroid surgery have undergone pre-operative examination of their vocal cords.
- The reoperation rate for postoperative haemorrhage after thyroidectomy is less than 5%.
- Patients with thyroid malignancy have been reviewed by the specialist multidisciplinary team.

Parathyroid

Standards

In patients who undergo first time operation for primary hyperparathyroidism:

- The indications for operation, risks and complications should be discussed with patients prior to surgery.
- The surgeon should identify and cure the cause of the disease in at least 95% of cases.
- All patients reporting voice change after parathyroid surgery should undergo examination of their vocal cords. Permanent vocal cord palsy should not occur in more than 1% of patients.
- All patients scheduled for reoperative parathyroid surgery should undergo preoperative examination of their vocal cords.
- Permanent hypocalcaemia should not occur in more than 5% of patients.

Outcome measures

There should be documented evidence to support that:

- The patient was informed of the indications for surgery and its risks and complications.
- After first time parathyroid surgery, at least 90% of patients are normocalcaemic without calcium or vitamin D supplements.
- The permanent postoperative vocal cord palsy rate is not more than 1%.
- All patients scheduled for reoperative parathyroid surgery have undergone preoperative examination of their vocal cords.

Adrenal

Standards

There should be multidisciplinary working to agreed diagnostic and therapeutic protocols that ensure an appropriate strategy is developed which includes the management of the pre-, per- and postoperative metabolic syndrome.

Outcome measures

There should be documented evidence to show that all patients have been discussed with the multidisciplinary team.

Biochemical cure should be evident in at least:

- 90% of patients with phaeochromocytoma
- 90% of patients with Conn's syndrome
- 90% of patients with Cushing's syndrome

Pancreas

Standards

- There should be multidisciplinary working to agreed diagnostic and therapeutic protocols that ensure an appropriate strategy is developed which includes the management of the pre-, per- and postoperative metabolic syndrome.
- Patients with familial endocrine disease should be identified prior to surgery.
- The aims of any surgical procedure must be clearly defined prior to surgery.

Outcome measures

There should be documented evidence to show that all patients have been discussed with the multidisciplinary team.

For *insulinoma*, surgery should result in a biochemical cure in at least 90% of cases, and for *gastrinoma*, surgery should result in a biochemical cure or clinically useful response in at least 60% of cases.

Training surgeons

Who should train the future endocrine surgeons and to what level of expertise?

Surgeons in training when appropriately supervised and assisted by their trainers can perform safe thyroidectomy.[11,12] Furthermore, surgeons who have completed a well designed training programme and who have become proficient in thyroid surgery will remain proficient when they practise as consultants.[13] In the UK, the higher surgical trainee should spend at least 1 year in an approved unit, which should consist of:

- One or more surgeons with a declared interest in endocrine surgery
- An annual operative workload in excess of 50 patients (verified by BAES audit)
- On-site cytology and histopathology services
- At least one consultant endocrinologist on site, holding one or more dedicated endocrinology clinics per week, with joint clinics or formal meetings held not less than once per month
- A department of nuclear medicine on site
- On-site magnetic resonance imaging and computed tomography scanning

In practical terms, flexible rotations between regions may be required for more specialised areas of endocrine practice, e.g. adrenal surgery.[14]

There is a clear need to improve the standards of care for patients with endocrine disorders requiring surgery in the UK, guidelines and audit will help surgeons pass the 'shadow line'[15] to achieve:

'…gains not only to oneself, but to the whole practice of surgery … not at the expense of overlooking how much there must always be to learn; the confidence and pride in one's own abilities that allows criticism from both within and without … a view of medicine as a whole that can allow all its surprises and uncertainties to be one's companions throughout one's career not as spectres reflecting inadequacy, but as impartial guides who point out the way forward…'.

Effective clinical governance will help define:

- The appropriateness and effectiveness of our interventions
- The lack of evidence that supports some of our current practice
- The needs for further research

Endocrine surgeons are not simply technicians; they must be both self-regulators and knowledgeable members of the endocrine team.

References

1. Lorenz W, Troidl H, Solomkin JS *et al.* Second step: testing-outcome measurements. World J Surg 1999; 23: 768–80.

2. Miccoli P. Minimally invasive endocrine surgery [editorial]. Acta Chir Austriaca 1999; 31: 195.

3. Vanderpump MP, Ahlquist JA, Franklyn JA *et al.* Concensus statement for good practice in the management of hypothyroidism and hyperthyroidism. The Research Unit of the Royal College of Physicians of London, the Endocrinology and Diabetes Committee of the Royal College of Physicians of London, and the Society for Endocrinology. BMJ 1996; 313: 539–44.

4. Asimakopoulos G, Loosemore T, Bowyer RC *et al.* A regional study of thyroidectomy: surgical pathology suggests scope to improve quality and reduce cost. Ann R Coll Surg Engl 1995; 77: 425–30.

5. Vanderpump MP, Alexander L, Scarpello JH *et al.* An audit of the management of thyroid cancer in a district general hospital. Clin Endocrinol (Oxf) 1998; 48: 419–24.

6. Chadwick DR, Harrison BJ. The role of fine-needle aspiration cytology and frozen section histology in management of differentiated thyroid cancer: the U.K. experience. Langenbeck's Arch Surg 1998; 383: 164–6.

7. Peacock T, Parrott NR. Variations in the surgical practice of thyroidectomy. Br J Surg 1997; 84: 1314.

8. Harness JK, van Heerden JA, Lennquist S *et al.* Future of thyroid surgery and training surgeons to meet the expectations of 2000 and beyond. World J Surg 2000; 24: 976–82.

9. Sosa JA, Bowman HM, Tielsch JM *et al.* The importance of surgeon experience for clinical and economic outcomes from thyroidectomy. Ann Surg 1998; 228: 320–30.

10. Miller BA, Moore S, Harrison BJ. Thyroid cancer management in North Trent. Case record review confirm the need for specialist care. Br J Surg 2000; 87: 1260.

11. Runkel N, Riede E, Mann B *et al.* Surgical training and vocal-cord paralysis in benign thyroid disease. Langenbeck's Arch Surg 1998; 383: 240–2.

12. Mishra A, Agarwal G, Agrawal A *et al.* Safety and efficacy of total thyroidectomy in hands of endocrine trainees. Am J Surg 1999; 178: 377–80.

13. Reeve TS, Curtin A, Fingleton L *et al.* Can total thyroidectomy be performed as safely by general surgeons in provincial centers as by surgeons in specialised endocrine surgical units? Making the case for surgical training. Arch Surg 1994; 129: 834–6.

14. A curriculum, organisation and syllabus for higher surgical training in general surgery and its sub-specialties. SAC in General Surgery, Joint Committee on higher Surgical Training, 1998. London: Royal College of Surgeons.

15. Hayward R. The shadow-line in surgery. Lancet 1987; 1: 375–6.

8 Medico–legal aspects of endocrine surgery

Anthony E. Young
Adam E. Young

Introduction

In this chapter we cover the steps needed to avoid complaint and litigation in endocrine surgery and suggest some responses to complaints or litigation, with an outline of the processes involved. We have tried to be as brief as possible and to avoid legal terminology except where it may be needed to interpret papers or events. We have based our views on an interpretation of English law and it should be remembered that in legal actions the jurisdiction that applies is that of the country in which injury occurred.

It is possible to go through a surgical career without ever being personally involved in litigation, although as practitioners become more senior they will almost invariably find themselves invited to give an expert opinion on the misfortunes of others. We have therefore described the role of expert opinion.

Litigation and complaint is on the increase and poor performance less readily forgiven than it was in the past. Therefore, the first step in approaching the issue of medical litigation is to look at the ways by which one's practice may be conducted so as to minimise, or even obviate, the risk of complaint and litigation.

Ensuring that things go smoothly

Risk management is the official title for ensuring that things go smoothly. It is a new phrase in most clinicians' vocabulary, and it neatly encapsulates the notion that all surgical activity involves some degree of risk and that the risk must be managed so as to achieve the best outcome for the patient. This is, and always was, an active process, but whereas in the past it was sufficient merely to be properly trained, caring and conscientious, against a background of optimism that does not now suffice. Not only must medical care be done effectively and carefully, but it must be seen to be done effectively and carefully. However cynical one might be about the mechanics of clinical governance and however self-confident one may feel as a professional, there is now a need to take public and documented steps to ensure that risk is being managed. This is not just defensive and reactive—there is already evidence that the risk management process has positive advantages in terms of delivering a higher quality of care, measured not only as an improved process of care but also better outcomes. Nevertheless whether the full bureaucratic processes of clinical governance can measurably improve clinical outcome so as to justify their considerable expense and disruption remains to be seen.[1] We will probably never know.

Risk management

Imagine yourself as the recently appointed clinical director of a department of surgery. What areas might be looked at to reassure yourself that risks taken by your endocrine surgeon are minimal? We suggest the following:

Staff issues

1. Are the consultants properly trained? Are they up-to-date with their postgraduate education in the field of endocrine surgery? Are you sure that other consultants are not undertaking endocrine surgery on an occasional basis because they enjoy it rather than because they are trained in it? If your hospital is a small one, are the consultants ready to refer complex patients to a specialist centre elsewhere?

2. Are the trainees appropriately engaged in the process? That is to say, if they are undertaking surgery has it been delegated by the appropriate person to the appropriate trainee in the full knowledge of the trainee's competence? In terms of their operative experience, is their supervision appropriate? It is not, for example, satisfactory to let new specialist registrars undertake a thyroidectomy just because they assert that they are capable of doing it. It is necessary first to supervise them undertaking thyroidectomy. This may mean cancelling cases when you are away or having a list take somewhat longer. Although the managerial side of the health service find the reduced service provision associated with this stance difficult to accept, one should not be abashed about insisting on it.

3. Are the working hours conducive to good practice? Are all staff working a sensible timetable that ensures that they will not be undertaking major surgery or making difficult decisions when they are tired or ill? Of course

such eventualities are not necessarily avoidable, but the directorate needs to have a plan in place to minimise it.

Communication issues

Are you comfortable that the patients are being properly informed about planned surgery and the alternative therapeutic options open to them (see informed consent below)? As a clinical director you will need to ensure that information sheets and procedure-specific consent forms are available and used.

Protocol issues

Are there agreed and shared protocols for dealing with specific clinical issues? Some of this will be to do with clinical decision taking, where adherence to, for instance, British Association of Endocrine Surgeons' guidelines will suffice, and some will need to be purely local. Examples of this latter situation are, for example, a written protocol for postoperative care of patients after thyroidectomy and a written protocol for house officers dealing with replacement medication after parathyroidectomy and adrenalectomy.

Record keeping

The NHS has a poor track record concerning record keeping. Hospital notes are usually disorganised and often lost or unavailable. If events are such that a legal case eventually develops, then the unavailability of records may be disastrous, wrecking an otherwise sound case. Clear and contemporaneous evidence must be available in the notes, showing that patients were properly counselled beforehand, were warned about the risks of surgery and that these were recorded in the notes. Similarly, the operation notes should be contemporaneous, written by the operating surgeons (or at the very least countersigned by them) and should confirm that, for example, during a thyroidectomy the recurrent laryngeal nerves were seen and spared and that parathyroid glandular tissue was retained.

Support services

You should check the quality of imaging and pathology services, especially cytopathology in relation to the thyroid. An increasingly common issue in litigation is delay in diagnosis or incorrect diagnosis, and in this context it is imperative that your cytologist should be known to be competent, not just in general cytology but in the specific and often difficult area of thyroid cytology.

Audit

Remember that simply keeping audit records and having regular audit meetings is not sufficient. The audit cycle must be seen to be occurring such that what has been learned from audit is applied and the whole cycle repeated. Of course this rarely happens. A National Audit Office report has found that only one formal audit study in six had gone round the whole audit cycle and was being repeated.[2]

Consent

A formal process of consent in surgery is essential as it is that consent that renders surgical intervention legal. Consent requires that the patient has the *capacity* to understand the process, has the *information* about the nature and the purpose of the surgery to allow informed consent and provides consent *voluntarily*. Failure to respect these principles means that there was effectively no consent, and the doctor is therefore open to charges of battery or to a claim of negligence. 'Battery' is the unlawful infliction of force on another person, negligence is the failure to take reasonable care. The courts have shown no enthusiasm for pursuing medical cases as battery and most concerning the adequacy of information giving are brought under the tort of negligence.

Lord Justice Dunn said in the hallmark UK case of Sidaway 'the concept of informed consent forms no part of English law.'[3] As in England, there is no explicit legal meaning to the term 'informed consent' that doctors use, and the topic exercises lawyers more than a little. The case of Sidaway revolves around a case in 1984 in which a patient experienced complications from spinal cord damage after an operation on a cervical vertebra as treatment for root pain. She had not been informed about this particular rare complication when she gave her consent, and she claimed that she would not have had the operation if more information had been available. The legal debate about consent revolves not around the necessity of it but the extent. In the Sidaway case, the patient was not warned because the neurosurgeon judged the risk to be remote, i.e. less than 1%. The problem is the potential gap between the 'patient standard,' which is what the patient might wish to know, and the 'professional standard,' which is what the doctor thinks the patient ought to or needs to know. Obviously patients who experience a complication from an operation will, with the wisdom of hindsight, wish they had been told about a rare but damaging complication, whereas surgeons in prospect might reasonably not tell patients of risks that occurred in only 1 of 200 patients (as was the case with Sidaway). In the matter of consent (as in most other medico–legal issues), case law in England and Scotland tends to reflect the application of the 'Bolam test' (see below), namely that the information that the surgeon needs to give is the information that a reasonable and responsible member of the medical profession would think it proper to give in the circumstances. The amount of information that is given to validate 'informed' consent is not defined in law. The rule of thumb is that it should be any risk that is likely to occur in more than 1–2% of cases, but it is important to remember that the quality of information given for consent in medical care is an ethical not a legal requirement of a doctor and is to do with the respect for the autonomy of the patient.[4] Ian Kennedy, not known for his sympathy to the medical view of events, describes the modern legal framework of consent on the basis of the Sidaway case as being 'unsupportable, both in principle and on its own reasoning'.[5] Sidaway puts the onus on doctors to decide what information to give, and the ethical requirement is merely to give what doctors' best judgement of patients defines as their need and to give it in terms appropriate to their understanding and their education. The American view of informed consent is based on what the prudent patient would wish to know rather than what the doctor judges is appropriate to tell. One suspects that practice will inexorably edge to the North American attitude to informed consent, which requires that far more risks are explained to patients and more explicitly. This trend is also likely to be encouraged by the Council of Europe's Convention on Human Rights: Biomedicine, 1997, which explicitly notes the 'need to restrain the paternalist approaches which might ignore the wishes of the patient.'[6] This all sounds very confrontational. It is better to look at the process of 'informed' consent as part of a shared decision-making process, founded in adult debate with patients about the management of their disease, such that the risks and consequences of the alternative treatment options are discussed in sufficient detail to be understood and in enough detail to allow them to make informed decisions.

As the need to inform prior to obtaining consent increases, this does not necessarily mean that the risks of being sued if things go wrong are also increasing. The 'doctrine of causation' is protective simply because it requires that the plaintiff (the suing patient) prove that if he or she had been told of the risks he or she would have refused the treatment. That, given the element of retrospection, is difficult to prove.

The chips are stacked against patients in both England and Scotland if an action is sought about the failure of the adequacy of consent. Successful negligence actions on the basis of flawed consent are virtually non-existent in the UK. One writer found only one case, Gookarni v Tayside Health Board 1991,[7] but to this might be added the case of Rogers v Whitaker in which a doctor was found negligent of failing to warn of the 1:14 000 risk of sympathetic ophthalmia after eye surgery, even though a responsible body of ophthalmologists would not have so warned.[8] The law may be changing its stance in favour of patients, as 'bilateralism'—respecting the autonomy of the patient—replaces a traditional paternalism.

- Obtain consent well before the operation
- Do not obtain consent after sedation has been given
- The person getting consent should be knowledgeable about the operation and its potential complications
- Explain 'material' risks
- Answer patients questions openly and honestly
- Do not subsequently alter the consent form
- Do not exceed the authority given. Additional procedures found necessary during the operation are covered only if they are necessary for the preservation of life or health

Table 8.1 *Check points for consent*

In practical terms the surgeon, or somebody who is familiar with the disease and its treatment, must sign the consent form together with the patient. Although we recommend the use of information sheets for patients (as illustrated in the British Association of Endocrine Surgeons' guidelines), their use does not obviate the need for detailed personal discussions between patients and surgeons.

We have dwelt at length on this seemingly straightforward topic because failure to inform appropriately of risks and to communicate effectively is perhaps the commonest starting point for litigation (**Table 8.1**).

When things do not go smoothly

Although many surgeons are anxious—even paranoid—about complaint and litigation, they need to remember that many things can and do go wrong during hospital admissions, and yet extremely few of them result in complaints and even fewer in litigation. The Harvard medical practice study found that 3.7% of admissions resulted in an adverse event, and in 1% of cases care was judged to be negligent and to have contributed to permanent disability or death.[9] This is probably a low figure, as an Australian study found that 16.6% of admissions resulted in an adverse event.[10] Only a tiny percentage of problems and errors mature into a complaint. It is clear that if complaints are handled effectively and promptly and if there is good and honest communication of facts, then the number of complaints that will mature into litigations will be few. The widely cited reason for this is that patients actively want to find out what happened when things do not turn out well, but once they are properly informed are less likely to be litigious. In reality one of the virtues of proper handling of complaints is that they often show that although everything did not turn out for the best, problems were within the boundaries of that experienced in medical care and were not a sign of negligence.

Handling complaints

After the Hospital Complaints Procedure Act, 1985, all hospitals now have a formal and structured process for dealing with complaints, and it is important that any complaint that has any degree of formality to it—and that normally means one made in writing—should be entered into this process. Informal complaints should be dealt with as promptly and as honestly as possible in the format of a normal communication, and it does no harm if there has been a degree of error to admit that and to apologise early. The authors, however, believe that if the surgeon or the person to whom the complaint has been made makes an honest and insightful assessment of the problem and considers that there has *not* been an error, there is no requirement to apologise simply because that is currently the politically correct thing to do. Any complaints that are dealt with orally should be recorded as a written or typed note and put in the patients' records. Nothing should be sent out in writing without first checking the text with the Trust's complaints officer and/or your defence organisation. This is invaluable if an informal complaint that is thought to have been dealt with satisfactorily turns subsequently into a formal one.

The formal handling of complaints

Local resolution of complaints

Procedures that came into force in April 1996 have defined in detail how, and how speedily, hospitals must respond to complaints. These processes have some key objectives:

- Ease of access to the complaints' system
- A simple, rapid, open process
- Fairness for complainants and staff alike
- Lessons from complaints to be used to improve patient services
- Investigation of complaints to be entirely separate from any subsequent disciplinary proceedings

Complaints must be made within 6 months of the event complained about or from the moment that patients realised that there had been a problem. The complaint can go through consecutive stages:

1. Local resolution;
2. Independent review;
3. Appeal to the health service ombudsman.

Details of these processes, which can be very cumbersome, can be found in your own hospitals' circulars or elsewhere.[11] These processes have been in place for over 4 years and most people (both staff and complainants) find them wanting. Staff feel that the process is too cumbersome and that so-called independent reviews are often not that but, by their reliance on lay members, tend to be too confrontational and too often lead to inappropriate disciplinary procedures. A review of the workings of the complaints' system noted that it was perceived as 'biased, closed and inadequate' and that 'patients feel suspicious, frustrated and let down' and clinicians 'undervalued and beset.'[12] The same survey characterised the present processes as tending 'to investigate superficially, to analyse defensively, and to jump to conclusions about the remedy, if any action is taken at all'; little wonder therefore that complaints can turn into litigation.

Complaints that turn into litigation

Many things about which formal complaints are made simply do not have the capacity to turn into litigation because there has been no measurable personal injury that could be connected to the problem about which the patients or their relatives complained. In some cases where you might think they had a case, such as delay in treatment allowing progression of the underlying disease to the point of incurability, experiencing pain while on a waiting list or being denied an expensive drug, all by a neat twist of the law cannot form the basis of a claim against the Trust, the NHS or the Secretary of State. As far as endocrine surgeons are concerned cases will be based in personal injury owing to an alleged breach of duty by them or their team. A complication of surgery or a delay in diagnosis will, from experience, be the probable reason. There are no published figures to indicate how often endocrine surgery in the UK has led to litigation in the past and how successful that has been. The best data although incomplete, comes from the USA. In a paper presented at the annual meeting of the American Association of Endocrine Surgeons in 1993, Kern identified 62 cases of malpractice from 21 states between 1985 and 1991, for analysis. In 54% of instances the problem arose from a surgical complication, almost all during thyroid surgery; 35% arose from delayed diagnosis, equally of thyroid and adrenal disease, and 11% were from morbidity attributed to radioiodine or propylthiouracil. It is sobering to see that even 10 years ago mean payouts for successful litigation for a recurrent nerve injury approached $1 million and the maximum was $2.5 million.[13] The number of endocrine cases currently passing through the system in the USA or the UK is not known.

The first intimation of litigation will usually be a letter from the solicitor to the hospital, and this may come without patients having troubled to go through a formal complaint process first, or patients may have been through some sort of formal or informal process and not been satisfied with the outcome. Once a problem turns into a formal process of litigation it is protracted, time consuming, distressing for all concerned and, from the NHS's point of view, expensive. It is important that clinicans handle them in as dispassionate and efficient a way as possible, however distressed they may feel by the complaint itself and by the process of dealing with it.

The solicitor's letter

The first manifestation will normally be a solicitor's letter asking for release of copies of all the notes, X-ray films, pathology reports, etc. In NHS practice the hospital complaints' or litigation officer should receive this, together with an indication that the request for release signifies or does not signify an impending action against the Trust (sometimes such requests are merely to do with insurance claims or actions against another party).

At this stage you may be asked by the hospital to confirm that you are happy for copies of the notes to be released. In effect you have no choice about this, but the solicitor requesting them must give sufficient detail, setting out the expected case against the doctor, to comply with the requirements of section 33 of the Supreme Court Act, 1981. Before the release of the notes you need to make sure that they are in sensible order, that copies of all the originals are retained by the hospital and that you have reviewed any part that you or your team had in the incident that has led to the litigation. You also need to check that it is the patient who indirectly is asking for release of the files. If it is not then you will need the patient's permission to release the file. The Medical Defence Union has produced a helpful pamphlet on this subject for its members.[14]

When reviewing the notes it is in order to ensure that the filing of the notes is logical, but you must not add anything, change anything or remove anything from the notes. Do, however, refresh your memory, as it may be several years since the events occurred. If you receive a request for notes in your capacity as a private practitioner, check the notes and photocopy them, but only release them to the patient's solicitors through your medical defence organisation.

The solicitors acting for the patient will now be finding an expert and getting an initial opinion. Additionally, experience shows that they will often be applying to the Legal Aid board for a certificate to confirm that this client's costs will be covered if they are eligible. It is a sad reflection on access to justice that medical negligence litigation is not realistically affordable by any but the very rich and those receiving legal aid. There will, in any event, be a lull, the extent of which is governed only by the limitation period of 3 years from the time that the plaintiff could reasonably have known that he or she had a cause for action. There are, however, situations where this time may be extended, but this requires a formal plea in court to disbar a defence plea that a plaintiff's action is disbarred by lapse of time.[15]

The next communication will probably be a writ and a statement of claim from the plaintiff's solicitors, outlining in detail the allegations and often enclosing the expert's report in the details of which the claim is usually grounded. The writ formally indicates the beginning of a legal action.

Most doctors become depressed, distressed, angry or all three of these at this point, and fortunately the handling of the process from here on is not in their hands but in those of the solicitors acting for the hospital, or the medical defence organisation if the matter relates to a private patient. The solicitors will want measured written responses to the allegations of negligence, of which there are often many (the 'scatter gun' approach). If you believe that the allegation of negligence is completely unfounded, it is important at this stage to ensure that the hospital is aware of the strength of your feelings and is prepared to defend the claim rather than simply settle to reduce costs (particularly in relation to plaintiff's receiving legal aid). You may want to liaise with your medical defence organisation about this, even if it is an NHS case. You may also wish to inform yourself about the process that is now under way. Many textbooks describe the detail of the legal processes and the details of the underlying laws, principles and customs. Currently, the two most readable of these books are *Medical Negligence, a Practical Guide*[16] (written by a barrister from the point of view of the plaintiff) and '*Medicine, Patients and the Law*'.[17]

Essentially the case will revolve around the fact that you, the surgeon, are claimed to have been negligent. Although negligence has lay meanings as a word, it has very specific legal meanings.

Medical negligence

Surgical cases come to court almost invariably as a result of patients suing in an action for negligence. This is a civil prosecution. Extremely occasionally, where a patient has died as a consequence of gross negligence, such as a surgeon operating while drunk, the authorities may undertake a criminal prosecution on a basis of involuntary manslaughter. Only negligence will be considered here.

Negligence is an area considered under the civil law called tort, i.e. civil wrongs. Any formal legal action in this area only succeeds if a particular legal formula is fulfilled. The components of this formula are:

(i)   A relationship must exist between the parties (the surgeon and the patient), which gives rise to a *duty of care*.

(ii)   The duty of care must have been *breached* in some way due to an unreasonable act or omission by one of the parties. This breach of the duty of care is the negligence.

(iii) In addition to the negligence the injured party must have experienced some '*damage*,' loss or injury of a type recognised by the law.

(iv) The damage must have been caused *by the other party*, in this case the surgeon.

(v) The action must be brought within a specified time after the injury has occurred (this is known as the *period of limitation* (see above).

Each of these categories will need to be looked at separately.

Duty of care

As the NHS surgical patient will already have come under the care of a hospital either as an outpatient or in-patient, the plaintiff will have no difficulty in establishing that the hospital Trust has a duty of care. In these circumstances the surgeon is merely acting as an agent of the Trust, which carries vicarious liability as the employer. In private practice (and this includes patients admitted to NHS pay beds) the relationship is primarily directly with the surgeon and separately with the other providers, such as the hospital, pathology laboratory, etc. The duty of care in this latter situation arises through the 'contract' that arises implicitly between the surgeon and patient.

Breaching of duty of care

A successful negligence claim requires that the patient claimant demonstrates that the defendant (Trust or surgeon) was in breach of its duty of care. In English law the breach or lack of it is determined by judging what an equivalent body of other doctors would have done in similar circumstances. This is known as the 'Bolam test.' The Bolam case refers to a patient who was given electroconvulsive therapy and sustained fractures. Negligence was alleged in that he was not given muscle relaxants and was not adequately restrained physically. From the medical evidence it became clear some doctors would have used relaxant drugs or restraints, but many would not. The judge found the doctor not guilty of negligence because he had acted:

> …in accordance with a practice accepted as proper by a responsible body of medical men skilled in that particular area … a man is not negligent, if he is acting in accordance with such a practice, merely because there is a body of opinion who would take a contrary view.[18]

Bolam[19] is the legal case cited in England. In Scotland it is Hunter *v* Hanley[20] where Lord Clyde's dictum was equally clear:

> 'To establish liability by a doctor where deviation from normal practice is alleged, three facts require to be established. First of all it must be proved

that there is a usual and normal practice; secondly it must be proved that the defender has not adopted that practice; and thirdly (and this is of crucial importance) it must be established that the course the doctor adopted is one which no professional man of ordinary skill would have taken if he had been acting with ordinary care.'

Essentially these cases have the same conclusion, which is generally favourable to the surgeon.

The more recent case of Bolitho *v* City and Hackney Health Authority, has slightly changed the principles behind the Bolam case. In this instance negligence was alleged because a paediatric registrar failed to attend a child with fluctuating respiratory difficulties. The child subsequently had a respiratory arrest, incurred brain damage and died. In this case the issue was to do with 'causation.' If the registrar had attended the patient when called would she have intubated the patient, thus avoiding the subsequent turn of events? Medical evidence from eight experts was divided between those who said she would and should have intubated and those who said the opposite. The judge accepted that both bodies of evidence were respectable and concluded that he was in no position to 'prefer' one view. This was in line with Lord Scarman's view in another case that:

> …a judge's preference for one body of distinguished opinion over another, also professionally distinguished, is not sufficient to establish negligence in a practitioner.[21]

The case was appealed eventually to the House of Lords who supported the trial judge's conclusion but added an important rider to the 'Bolam test' in that it was no longer sufficient for experts to aver that something was acceptable practice but needed to show that in 'forming their view, the experts have directed their minds to the question of comparative risks and benefits and have reached a defensible conclusion on the matter.'[22]

Courts in the Republic of Ireland have in general also accepted the Bolam test but have spelled out the same limitations, that the treatment supported must be logical. Judge Finlay in the case of Dunne *vs* National Maternity Hospital said:

> 'If a medical practitioner charged with negligence defends his conduct by establishing that he followed a practice which was general and which was approved of by his colleagues of similar specializations and skill, he cannot escape liability if in reply the plaintiff establishes that such practice has inherent defects which ought to be obvious to any person giving the matter due consideration.[23]

Experts supporting or rejecting a particular course of action must therefore ground their views in a defensible clinical assessment of the pros and cons of any particular course of action.

A recent twist to this has been the position of guidelines and protocols. Many surgeons are apprehensive that they may not, on the basis of their own experience and reading, agree with protocols that are promulgated either nationally or within their own organisation, and therefore they might feel particularly threatened if they departed from those guidelines. Guidelines and protocols hold no special status legally and they should merely be regarded as an extension of the Bolam principle, as defining the views of other reputable practitioners. A guideline should not be published unless the authors can justify their joint view with reference to normal good clinical practice and the literature. Similarly, surgeons who depart from guidelines must be able logically and clinically to defend their departure from those guidelines. It is the courts who retain the right to decide whether a particular clinical practice is acceptable or not. Expert evidence of professional habits will carry the day in most cases, but surgeons cannot rely on this with complete certainty. There seem to be only a tiny number of cases where the court has chosen not to accept the expert medical evidence.

It is hardly surprising that doctors have a duty to keep themselves informed of major developments such as might be encompassed by guidelines. That duty cannot extend to a requirement that they know everything there is to know. For example, in the case of Crawford *v* the Board of Governors of Charing Cross Hospital, the plaintiff had developed a brachial palsy because of his position on the operating table. Six months prior to the event, an article had appeared in the *Lancet* warning of this danger, but the anaesthetist involved in the case had not read the article. The Court of Appeal found in favour of the anaesthetist. Lord Denning stating that:

'It would I think be putting too high a burden on a medical man to say he has read every article appearing in the current medical press; and it would be quite wrong to suggest a medical man is negligent because he does not at once put into operation a suggestion which some contributor or other might make in a medical journal. The time may come in a particular case where a new recommendation may be so well proved, and so well known, and so well accepted that it should be adopted, this was not so in this case.'[24]

A widely promulgated guideline could, however, in Lord Denning's terms fall into a recommendation 'so well proved and so well known and so well accepted that it should be adopted.'

Damage

Damage cited by plaintiffs must have been caused directly by the defendants' negligence, not, for example, simply by progression of underlying disease.

Damages subsequently awarded in the UK simply aim to place defendants in the position they were in before the damage was sustained, plus an element for pain and suffering. The situation in the UK is totally different from that pertaining in the USA, where juries, not judges, decide damages, and a strong punitive element is often included.

Causation

Letters from solicitors will often use the term 'causation,' a term not immediately understood by doctors (**Table 8.2**). In the legal setting 'causation' is merely the establishment of a factual and legal link between the breach of duty and the damage caused. This is often difficult to prove. Normally the 'but for' test is used. For example, 'but for the failure to take a fine needle biopsy at the first outpatient visit the patient's thyroid carcinoma would have been diagnosed 6 months earlier.' In the much discussed case of Bolitho described above, the failure to attend the child with a breathing problem was admitted by the defence as negligent, but the whole allegation of negligence failed because causation could not be shown on a balance of probability that 'but for the failure to attend the patient he would have survived.' Note that in negligence cases guilt or innocence is decided on grounds of 'balance of probability' rather than 'beyond reasonable doubt,' as applies in criminal cases.

The outcomes of litigation

The first duty of solicitors and barristers involved in litigation is to prevent cases going anywhere near court. The reasons for avoiding a formal contest in court

Causation	No causation
A patient comes into hospital for thyroidectomy. The cords are checked preoperatively and both move. After the operation, the patient is hoarse and laryngoscopy shows one cord is not moving. The plaintiff's barrister could readily show that there was a duty of care, that there was damage and could prove causation. But it would be hard to prove negligence. Laryngeal nerve palsy *ipso facto* is not evidence of negligence.	A patient comes to the outpatient department with a longstanding mass in the neck. The mass is fixed to the surrounding structures. The surgeon neither biopsies the mass nor operates. Two weeks later the patient dies and the post mortem shows an anaplastic carcinoma obstructing the airway. There was a duty of care but there was no causation in that on a balance of probability failure to biopsy the mass or arrange treatment did not alter the outcome.

Table 8.2 *Examples of causation and no causation*

are primarily to do with cost. Only rarely do the potential injuries in financial terms justify the costs of a full court hearing.

If you or your legal advisors lose the case or settle the case then the costs of that will, if you are in private practice, be met by your medical defence organisation. If you are practising in the NHS the costs will be met by the health services, sometimes by your Trust but normally by the Clinical Negligence Scheme for Trust (CNST). The inclusion of clinicians in the NHS indemnity scheme has been in place since 1990 so there should now be no cases pending, reflecting the time when clinicians were responsible for their own insurance arrangements.

Expert opinions

Although it is for the court to decide on matters put before it, right or wrong, true or false, negligent or not negligent, it can only do so in medical cases by drawing on expert advice from clinicians and others. More importantly—and more commonly—expert advice is also used to determine whether a case needs to be put before the court or should be abandoned or settled out of court. In the recent past there was very little oversight concerning the choice of expert. Experts tended to be identified as plaintiff's experts or defendant's experts and were as likely to be chosen for their experience in writing reports and their performance skills in court as for their personal expertise in the detailed clinical problem under scrutiny. There was no real attempt to bring the experts from two sides together to sort out differences in opinion early in the process. This encouraged the confrontational style of litigation that has tended to make medical litigation both protracted and expensive. New guidance for expert opinions has recently been promulgated and must now be adhered to by any clinician asked to provide a report. Anyone asked to provide an expert report will now usually receive with that request guidance notes advising that the expert's duty is to the court and not to the plaintiff, the defendant or the solicitor that has instructed him. Therefore:

- The report is addressed to the court
- It contains a statement that experts understand that their duty is to the court
- Experts may if they wish file a written request to the court for directions to assist them in carrying out their function as an expert. They do not need to give the claimant, defendant or the instructing solicitor any notice of such a request.

The report must:

- Give details of the experts' qualifications. This should include information that confirms their position as experts in a particular field

- Give details of any literature or other material which experts have relied on in preparing reports and ideally include copies of that material
- If there is a range of opinion about a particular issue, the experts should summarise that range of opinion and give reasons for their own position within that spectrum
- Set out a list of all facts and material instructions (either written or oral) which the experts have received and which are germane to the opinions subsequently expressed in their reports
- End with a statement of truth in the following terms: 'I believe that the facts I have stated in this report are true and that the opinions I have expressed are correct'.

When the solicitors have exchanged experts' reports, either side may, within 28 days, submit written questions on a report to its author, the answers to which will form part of the report. If, following these reports, the matter remains unresolved and proceedings are started, the various experts may be required to meet to identify the issues in the case, where possible to reach agreement and potentially to assist in the preparation of a joint report for the court, summarising which issues have been agreed and which not. In the latter case the reasons behind the disagreement will need to be summarised. The content of this experts' meeting will not be referred to at any trial unless the claimant and the defendant agree.

Reforms

The surgeon should be aware of several changes that will affect medical litigation over the next 10 years:

1. Conditional/contingency fees ('no win, no fee').
2. The recommendations of the Woolf report.
3. Attempts to control the cost of legal aid.
4. The use of mediation.

No win, no fee

The legislation to allow lawyers and their clients to come to conditional agreements about fees—the fee being conditional on the outcome of the case—came into effect in July 1995. There was alarm that this would allow the 'ambulance chasing' and speculative litigation common in the USA to appear in the UK. Fortunately, there are other differences in the law between the UK and the USA that make this unlikely. In the USA, the plaintiff and the defendant pay their own costs regardless of the outcome, whereas in the UK the loser must pay the other party's costs. The option, therefore, of not having to pay your lawyer if you lose does not guarantee a risk-fee exercise for the plaintiff, although in theory it is possible to insure for the other party's costs if you lose but the uncertain outcomes of medical litigation tend to make this prohibitively expensive. The 'no win, no fee' arrangement also puts greater pressure on the claimant's solicitor to check that the case is worth pursuing, and that pressure is much greater than it is in cases supported by legal aid. Overall, the system will probably reduce rather than increase the number of vexatious and speculative claims.[25] Doctors in the UK also retain the continuing privilege of the application of the 'Bolam test'.

The Woolf report

The Woolf report[26] reviewed the whole of the civil justice system in England and Wales and recommended radical change. Medical negligence litigation did not escape Lord Woolf's attentions because he considered most cases currently to be unduly long, complex and expensive. In a sample of medical negligence cases that were reviewed for the report, his commission found that the average time from first contact with a lawyer to resolution was 65 months and that for claims worth less than £12 500 the legal costs of just one side averaged 137% of the claim's value! Lord Woolf also found that unmeritorious cases were pursued too long and that the degree of lack of cooperation and mutual suspicion was greater than in any other class of litigation. The recommendations of the report have been summarised as follows:

1. Greater effort at prevention and early resolution of disputes. As steps towards this, Lord Woolf recommended that medical record keeping should be better, the procedures for local resolution of problems should be clearer and that there should be more use of mediation with jointly instructed experts where possible and a greater use of experts' meetings. Overall though, he recommended a more sparing use of experts.

2. An improved summary disposal procedure to weed out weak claims and weak defences.

3. The introduction of a system of plaintiff 'offers to settle,' with sanctions where a defendant unreasonably refused to cooperate.

4. Claims of £10 000 or less to be handled by a slimmed down procedure with a limited range of legal processes conforming to tightly controlled timetables and costs.

5. Large and complex claims to be handled by a 'multitrack' process, where the management of each case legally is decided by the courts themselves rather than by lawyers.

Much of this was welcomed, although there was considerable scepticism about the prospect of only a single medical expert being involved in some cases. Lewis, in a considered assessment of the Woolf reforms, thinks there is no reason to expect that they would improve the cost or pace of the legal process and considers that using judges to manage the process may be unfair as few judges have much experience of medical negligence litigation and the particular needs and procedures relevant to a claim. He noted that the use of judges to manage the outline and conduct of cases in the context of general civil litigation led to chaos in the Court of Appeal because of the number of appeals against judges' processing of the cases, and he quoted a judge in another case as observing that 'it is easy to dispense injustice quickly and cheaply, but it is better to do justice, even if it takes a little longer and costs a little more.'[27]

Changes to legal aid legislation

The costs of legal aid are rising annually, and this is a cause of concern for the Government. Recent changes to the rules to reduce access to legal aid excluded medical negligence cases. Curiously, instead of addressing the problems within the system, the Secretary of State for Health and the Lord Chancellor merely put their efforts into 'naming and shaming' those lawyers who were earning most from the system, which did not move the debate forward at all. Subsequently there have been more definite steps to limit the management of medical negligence cases to legal practices with proven expertise.

Mediation

Mediation is not simply a way of avoiding the expense of full blown litigation, it is a means to resolve disputes more simply and humanely. It requires the services of trained and committed mediators. Pilot projects for mediation are underway at present and mediation is likely to form a more common way of resolving allegations of negligent care in the future. It is certain that there will be in it a large role for the independent, informed clinical expert to assist arbitrators.

Conclusions

Complaint and litigation is not going to go away. An increase in individualism, loss of respect for professionals, more mechanical medical processes and a good supply of well trained, proficient lawyers is going to ensure that whatever the changes in legislation and clinical practice, litigation will continue. Surgeons can do their bit to minimise this by ensuring more sophisticated and better documented consent and informing of patients. Adherence to protocols, sound postgraduate education and proper training of trainees will reduce the incidences of harm to a largely unavoidable minimum. When complaints arise they can perhaps be better managed at the early stages. The complaints that are not satisfactorily resolved may be better handled by processes of arbitration or mediation rather than the traditional confrontationalism of the legal process. It would be in everybody's interests to have speedier resolution and for there to be less financial incentive for lawyers to support the vexatious or unbelievable cases. The legal aid process is already attempting to weed out such cases.

It may be that some form of 'no fault' compensation such as exists in New Zealand will be instituted, in which compensation is paid to victims of medical mishaps without recourse to negligence actions. Appealing as this may be both for patients and clinicians, it still leaves unresolved problems, particularly in relation to distinguishing between effects that are simply disease progression rather than harm from the medical process and the difficulties of defining the difference between misadventure and negligence. Indeed, it is the placement of that fine boundary between misadventure and negligence that is behind most medical litigation in endocrine surgery as in all other branches of medicine.

A complementary chapter on medico–legal aspects of breast disease is to be found in *Breast Surgery* 2nd edition.

References

1. Goodman NW. Accountability, clinical governance and the acceptance of imperfection. J Roy Soc Med 2000; 93: 59–61.

2. National Audit Office. Clinical audit in England. London: Stationery Office, 1995.

3. Sidaway *v* Board of Governors of the Bethlehem Royal Hospital. [1984] QB493 at 517, [1984] 1 All ER 1018 at 1030, CA.

4. Davies M. Textbook on medical law. London: Blackstone Press, 1996; pp. 166–74.

5. Kennedy I. Treat me right. Essay in medical law and ethics. Oxford: Clarendon Press, 1988; p. 177.

6. Medical Law Monitor, 1997; 4 (10): p. 6.

7. Mason JK, McCall Smith RA. Law and medical ethics. London: Butterworths, 1994; p. 247.

8. Rogers *v* Whitaker [1992] 67 AWR 47.

9. Hiatt HH, Barnes BA, Brennan I *et al.* The study of medical injury and medical malpractice; an overview. N Engl J Med 1989; 321: 40.

10. Wilson RM, Runciman WB *et al.* The quality in Australian health care study. Med J Aust 1995; 163: 458–71.

11. Young AE. The medical manager, a practical guide for clinicians. London: BMJ Publishing, 1999; pp. 257–63.

12. Hill AP, Baeza J. Dealing with things that go wrong. Lancet 1999; 354: 2099–100.

13. Kern KA. Medicolegal analysis of errors in diagnosis and treatment of surgical endocrine disease. Surgery 1993; 114: 1167–74.

14. Hoyte P. Can I see the records? London: Medical Defence Union, 1996.

15. Finch J. Spellers law relating to hospitals, 7e, section 5.2. London: Chapman & Hall Medical, 1993.

16. Lewis C. Medical negligence, a practical guide, 4e. London: Butterworths, 1998.

17. Brazier M. Medicine, patients and the law. London: Penguin, 1992.

18. Bolam *v* Friern HMC [1957] 1 WLR 582, 587–8.

19. Bolam *v* Friern Hospital Management Committee [1957]; 2 All ER 118, [1957] 1 WLR 582.

20. Hunter *v* Hanley. 1955 SC 200.

21. Maynard *v* West Midlands Regional Health Authority [1984] 1 WLR 634 at 639.

22. Bolitho [1997] 4 All ER 771.

23. Dunne *v* National Maternity Hospital [1989] ICRM 735.

24. Cited by Mason JK and McCall Smith RA. Law and medical ethics. London: Butterworths, 1994; p. 202.

25. Barton A. Conditional fees: access to justice for all. Clin Risk 1997; 3: 130–1.

26. Lord Woolf. Access to justice. London: Stationery Office, 1996.

27. Lewis CJ. Medical negligence. London: Butterworths, 1998; pp. 7–9.

9 The salivary glands

Z. Rayter

The parotid gland

Diseases of the parotid gland are relatively uncommon, but it has one of the greatest diversities of pathology. Most lesions are of an inflammatory nature although some arise from a post-traumatic, systemic or uncertain pathogenesis. There is also a wide spectrum of neoplastic conditions, some of which are unique to the parotid gland. The differential diagnosis of a parotid mass remains an important aspect of a surgeon's training.

Embryology

The mouth is developed partly from the stomodaeum and partly from the cephalic portion of the foregut. By the growth of the head end of the embryo and formation of the head fold, the pericardial area and the oral or buccopharyngeal membrane come to lie on the ventral surface of the embryo. With the further expansion of the brain and the bulging of the pericardium, the oral membrane comes to lie at the bottom of the depression bounded by these two prominences.[1] This depression constitutes the stomodaeum or primitive mouth (**Fig. 9.1**). The parotid gland can be recognised in human embryos 8 mm long and arises from the epithelial lining of the mouth, appearing as an elongated furrow running dorsally from the angle of the mouth between the mandibular arch and maxillary process. The groove, which is converted into a tube, loses its connection with the epithelium of the mouth[1] (except at its anterior end) and grows dorsally into the substance of the cheek. This tube persists as the parotid duct, and its blind end proliferates to form the gland. Subsequently, the size of the oral fissure is reduced, and the parotid duct opens on the inside of the cheek at some distance from the angle of the mouth. The epithelial buds enlarge, elongate and branch, initially forming

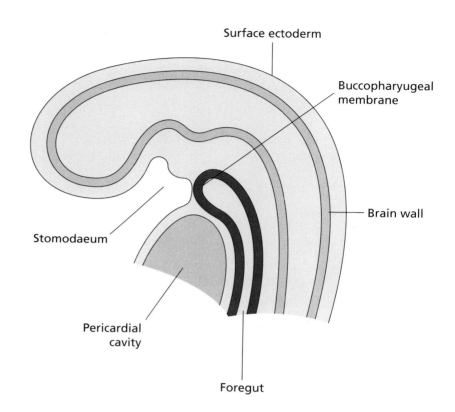

Figure 9.1
Sagittal section of the caphalic end of a 25 day embryo illustrating the development of the mouth prior to the appearance of the parotid gland.

Surface ectoderm

Buccopharyugeal membrane

Brain wall

Stomodaeum

Pericardial cavity

Foregut

solid structures, but they eventually cannalise, creating lumina. The lining epithelial cells of the ducts, tubules and acini then differentiate both morphologically and functionally, and the contractile myoepithelial cells become placed around the acini.[2] The interaction between the parenchymal and stromal elements with the autonomic system is necessary for normal salivary gland development and function; sympathetic nerve stimulation leads to acinar differentiation whereas parasympathetic nerve stimulation is required for overall glandular growth.[2]

Prior to the complete development of the parotid gland, the lymphatic system begins to emerge in the mesoderm. Because of this, in the adult there are unique intraglandular lymph nodes and lymphatic channels. In addition, salivary epithelial cells can be included within these lymph nodes. This unusual situation is believed to have a role in the development of Warthin's tumours and possibly lymphoepithelial cysts.[3] As parotid epithelial buds grow and branch, they extend between and around the division of the facial nerve, incorporating the distal portion of this nerve within the gland.[2]

Anatomy

The parotid gland occupies the irregular space bounded behind by the external auditory meatus, the mastoid process and the sternomastoid muscle, in front by the mandible and its attached muscles and medially by the styloid process and its attached muscles. It extends upwards as far as the zygomatic arch and forwards, both deep and superficial to the ramus of the mandible. The gland is separated from the skin by the general investing layer of the deep fascia of the neck, which above the angle of the mandible passes over the gland and fuses with the masseter muscle on the outer aspect of the ramus of the mandible. The fascia is attached to the zygomatic arch and becomes continuous with the temporal fascia. There is no true capsule to the parotid gland, and the lobules of gland substance fill the available space and conform to the shape of the surrounding structures. The duct of the gland (Stensen's duct) follows the masseter muscle to its anterior edge, where it turns medially through buccinator to open on to the mucous membrane of the cheek opposite the crown of the upper second molar tooth. As Stensen's duct passes over the masseter, it may receive the duct of an accessory parotid gland, which is found overlying the masseter muscle in approximately 20% of people, usually related cranial to Stensen's duct.

The facial nerve emerges from the mastoid at the stylomastoid foramen lateral to the styloid process and almost immediately enters the parotid. Before entering the parotid gland, the facial nerve gives off branches to the stylohyoid, the posterior belly of the diagastric muscle and the occipitalis muscles. The main trunk of the nerve (the pes anserinus or goose's foot) then usually divides into its upper and lower divisions two thirds of the way to the mandible. The two divisions are the temporozygomatic and the cervicofacial branches, which pass through the parotid gland superficial to the retromandibular vein.[4] The two divisions divide into peripheral branches. The nerves to the forehead muscles and the upper and lower eyelids arise from the temporozygomatic branch, and the buccal branch and nerves to the upper and lower lips arise from the cervicofacial branch (**Fig. 9.2**). Variations to this pattern are common. This division of the parotid gland by the facial nerve into superficial and deep lobes is important when operating on parotid lesions.

The external carotid artery enters the deep surface of the parotid and divides at about the level of the neck of the mandible into the superficial temporal artery, which emerges from the upper edge of the gland, and the maxillary artery, which passes medially out of the gland. In the substance of the gland are numerous lymph nodes. The anterior surface of the gland is in contact with the mandible and the masseter and medial pterygoid muscles. The posterior surface is in contact below with the mastoid process and the sternomastoid and digastric muscles and above with the external auditory meatus. Medially, the gland is separated by the digastric muscle from the internal jugular vein and the styloid process and stylohyoid muscle from the internal carotid artery. Above, the gland is in contact with the capsule of the mandibular joint. The postganglionic nerve supply of the gland runs in the auriculotemporal nerve from the otic ganglion. The preganglionic fibres arise in the inferior salivary nucleus in the medulla

Figure 9.2
Surgical anatomy of the parotid salivary gland.

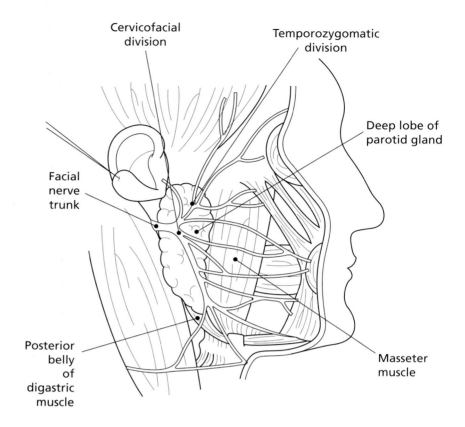

oblongata, run in the glossopharyngeal nerve and its tympanic branch to the lesser petrosal nerve and so enter the otic ganglion. The parotid and periparotid lymph glands drain primarily into the internal jugular chain nodes, with some drainage going to the upper spinal accessory chain of nodes.

Physiology

The physiological control of parotid gland secretion is almost entirely by the autonomic nervous system. If the parasympathetic innervation is interrupted, glandular atrophy occurs. If sympathetic innervation is interrupted, there is little effect.[5] Normal saliva is 99.5% water but contains salts and mucins, amylase and maltase. The total volume of saliva produced may be up to 1500 ml per day, 45% of which is produced by the parotid glands. Saliva moistens food allowing it to be swallowed easily. Other functions of the salivary glands are to moisten mucous membranes and to inhibit bacterial invasion, which is mediated by the secretion of secretory immunoglobulin A. Finally, the salivary glands assist in the excretion of heavy metals and inorganic and organic materials and in the maintenance of water balance.

Developmental abnormalities

Developmental abnormalities of the parotid glands are rare. When they do occur, other facial abnormalities may be present and are associated with xerostomia, sialodenitis and dental caries. Parotid gland agenesis has been reported with hemifacial microstomia, mandibulofacial dysostosis, cleft palate and anophthalmia.[6] Recently, agenesis of one parotid gland has been reported with sialosis of the contralateral parotid.[7] Hypoplasia of the parotid gland has been reported in the Melkerson–Rosenthal syndrome, and congenital fistula formation of the ductal system has been associated with branchial cleft abnormalities, accessory parotid ducts and diverticula.[8]

Ectopic location of salivary gland tissue can occur in many sites, including the external auditory canal and middle ear cleft, the anterior mandible, the inner-posterior mandible (Stafne cyst), the pituitary gland and even the cerebello-pontine angle.[8]

Investigation of the parotid gland

Clinical evaluation

Most lesions of the parotid gland are either due to tumour, inflammatory conditions or obstruction of Stensen's duct. The commonest presentations of parotid pathology are therefore swelling of the whole gland (in inflammatory conditions and obstructions of the duct) or a solitary mass in the parotid region. It should be possible for the clinician to make this distinction,[9] which is important as a mass nearly always implies a neoplasm. In the assessment of a parotid mass, particular attention should be paid to the presence or absence of facial palsy, as its presence strongly suggests malignancy.[10] Other important aspects of the clinical examination are fixity and site of the lesion within the parotid. Thus, a recent study concluded that 96% of tumours in the tail of the gland (that region lying inferiorly) were benign if there was no facial palsy, pain, trismus or fixation.[10] This may be useful in the assessment of frail elderly patients in whom fine needle aspiration is not performed.

In assessing any parotid mass, the patient should be asked to clench teeth to contract the masseter muscles; this allows the examiner to assess if the swelling is due to hypertrophy of the masseter or whether the mass is in the substance of the muscle (haemangioma or myxoma). Complete examination of all the other salivary glands should be performed to ascertain whether multiple masses are present (as in Warthin's tumour) or whether other glands are involved in a systemic disease (as in Sjögren's syndrome). All glands should be examined bimanually and each duct orifice inspected and palpated. No examination is complete without examination of the pharynx to ascertain the presence of a parapharyngeal tumour,

Sebaceous cyst
Enlarged preauricular lymph node
Branchial cyst
Dental cyst
Lipoma
Lymphangioma
Mandibular tumours
Myxoma of the masseter
Neuroma of the facial nerve
Facial vein thrombosis
Temporal artery aneurysm
Mastoiditis
Hypertrophic masseter
Winged mandible

Table 9.1   *Differential diagnosis of a parotid mass not caused by a parotid tumour*

which may be shaped like a dumb-bell and present as a parotid mass. The diagnosis of a parotid mass is not usually difficult, but clinicians should bear in mind the rarer causes of an apparent parotid mass (**Table 9.1**).

Radiology

The choice of imaging modalities has increased dramatically recently and the emphasis is now on ultrasonography, computed tomography (CT) and magnetic resonance imaging (MRI). As a general rule, inflammatory lesions are probably best imaged using CT, whereas tumours are best imaged by MRI. Ultrasonography is also useful for the evaluation of both parotid lesions in children and tumours.[11]

Plain X-ray films

These are rarely used now as most parotid calculi are radiotranslucent and are better visualised by ultrasonography or CT. Plain films may be useful in differentiating some of the extra-salivary causes of sialomegaly.

Sialography

This remains the most detailed method of visualising the duct system but is now rarely used except in the assessment of suspected sialectasis. In congenital saccular sialectasis, the characteristic snowstorm appearance is seen, and strictures and clubbing of the duct system may be demonstrated. In advanced cystic sialectasis, large collections of contrast may be seen. It can occasionally be useful for identifying a stenosis of the duct, which can be dilated with an inflatable balloon. Sialography is contraindicated in the presence of active infection or allergy to the contrast medium.

CT

If the patient's history is suggestive of inflammatory disease, CT will identify the actual disease and may also identify the calculi responsible.[12] Usually, little extra information is obtained with the use of contrast.[11]

MRI

This is probably the preferred method of imaging a mass suspected of being a tumour. This is sometimes combined with contrast and is useful in assessing perineural tumour spread in parotid malignancies.[13] MRI studies are usually performed as 3 mm-thick slices with a 1 mm interslice gap. Non-contrast T1 and T2 weighted sequences and then T1 weighted, postcontrast, fat-suppressed images are obtained. Axial views are obtained for all sequences and sagittal and coronal views obtained as required.[11,14] Normally, the facial nerve is not imaged. The recent use of high-resolution three-dimensional Fourier transformed MRI has allowed the facial nerve to be consistently visualised on contiguous scans.[15] MRI is also particularly useful in lesions situated within the deep lobe of the parotid.

Ultrasonography

This was traditionally used to differentiate between solid and cystic masses in the parotid gland and to identify salivary calculi. It can also be used to identify the more advanced stages of autoimmune disease (Sjögren's syndrome) and to differentiate between lymphomatous and non-lymphomatous nodes,[16] although not with sufficient accuracy to avoid biopsy. Ultrasonography is particularly useful in children in whom exposure to radiation is to be avoided. For lesions that have spread beyond the capsule, it does not provide the detailed anatomical information obtained with CT and MRI.[17–19]

Other radiological techniques

Radionuclide salivary gland scans are based on the fact that salivary glands normally concentrate technetium pertechnetate (^{99m}Tc) and some masses excessively accumulate the radionuclide, especially Warthin's tumours and oncocytomas.[20,21] Radionuclide scans are rarely used now that CT and MRI are freely available. Angiography was useful in the investigation of tumours situated in the parapharyngeal space to differentiate salivary gland tumours from chemodectoma of the carotid or from a nerve sheath tumour. Its use has also been superseded by CT and MRI. MRI spectroscopy is still a relatively new procedure and is based on the fact that salivary tumours express increased quantities of phosphates compared with normal. This is detectable by means of 31-phosphorus spectroscopy,[22] but this is primarily an investigative and research tool.

Fine needle aspiration cytology

Fine needle aspiration cytology (FNAC) of a discrete parotid mass remains controversial.[23] Its proponents argue that it has a high diagnostic accuracy, may influence the decision to operate, may allow planning of the most appropriate operative procedure and allows better-informed preoperative counselling.[24-27] Its detractors argue that it is not sufficiently accurate at diagnosing low-grade malignant lesions, that the decision to operate is clinically based and the extent of the surgery is not influenced by the cytology, as in the parotid gland more radical surgery for a malignant lesion does not influence outcome.[23] However, all authorities are agreed that FNAC does not cause tumour seeding and that it is free of any major morbidity. A recent survey of 34 institutions with a major interest in salivary gland tumours concluded that approximately one third of surgical oncologists did not employ FNAC, one third always employed it and one third employed it selectively.[23]

Numerous series now attest to the accuracy of FNAC (**Table 9.2**). FNAC is particularly accurate in the diagnosis of pleomorphic adenoma,[24] and a recent study highlighting the features of infarction and squamoid metaplasia achieved an accuracy of up to 88% for adenolymphoma.[26] Even proponents of the technique have emphasised the pitfalls in diagnosis and have concluded that atypical pleomorphic adenoma is difficult to distinguish from monomorphic adenoma, mucoepidermoid carcinoma and adenoid cystic carcinoma.[28]

FNAC is useful if lymphadenopathy is suspected due to sarcoid, tuberculosis[24] and lymphoma. It may assist in distinguishing a parotid lesion from other local structures such as a branchial cyst, lymph node or even submandibular gland. It can often confirm a benign neoplasm in an elderly, unfit patient for whom surgery would carry significant risk. It is essential to discriminate between a parotid lesion and a secondary deposit from a melanoma or squamous cell lesion.

Authors (ref)	No of patients	No with histology	Sensitivity (%)	Specificity (%)	Accuracy (%)
Eneroth et al.[29]	1000	690	64	95	89
Layfield et al.[30]	171	171	91	98	92
Lindberg and Akerman[31]	860	461	67	85	81
O'Dwyer et al.[32]	341	341	73	94	93
Persson and Zettergren[33]	362	216	86	99	70
Qizilbash et al.[34]	160	101	88	99	95
Shaha et al.[24]	160	NS	95	98	97
Filopoulos et al.[35]	129	121	95	97.6	96.7

NS = Not stated.

Table 9.2 *Accuracy of fine needle aspiration cytology (only series of more than 100 patients)*

In the current climate of informed consent, the most useful role of FNAC may be in preoperative counselling of the patient.

Sialometry

Salivary gland output can be determined from individual major salivary glands or from the aggregate fluid in the oral cavity (termed whole saliva). Secretions can be collected in a resting (unstimulated) state or after gustatory or mechanical stimulation. Whole saliva collection is a useful screening technique to determine overall gland function in patients suspected of xerostomia (dry mouth) and may be particularly useful in the diagnosis of Sjögren's syndrome (see below).

Infections of the parotid gland

Bacterial infections

Bacteria usually reach the gland by retrograde infection from the mouth, although rarely infection may be blood borne. The commonest causative organisms are *Staphylococcus aureus, Streptococcus viridans, Streptococcus pyogenes. Haemophilus influenzae, Escherichia coli* and *Streptococcus pneumoniae.*[36] Infection is usually unilateral and may involve intraparotid and periparotid lymph nodes. The aetiology of acute parotitis is usually due to debility and dehydration after major surgery or due to serious medical disease but may be idiopathic, secondary to obstruction of Stensen's duct (usually due to calculi) or a complication of septicaemia.

The clinical features are of a painful swelling of the side of the face and fever. Pus or purulent fluid may be expressed from Stensen's duct. Untreated, the condition may progress to a parotid abscess, which may subsequently extend to the upper neck or to the parapharyngeal space. The treatment of acute bacterial parotitis consists of oral hygiene, correction of dehydration and appropriate antibiotics. Signs of improvement are usually evident within 48 hours. If no improvement after this time has occurred, a parotid abscess should be suspected. CT[37] not only confirms the diagnosis but allows planning of the most appropriately sited incision to drain the abscess to spare the branches of the facial nerve. If no abscess is present and fulminating parotitis is suspected, decompression of the parotid gland should be considered.[38] Recurrent subacute and chronic parotitis is more common than an acute infection and is usually due to parotid calculi (see below).

Viral infections

The commonest infection of the parotid glands is mumps.[39] It can also occur in the submandibular and sublingual glands. Mumps is most reliably diagnosed during epidemics or by measuring serum antibody titres.[3] It usually affects children between the ages of 4 and 12 years. Common manifestations of active disease include bilateral or occasionally unilateral parotid swelling, fever, chills, joint pain and myalgia. Uncommon manifestations include epididymitis, orchitis, pancreatitis, thyroiditis, meningoencephalitis and unilateral sensorineural hearing loss. The treatment relies on isolation of the patient, adequate hydration and nutrition and measures to relieve symptoms.

Other viruses that can cause acute viral parotitis include Coxsackie viruses, parainfluenza viruses (type 1 and 3), influenza virus type A, herpesvirus, echovirus and choriomeningitis virus.[36,40] Although Epstein–Barr virus and cytomegalovirus can be found in saliva, they do not seem to directly infect the major salivary glands. The same seems to pertain to the human immunodeficiency virus.[41]

Granulomatous and other diseases

These diseases may affect the intraparotid and extraparotid lymph nodes, and the parenchyma of the parotid gland can also be affected. The chief granulomatous diseases affecting the major salivary glands include sarcoidosis, tuberculosis, atypical mycobacterial infection, syphilis, cat-scratch fever, toxoplasmosis and actinomycosis.[43] In practice, not all of these diseases produce histologically recognisable granulomata.

Sarcoidosis

This is a systemic disease characterised by non-caseating granulomas involving many organs. Its presumed aetiology is infectious. The parotid glands are affected in 10–30% of patients and occasionally may be the only manifestation of the disease. It usually presents as a non-tender, painless, chronic enlargement of the gland, which may mimic malignancy. CT and MRI reveals multiple, benign, non-cavitating masses. The major differential diagnosis is lymphoma, although if the lesion is solitary it may be difficult to distinguish between other benign lesions. If FNAC excludes a neoplasm, incisional biopsy may be performed and will confirm the diagnosis.[43] Most cases resolve with treatment of the generalised condition.

Tuberculosis

Primary involvement of the salivary glands is rare. Usually, the salivary gland disease arises from a focus in the tonsils and spreads to the salivary gland via the regional lymph nodes. FNAC is often a helpful diagnostic procedure. Treatment is with appropriate antituberculous chemotherapy, and surgery is rarely necessary.

Cat-scratch fever

This diagnosis is suggested by a history of cat scratch followed by fever, malaise and enlargement of the salivary glands and lymph nodes. Identification of the causative organism is often difficult. Treatment consists of incision and drainage of any abscess and antibiotic chemotherapy of secondary infection.

Toxoplasmosis

Infection by *Toxoplasma gondii* causes asymptomatic lymphadenopathy and in the parotid gland may be indistinguishable from the above granulomatous diseases. Active and previous infection can be confirmed on serological testing.

Actinomycosis

Infection by *Actinomyces israelii* is usually caused by spread of the organism from dental, periodontal or intestinal disease. Parenchymal disease is characterised by granulomatous inflammation with abscess and fistula. 'Sulphur granules' may also be found. The treatment of choice is with long-term penicillin.

Autoimmune disease

Autoimmune disease affecting the salivary glands is best considered as Sjögren's syndrome. This is a systemic disorder of the exocrine glands that occurs either alone (primary Sjögren's syndrome) or with any other connective tissue disease (secondary Sjögren's syndrome). The diagnosis is suspected when two or more of the following clinical features are present: keratoconjunctivitis sicca, xerostomia and a connective tissue disease, which is usually rheumatoid arthritis.[44] Usually the lacrimal and salivary glands are affected but other exocrine glands can also be involved.[45]

The incidence of Sjögren's syndrome is difficult to establish, but among the autoimmune diseases it is probably second in frequency only to rheumatoid arthritis.[45] The adult form of the disease is 10 times more common than the childhood form, and children are less likely to develop the advanced features.[46] It is important to establish the diagnosis early in children because many cases may spontaneously resolve by puberty, and this knowledge may avoid unnecessary surgery.

The adult form of the disease is most common between the ages of 40 and 60 years with a male to female ratio of 1:9. It tends to be progressive. The incidence of parotid enlargement varies from 25 to 55% of cases, and either parotid or submandibular gland enlargement occurs in 80% of all cases of Sjögren's syndrome. The risk of developing non-Hodgkin's lymphoma is estimated to be 44 times greater than in normal controls.[8] Local radiotherapy or immunosuppression may further increase this risk.

Two types of pathological appearance are evident in the salivary glands: the benign lymphoepithelial lesion, occurring primarily in the parotid glands, and focal lymphocytic sialodenitis, occurring in the other major and minor salivary glands.[47] Studies with monoclonal antibodies have shown that lymphocytes in labial salivary glands contain more than three times as many T-helper cells (CD4[+]) as T-suppressor cells (CD8[+]).[48]

The diagnosis is most reliably made by labial salivary gland biopsy, and usually biopsy of the parotid gland is not required unless this is the only gland affected.[43,47] The suspicion of malignant lymphoma should be borne in mind in this subset of patients. Sialography is the most useful radiological adjunct to diagnosis, showing a normal central duct system and numerous peripheral punctate collections of contrast material uniformly scattered throughout the gland. Eventually, larger globular collections of contrast material may also be seen scattered uniformly throughout the gland, and MRI findings of these globular changes are diagnostic.[37]

The management of patients with Sjögren's syndrome involves reducing the patient's symptoms and preventing irreversible damage to the teeth and eyes. Thus, attention should be paid to treating and preventing dental caries, treating oral candidiasis, stimulating the remaining salivary glands to produce more saliva and selectively using saliva substitutes.[47] Stimulation of the salivary glands may be accomplished by local gustatory stimuli such as mints or chewing gum or by systemic sialogogues. More recently, immunosuppressive therapy with cyclosporin A has shown some promise.[49] The combination of prednisolone and chlorambucil has recently been shown to decrease disease progression.[50] Finally, corticosteroid irrigation of the parotid duct has been shown to significantly increase salivary flow rate compared with saline irrigation in a controlled study, and this benefit seemed to be sustained for a mean of 8.4 months.[51]

Obstructive parotid gland disease

Stricture of Stensen's duct

This may be caused by repeated infection, iatrogenic injury, congenital abnormality or trauma or through compression by a tumour. The clinical features are of pain and swelling of the parotid gland associated with eating. The diagnosis is established by sialography, which may also establish whether calculi are present. Distal duct or orifice stricture can now be treated by repeated duct dilatation, and surgery is seldom indicated. In patients who fail to respond, a formal stenotomy or marsupialisation of the duct orifice may be required. Duct reimplantation or excision of the gland are rarely required. Proximal duct stricture is more difficult to deal with, and alternative forms of treatment may be duct ligation (usually leading to atrophy of the gland) or rarely radiotherapy.

Sialolithiasis

Stone formation in the parotid gland is less common than in the submandibular gland. It may be primary or secondary. Stasis or slow clearance of salivary gland secretions occurs with one or more predisposing factors, including anatomical alterations in the duct, damaged duct epithelium from infection or trauma, stricture, alteration of the physicochemical composition of salivary secretions and systemic metabolic disease (particularly hyperparathyroidism and hyperuricaemia). A history of recurrent progressive glandular swelling, initially associated with meals, is common. The stone may occasionally be palpated along the course of Stensen's duct. Diagnosis is best made by sialography. Treatment depends on the location of the stone. If located superficially in the cheek, the stone may be removed via the oral cavity. If located in the proximal duct or in the hilum of the gland, the stone may be removed by parotidectomy. Multiple small stones may be dealt with by irrigation, stenting and ductoplasty.

Sialectasis

This is a disease of unknown aetiology in which progressive destruction of the alveoli and parenchyma of the gland are accompanied by duct stenosis and cyst formation as the alveoli coalesce. Most patients are thought to have congenital sialectasis and in children it may mimic mumps, although mumps seldom recurs. Approximately 50% of children have no symptoms by the time they reach adulthood, and only a small proportion require treatment.[52] The typical presentation is painful enlargement of one salivary gland after eating. The attack regresses after a few hours but is made worse by eating again. Attacks vary in frequency and are due to the main ducts being blocked by stones or epithelial debris. The diagnosis may be confirmed by sialography. Surgery to remove stones may be necessary, and occasionally the gland may require excision.

Cysts in the parotid gland

Cystic lesions account for up to 5% of parotid masses, but if neoplasms are excluded then the number of true cysts is greatly diminished.[3] Cystic lesions may be solitary or multiple. Solitary cysts may be due to obstruction of the ductal system from any cause[8] or may be a lymphoepithelial cyst probably formed owing to intranodal inclusions.[3] Rarer causes of solitary cystic lesions of the parotid are dermoid cyst, necrotic metastatic lymph node or cystic degeneration in low-grade mucoepidermoid carcinoma, papillocystic variant of acinic cell carcinoma or oncocytic cystadenoma. Lymphoepithelial cysts have occasionally been reported in association with Castleman's disease or angiofollicular lymph node hyperplasia.[53] Multiple cysts most often occur in Warthin's tumour and in HIV infection when they are associated with multiple cervical lymphadenopathy.[37]

Post-irradiation sialadenitis

This is due to irradiation of the gland as part of the planned treatment for head and neck malignancy. After 4000 cGy, the gland atrophies and xerostomia results.

Characteristic findings on CT and MRI have been described.[37] External beam irradiation is a tumour promoter, and an increased incidence of malignancy of the parotid gland occurs after 10 to 25 years.[45]

Tumours of the parotid gland

Classification and staging

There have been a variety of classifications of salivary gland tumours but the most widely used is the World Health Organization's (WHO) classification based on the classic work by Thackray and Sobin (**Table 9.3**).[54] The TNM staging of parotid tumours is illustrated in **Table 9.4** and is based on that described by Hermanek and Sobin.[55]

Benign epithelial parotid neoplasms

Pleomorphic adenoma

This is the most common salivary gland tumour (50% of all salivary gland tumours and approximately 80% of parotid tumours) and is so called because of

Tumour type	Approximate % of all salivary tumours
Benign epithelial tumours	
Pleomorphic adenoma	48
Adenolymphoma (Warthin's)	18
Monomorphic adenoma	<1
Malignant epithelial tumours	
Mucoepidermoid tumour	4
Acinic cell tumour	2
Carcinomas	16
Adenoid cystic	
Carcinoma ex-pleomorphic adenoma	
Adenocarcinoma	
Epidermal carcinoma	
Undifferentiated carcinoma	
Non-epithelial tumours	4
Haemangioma	
Lipoma	
Neurofibroma	
Unclassified tumours	8
Tumours from neighbouring organs or metastases	
Lymphomas	
Allied conditions	
Benign lymphoepithelial lesions	<1

Table 9.3 *WHO classification of salivary gland tumours*[54]

T	Primary tumour
TX	Not assessible
T0	No evidence of primary tumour
T1	Tumour ≤2 cm without extraparenchymal extension
T2	Tumour >2–4 cm without extraparenchymal extension
T3	Tumour >4–6 cm or tumour with extraparenchymal extension without seventh nerve involvement
T4	Tumour >6 cm or tumour invading skull base or seventh nerve

N	Regional lymph nodes
NX	Not assessible
N0	Regional nodes not involved
N1	Metastasis in a single ipsilateral node, ≤3 cm
N2	Metastasis in a single ipsilateral node >3–6 cm
	Metastases in multiple ipsilateral nodes, none >6 cm
	Metastases in bilateral or contralateral nodes, none >6 cm
N3	Metastasis in a lymph node, >6 cm

M	Distant metastases
MX	Not assessible
M0	No distant metastases
M1	Distant metastases present

Stage			
1	T1/2	N0	M0
2	T3	N0	M0
3	T1/2	N1	M0
4	T4	N0	M0
	T3/4	N1	M0
	Any T	N2/3	M0
	Any T	Any N	M1

Table 9.4 *TNM classification of parotid tumours*[55]

its mixed epithelial and mesenchymal elements. A recent study has suggested that epithelial–mesenchymal transition occurs within this tumour.[56] The annual incidence of parotid pleomorphic adenoma in the UK is approximately 1.4 per 100 000 people.[57,58] The peak age of incidence is in the fifth decade, and women are more commonly affected than are men. The commonest site within the parotid gland is in the tail,[10,57] with most tumours lying superficial to the facial nerve. The history is usually that of a slowly growing painless mass in the parotid, and pain and facial palsy are rare. The latter should prompt consideration of a malignant lesion. Fortunately, malignant transformation of a previously benign pleomorphic adenoma is rare.[57]

The diagnosis is primarily clinical, and it has been argued that radiological and cytological investigations are unnecessary,[23,57] although FNAC is useful in distinguishing between benign and malignant neoplasms and in determining pleomorphic adenoma from Warthin's tumour.[26] Radiological confirmation of a truly single lesion may be performed using ultrasonography or MRI and may show the depth of the neoplasm. The value of this is in preoperative counselling of the patient in the likelihood of a neuropraxia. Treatment is usually by some form of superficial or total conservative parotidectomy, with identification of the facial nerve during surgery (see techniques of parotidectomy).

Recurrence of pleomorphic adenoma occurs and the reasons for this have been hotly debated. When the surgical management in the early 20th century was local excision (for fear of damaging the facial nerve), local recurrence was in the order of 20–45%.[57] By the 1940s, superfical parotidectomy with dissection of the facial nerve was being advocated, and this reduced local recurrence. In 1957, Patey and Thackray demonstrated that small tumour buds protrude from the tumour surface into the surrounding tumour capsule.[59] This came to be accepted as the cause for local recurrence but was disproved by Nicholson and Gleave who practised the technique of 'extracapsular dissection' for 45 years with results that were equally as good as those for superficial parotidectomy.[60] It is therefore clear that the main factor regarding recurrence was incomplete surgical excision, and the same group confirmed a recurrence rate of only 1.6% after a median follow-up of 12.5 years. This low rate of local recurrence has also been achieved by other groups.[61] This also explains the paradox that preserving the facial nerve did not increase the risk of tumour recurrence despite the observation that in 50% of patients, a branch of the nerve was in direct contact with the tumour capsule.[57] Other factors said to contribute to local recurrence are young age at presentation[62] and inadequate surgical margins.[63, 64] Rupture of the capsule as a cause of local recurrence has recently been disputed.[64] Radiotherapy in such patients is regarded as unhelpful.[63] Most pleomorphic adenomas are probably best treated by superficial parotidectomy with identification and preservation of the facial nerve.

Local recurrence of pleomorphic adenomas may be uninodular or multinodular,[62] and this distinction is important. When uninodular disease is treated by surgery alone there is a failure rate of 15% at 15 years; with multinodular disease the failure rate is 43% but is reduced to 4% by the addition of postoperative radiotherapy,[62] although no randomised studies exist to examine which patients may benefit from this treatment. The type of surgery, not surprisingly, is not standardised for such an uncommon procedure and depends on the type, site and extent of the local recurrence. It is not surprising that the incidence of temporary and permanent facial nerve damage is greatly increased in this situation.

Adenolymphoma (Warthin's tumour)

Warthin described only two patients over a 35-year period, and first described them as papillary cystadenoma lymphomatosum.[65] It is apparent that its incidence has been increasing since its description and may now constitute 18% of all salivary gland neoplasms (Table 9.3) and up to 33% of all parotid neoplasms.[66,67] The highest incidence of those confined almost entirely to the parotid gland occurs in the sixth and seventh decades, with a male:female ratio of 1.6:1.[67] Smoking has been noted to be a strong aetiological factor and may explain the increasing incidence of this tumour and the change in its sex distribution over the past 70 years.[67, 68]

Clinically, this tumour presents as an ovoid, smooth lump containing cystic spaces filled with fluid and lined by papillary epithelium set in a lymphoid stroma. The epithelium develops from parotid duct cells as a result of metaplasia, forming two layers. Lining the cysts, the inner layer of epithelium is formed largely by tall columnar cells called oncocytes, whereas the basal layer of epithelium is formed by small, elongated irregular cells containing oval vesicular nuclei.[67] The most satisfactory explanation for the inclusion of lymphoid stroma lies in the embryological development of the parotid gland (see embryology) and that the tumour is due to a cellular response to the epithelium by the included residual lymphatic tissue. It has been proposed that adenolymphoma is not a benign neoplasm but a manifestation of a delayed hypersensitivity reaction, and that the trigger for the reaction is metaplasia of the ductal epithelium secondary to a metabolic or nutritional defect,[69] such as caused by smoking.[67] In up to 10% of patients, the lesions are multiple and occasionally bilateral, either synchronously or asynchronously.

Preoperative diagnosis has recently been improved by attention to specific cytological features of squamoid metaplasia and infarction.[26] Ultrasonography allows the detection of previously unsuspected multiple lesions within the same gland and occasionally identifies occult contralateral lesions. A correct preoperative diagnosis allows the correct surgical procedure to be planned. Because these tumours are benign and do not recur locally, a conservative surgical approach to their excision has been advocated in the form of 'controlled enucleation.'[67, 70] This allowed a reduction in temporary facial neuropraxia from 43% for superficial parotidectomy to 8% for controlled enucleation.[67] This procedure is unsuitable for multiple lesions and identification of the facial nerve is then required, especially for lesions in the deep portion of the gland.

Monomorphic adenoma

This is a rare benign tumour characterised by a proliferation of epithelial elements in the absence of cells of mesenchymal origin. In practice, preoperative diagnosis is difficult and distinction between a low-grade acinic cell carcinoma may be impossible. Treatment should ensure an adequate margin of excision, and most are therefore treated by superficial parotidectomy.

Oncocytoma

This rare, benign tumour usually affects elderly people and may originate in the salivary glands. It presents as a slow-growing painless lump that is well circumscribed and soft. Histologically, this tumour is characterised by tetrahedral cells with eosinophilic cytoplasm, and treatment is by surgical excision.

Malignant epithelial parotid neoplasms

Tumours of variable malignancy

1. Mucoepidermoid tumours

Since their description in 1945, there has been some debate as to the true biological nature of these tumours. One view has been that their biological nature is related to grade. Thus, low-grade tumours behave more like pleomorphic adenomas whereas high-grade tumours behave more aggressively and metastasise. A more recent view is that their behaviour is not related to histological appearance and that apparently even low-grade tumours may metastasise and even initially aggressive tumours may be cured with appropriate treatment.

Mucoepidermoid tumours can arise in any salivary gland, but 90% occur within the parotid (Table 9.3). The age of presentation is wide and may even occur in childhood, although the peak incidence lies in the fourth decade. The sex distribution is equal. These tumours may in addition be subdivided according to grade, which has a bearing on survival.[71, 72] Thus, if all grades of tumour are included, mortality may be as low as 8.7%.[71] Spiro has shown that the overall survival of 434 patients with mucoepidermoid tumours was of the order of 70%.[72] For intermediate- and high-grade tumours, survival may fall to as little as 40%.

2. Acinic cell tumours

This accounts for approximately 2% of all parotid tumours, and like Warthin's tumour, it may be bilateral in 3% of patients. It is uncommon outside the parotid gland. It occurs in childhood, but its peak age of incidence is in the fifth decade. It may also occur in intraparotid lymph nodes. Its biological behaviour is variable, but in general it has a better prognosis than mucoepidermoid tumours, and survival over 20 years has been reported to be between 75 and 84%.[71,72] Approximately 10% metastasise.

Carcinomas of the parotid gland

1. Adenoid cystic carcinoma

This histological type of cancer accounts for only 10% of salivary neoplasms. Only about 20% arise within the parotid, and they form only 2% of all parotid tumours.[73] The median age of presentation for patients with tumours arising in the parotid gland is 43 years, 10 years younger than for patients whose tumours arise in other salivary glands.[73] Histologically, these tumours contain round or oval cells forming strands or clusters in a myxomatous connective tissue matrix. The islands or strands of tumours cells interconnect to enclose characteristic cystic spaces, presenting a cribriform, cylindromatous pattern of growth. Classification into three grades is feasible but has not been found to be clinically useful.[74,75] This tumour has a predilection for neural spread, and this may account for the high proportion of patients (18%) who present with some degree of facial weakness. The incidence of lymph node spread is relatively low (6–10%),[73,74] and the incidence of distant metastases is high (40%).[75] Survival from adenoid cystic carcinoma tends to be better for parotid sites compared with other salivary gland sites, with 5-year and 10-year survival in the order of 42% and 25%, respectively. Local recurrence seems to be improved with the addition of postoperative radiotherapy but overall survival seems not to be affected.[73] The most important factor that influences survival seems to be stage at presentation,[73,75] and the previously reported finding that grade of tumour is an important determinant of survival of adenoid cystic carcinoma[76] has not been confirmed by later studies.[73,75]

2. Carcinoma ex-pleomorphic adenoma

This is sometimes described as a malignant mixed parotid tumour,[74] because the histological features show some characteristics of a benign mixed tumour (pleomorphic adenoma) with other areas containing carcinoma cells. These tumours comprise 18% of parotid cancers[74] and may arise as either malignant transformation in a longstanding pleomorphic adenoma (occurring in 10% after 15 years) or as a carcinoma arising in a mixed cell tumour. Lymph node metastases occur in approximately 20% of patients, and survival at 5 and 10 years has been reported to be 63% and 39%, respectively.[74]

3. Adenocarcinoma

This comprises 10% of malignant tumours of the parotid and approximately 3% of all salivary gland tumours. The sex incidence is equal and occasionally occurs in children. The histological pattern varies from trabecular to tubular, solid, papillary or mucus-secreting varieties without epidermoid differentiation. They may be low, intermediate or high grade and this, along with stage at presentation, influences survival, which may be as low as 19% at 10 years with high-grade lesions.[72,74]

4. Epidermoid carcinoma

This is rare, occurring in only 3% of malignant parotid tumours, and is characterised by exhibiting epidermoid or squamous differentiation. It may be difficult to differentiate from squamous cell carcinoma arising in other sites.[74] It is an aggressive tumour, presenting clinically with pain, skin fixation, ulceration, facial nerve palsy and metastatic spread to lymph nodes in 50% of patients.[74] Survival is poor and depends on grade of tumour and stage at presentation.

5. Undifferentiated (anaplastic) carcinoma

This is a rare tumour, invariably of high grade and with a poor prognosis.

Benign non-epithelial parotid neoplasms

Within the parotid gland, these tumours are rare. *Haemangiomas* of the parotid may be primary or secondary, involving the parotid from a primary site nearby such as the skin overlying the gland or the infratemporal fossa.[3] Some tumours may spontaneously regress, and treatment by embolisation is preferable to surgery.[77] *Lipomas* usually lie lateral to the parotid gland and are unilateral. They need to be distinguished from fatty infiltration of the parotid, which is usually bilateral. There are three types of *lymphangiomas*; simple lymphangioma, cavernous lymphangioma and cystic hygroma. Cavernous lymphangiomas are prone to recur after excision because they are almost impossible to remove completely. Cystic hygromas almost always involve the parotid gland and submandibular space and may require several excisions for complete removal.[77]

Lymphomas of the parotid

Malignant lymphoma of the parotid is a rare condition, occurring in only 2% of lymphomas of the head and neck.[78] They are usually described as mucosa associated lymphoid tissue (MALT) lymphomas, which histologically exhibit centrocyte-like cell proliferation surrounding B-cell reactive follicles. They may be surgically excised, but successful treatment with radiotherapy alone has been described, with a good prognosis.[78]

Management of patients with a parotid neoplasm

Since most benign tumours occur in the superficial lobe of the parotid, the standard operation since the 1950s has been superficial parotidectomy with dissection and preservation of the facial nerve. This is also true for low-grade parotid carcinomas such as the mucoepidermoid tumours and acinic cell tumours, which uncommonly present with lymph node metastases.[57] Total conservative parotidectomy (with facial nerve preservation) may be indicated for these tumours depending on the size of the tumour and its position within the parotid gland, especially if located in the deep lobe. The aim of the surgery is to achieve a clear margin of excision around the tumour to minimise the risk of local recurrence. A variation on this procedure is subtotal parotidectomy, which has been described as a conservative resection of the superficial lobe with less than a full facial nerve dissection.[79] The merits of this procedure are that for benign and low-grade malignant lesions, surgical clearance is adequate with the advantage of a reduction in the postoperative complication rate, especially that of facial nerve paresis.

Postoperative radiotherapy may be given after excision of a low-grade carcinoma if the surgical margin is involved by tumour,[57] but its use after surgery for pleomorphic adenoma is controversial.[80] Postoperative radiotherapy may have a place in the management of patients with recurrent pleomorphic adenoma, especially in patients in whom recurrences are multinodular. In this situation, the addition of postoperative radiotherapy is associated with a significantly improved rate of local control.[62]

The treatment of Warthin's tumour has hitherto also been by superficial parotidectomy, but increasingly some authorities have advocated an even more conservative approach and have recommended enucleation.[68,70] The rationale for this approach has been the zero recurrence rate after complete excision and the greatly reduced incidence of facial nerve paresis compared with superficial parotidectomy (8% vs. 43%, respectively).[67]

The management of patients with overtly malignant tumours is primarily surgical, the extent of surgery depending on the stage of presentation. Facial nerve paresis and clinically detectable lymphadenopathy both occur in approximately 20% of patients,[72–74] and careful clinical staging is essential. An accurate preoperative diagnosis is also highly desirable using either FNAC or even a Tru-cut biopsy.[81] Imaging of the head and neck, as well as the chest, with CT scanning has been advocated,[81] although MRI is probably better for evaluating tumours.[37] This allows better visualisation of the primary tumour—notably any deep-lobe extension—and may identify fixity to surrounding structures. It is also useful in identifying clinically occult lymph node metastases. Finally, MRI allows for better preoperative counselling of the patient, especially if the extent of the surgery is likely to sacrifice the facial nerve or if immediate reconstructive surgery is contemplated. Prophylactic radical cervical lymphadenectomy has been advocated in the past and is much more controversial.[82] It is unnecessary in all patients in whom lymph node metastases are only suspected, and studies suggest that local recurrence is unlikely if a jugulodigastric lymph node examined by frozen section at operation is free from tumour.[83] Postoperative radiotherapy may be required, and an oncologist should be involved early in the management of these patients.

Surgery of the parotid gland

Superficial conservative parotidectomy

Superficial conservative parotidectomy is indicated for benign tumours and low-grade malignant tumours confined to the superficial lobe of the parotid.

The patient is positioned in the supine position with the neck slightly extended and the head turned away from the surgeon. The table is inclined in a slightly head-up position to reduce venous congestion, and a small 'peanut' swab is placed in the external auditory canal to protect the tympanic membrane. The towels are arranged so that the ipsilateral eye and corner of the mouth can be viewed when necessary during stimulation of the facial nerve. During general anaesthesia, muscle relaxants should be avoided.

The incision begins near the top of the pinna in the preauricular crease, runs inferiorly until the point at which the ear lobe joins the face and then sweeps posteriorly and upwards beneath and behind the ear lobe. The incision is then extended inferiorly along the anterior border of the sternomastoid for 2 cm. The incision is then deepened through the superficial fascia and platysma, and the anterior skin flap is mobilised superficial to the parotid gland as far as its anterior border. The skin flap and the ear lobe may then be retracted out of the operative field with sutures. The great auricular nerve is identified lying on the deep cervical fascia investing the sternomastoid muscle. The sternomastoid muscle is separated from the posterior border of the parotid gland, and the great auricular nerve is divided at the point where it crosses on to the parotid gland. The posterior border of the parotid gland is then separated from the mastoid process and the cartilaginous external meatus, opening up a sulcus between the parotid gland and these structures, which is extended inferiorly between the gland and the sternomastoid muscle. This sulcus is further deepened to expose the posterior belly of the digastric muscle, which is then followed upwards to a point where it dips beneath the mastoid process. Great care must be taken to avoid damage to the facial nerve at this point.

The sulcus between the posterior border of the parotid and the external meatus and mastoid process is deepened by carefully dividing the fibrous septa bridging it, and the main trunk (pes anserinus) of the facial nerve is identified. Identification of the facial nerve is facilitated by the use of a nerve stimulator, but even so, great caution must be maintained during this and the subsequent dissection. The nerve has a characteristic appearance and usually has a tiny blood vessel on its surface. The parotid gland is then retracted forwards, and the plane between the nerve and the superficial lobe is dissected forwards until the bifurcation of the nerve is identified. A haemostat is now slid over the upper division of the nerve and the blades opened. Glandular tissue overlying the posterior blade is divided with a knife or scissors to divide the posterior border of the gland. Keeping the superficial lobe retracted, the plane between the nerve and the superficial lobe is gently dissected so as to eventually identify all the branches of the nerve, keeping the scissors used for dividing the septa of the gland in a forward direction. It is important to remember that the smaller branches of the facial nerve become more superficial as the dissection proceeds distally, and great care is needed to ensure that one of the peripheral branches of the nerve is not damaged as the superficial lobe is dissected away from the nerve. The superficial lobe can then be mobilised sufficiently to allow it to be pedicled anteriorly.

The buccal branch or branches are then traced downwards and the superficial lobe eventually severed. Small bleeding vessels may be tied off with a fine absorbable suture. It is usual to see the retromandibular vein lying vertically deep to the branches of the facial nerve and emerging from the tail of the remaining gland just posterior to the mandibular branch.

The platysma may be sutured as a separate layer but is often deficient in the superior part of the wound. A small suction drain is used to drain the cavity, and the skin is sutured with a subcuticular absorbable suture. The drain may be removed on the first postoperative day and the patient discharged.

Variations to this procedure are the partial superficial parotidectomy[84] and the conservative parotidectomy by the peripheral approach, in which the branches of the facial nerve (usually the cervical branch) are identified first, with subsequent proximal dissection to the main trunk of the nerve.[85]

Total conservative parotidectomy

Total conservative parotidectomy is indicated for benign neoplasms arising in the deep lobe of the gland, chronic parotitis secondary to longstanding duct obstruction and tuberculous parotitis. It may also be indicated for recurrent pleomorphic adenoma, low-grade malignant tumours and, only occasionally, high-grade tumours in which the facial nerve is not involved. It is contraindicated for tumours in which the nerve is involved.

The operation involves removal of the superficial and deep lobes of the gland, with preservation of the facial nerve. A superficial parotidectomy is first performed. The branches and main trunk of the facial nerve are dissected off the underlying deep lobe using small scissors to divide the fascial attachments of the nerve to the underlying gland. This manoeuvre is facilitated by lifting the branches with a nerve hook. The deep lobe is separated with scissors from the posterior border of the ascending ramus of the mandible and from the temporomandibular joint. The deep aspect of the gland is gently separated from its underlying bed with small scissors, which are introduced above and below the main trunk of the nerve. Any attachments of the gland to the styloid process are divided. The upper and lower ends of the retromandibular vein and any anterior branches are divided between ligatures. The more deeply placed external carotid artery may not have to be interrupted if it does not actually penetrate the gland but lies deep to it. However, it often perforates the deep lobe, and that portion may have to be excised with the specimen. If so, the artery is divided at the lower border of the gland above the posterior belly of digastric and stylohyoid muscles and superiorly where it becomes the superficial temporal artery. The internal maxillary and transverse facial branches of the external carotid artery are then also divided, enabling the deep lobe to be dissected off its bed in a downward direction. The wound is closed as described for superficial parotidectomy.

Radical parotidectomy

High-grade carcinoma of the parotid gland is the primary indication for radical parotidectomy. It is only occasionally indicated for recurrent pleomorphic adenoma when, for technical reasons, there is little chance of preserving the facial nerve. Histological confirmation of malignancy is desirable prior to surgery and this may be performed preoperatively with a Tru-cut biopsy.[81]

The patient is positioned as described for superficial parotidectomy. In some patients, radical parotidectomy may be accompanied by a radical or functional neck dissection to remove regional lymph nodes also involved by tumour. An incision similar to that described for superficial parotidectomy is performed. This may need to be extended inferiorly to accommodate a radical neck dissection. The description which follows applies to the parotid gland and does not take into account radical neck dissection in-continuity. The posterior limits of the dissection are defined in the same way as for superficial parotidectomy, thus dissecting the posterior border free from the sternomastoid muscle to expose the posterior belly of the digastric muscle. The gland is freed superiorly from the mastoid process and external auditory meatus. The retromandibular vein is then ligated and divided at the tail of the parotid. The parotid gland is then elevated to reveal the posterior belly of the digastric and the stylohyoid muscles, and the external carotid artery is ligated and divided just before it enters the deep aspect of the gland above the stylohyoid muscle. The soft tissues at the tail of the parotid gland are further incised in a forward direction until the angle of the mandible is reached. Starting at the lower border of the mandible and dissecting upwards along a vertical line anterior to the parotid gland, the soft tissues overlying the ascending ramus are divided down to bone all the way up to the zygomatic arch. The structures divided during this dissection include subcutaneous fat, branches of the facial nerve, the transverse facial artery and veins, the parotid duct and the masseter muscle. The cut peripheral branches of the facial nerve may be tagged with a suture for ease of identification if a nerve graft is contemplated.

A periosteal elevator is used to push the soft tissues of the specimen backwards to the posterior border of the ascending ramus of the mandible. The soft tissues overlying the zygomatic arch are incised down to the bone as far back as the pinna. Branches of the upper division of the facial nerve are divided during this step and may also be tagged with a suture. The superficial temporal artery and vein are divided at the point where they cross the arch. The incision is now carried inferiorly between the parotid gland and the cartilage of the external auditory meatus to join the earlier line of separation of the posterior border of the parotid gland.

By retracting the tail of the specimen superiorly, the gland is dissected away from its bed with scissors, starting from below and working upwards. It is separated from the posterior border of the mandible, from the styloid process which lies deep to it and from the anterior aspect of the bony external meatus, below which the facial nerve is divided as it emerges from the stylomastoid foramen. The specimen can now be retracted downwards and laterally sufficiently to expose the maxillary artery and veins so that they can be divided between ligatures or clamps. A nerve graft consisting of branches of the cervical plexus derived from a common stem can now be inserted between the divided trunk and branches of the facial nerve and sutured in place. The wound is closed as described for superficial parotidectomy.

Locally advanced tumours may require resection of adjacent tissues such as muscle, bone or overlying skin (extended radical parotidectomy), and this may necessitate soft tissue reconstruction such as a cervical cutaneous flap or pectoralis major, latissimus dorsi and trapezius flaps. A free flap such as the radial forearm flap provides a good cosmetic result.

Postoperative complications

Facial nerve injury

After superficial parotidectomy, permanent nerve injury only occurs in 1% of patients.[60] Transient nerve paresis occurs much more commonly—30–43%.[60,67] After total conservative parotidectomy, permanent and transient nerve paresis increases to 6% and 60%, respectively,[62] and 90% of transient injuries recover within 12 months.[57] Clearly, more limited resection of the parotid gland is associated with a marked reduction of transient facial paresis to approximately 8%.[67]

Several techniques have been described to repair a divided facial nerve and consist of faciohypoglossal transposition, end-to-end anastomosis and cable graft anastomosis. The comparison of the results of such surgery has been facilitated by the development of facial function scoring systems such as the House–Brackmann scale.[86] Results of these techniques indicate an improvement in facial function in two thirds of patients.[87]

Frey's syndrome

This consists of discomfort, sweating and occasionally redness of the skin overlying the parotid area, which occurs during and after eating. It is due to the severed ends of the parasympathetic secretomotor fibres growing into the skin, which are then stimulated by eating, causing vasodilation and sweating. It may occur in up to 60% of patients postoperatively, but only 20% of patients actually complain about it.[77] The condition usually resolves spontaneously but if persistent it may be treated by tympanic neurectomy, which divides the parasympathetic pathway. A variety of topical agents have been tried to alleviate these symptoms and a clinical trial using 1% glycopyrrolate roll-on lotion or cream has been found to be effective in controlling gustatory sweating for up to 3 days.[88] It is claimed that the incidence of clinical Frey's syndrome can be reduced to 3% with the use of a synthetic implant (expanded polytetrafluoroethylene) placed in the cavity after superficial parotidectomy.[89]

Salivary fistula

This is uncommon and due to the excessive production of saliva from the remaining deep lobe after superficial parotidectomy. In most patients, it resolves spontaneously after a few weeks, but if it does persist, the deep lobe of the gland may be removed; an alternative to this is to irradiate the remaining parotid gland. The use of a fascial flap has been advocated to prevent this complication.[90]

Hypoaesthesia of the ear lobe

It is common for patients to experience some hypoaesthesia of the preauricular region and the lower half of the pinna due to division of the posterior branch of the great auricular nerve. This usually improves with time and does not require any specific treatment.

Neuroma

Occasionally a neuroma may arise from the cut end of the posterior branch of the great auricular nerve. This complication should be borne in mind before concluding that the swelling is a recurrence of a parotid tumour.

Radiotherapy

A major proportion of parotid tumours are radiosensitive.[91] Postoperative radiotherapy has been recommended for all patients with malignant salivary tumours[71] but local recurrence is rare after complete excision of low-grade tumours, and radiotherapy is probably best reserved for those patients with high-grade tumours.[92] Radiotherapy alone may achieve temporary local control in approximately 30% of patients and may produce a sufficient reduction in tumour bulk to facilitate subsequent excision.[93,94]

The submandibular gland

Diseases of the submandibular gland are less common than those of the parotid. Furthermore, the pattern of disease is slightly different, with stones in the gland or its duct being more common than tumours, which are also less diverse in their histological features. The submandibular gland may be affected by the same infections and autoimmune diseases as the parotid and will not be described again.

Embryology

The submandibular gland develops as an epithelial outgrowth from the floor of the alveololingual groove. It increases rapidly in size by giving off numerous branching processes, which later acquire lumina. At first, the connection of the submandibular outgrowth with the floor of the mouth lies at the side of the tongue, but the edges of the groove in which it opens come together from behind forwards and form the tubular part of the submandibular duct. As a result, the orifice of the duct is shifted forwards until it comes to lie below the tip of the tongue, close to the median plane. The submandibular gland becomes encapsulated before the emergence of the lymphatic system in the mesoderm, and this explains why the spectrum of benign tumours differs from that of the parotid.[2]

Anatomy

The submandibular gland is the second largest salivary gland, being about one half the weight of the parotid. It occupies most of the submandibular triangle of the neck and is folded around the dorsal free edge of the mylohyoid muscle. Although there are no separate lobes to the gland, by convention it is often described as having a superficial and deep lobe. The larger superficial lobe lies in the submandibular triangle, superficial and caudal to the mylohyoid. It lies deep to the skin and platysma and is crossed superficially by the cervical branch of the facial nerve. This is extremely important to know as the nerve may be damaged by an incision placed too high in the neck when excision of the gland is to be performed. The smaller, deep lobe lies between the mylohyoid and hyoglossus muscles. The duct (Wharton's duct) arises from this deep portion and passes forwards adjacent to the sublingual gland to the papilla in the floor of the mouth to the side of the frenulum of the tongue. Posteriorly, the gland is grooved by the facial artery. The lingual nerve lies on the hyoglossus above the gland but crosses the duct first on its outer (mandibular) aspect and then recrosses it on its deeper (lingual) aspect. The hypoglossal nerve lies between the gland and the hyoglossus and then runs forward, inferior to the duct. In front of the hyoglossus, the nerve passes deep to the duct to reach the muscles of the tongue. The digastric and stylohyoid muscles lie inferior to the more superficial part of the gland.

The arteries supplying the submandibular gland are branches of the facial and lingual arteries, and the venous drainage follows that of the arteries. The nerves are derived from the submandibular ganglion, through which the gland receives parasympathetic fibres from the chorda tympani branch of the facial nerve, the lingual branch of the mandibular nerve and sympathetic fibres. Lymphatic drainage is to the submandibular and upper deep cervical lymph nodes.

The submandibular gland is a mixed serous and mucous gland, with about 10% of the acini being mucinous. By contrast with the parotid, adipose tissue is not a prominent component of the glandular parenchyma.

Physiology

The submandibular glands contribute approximately 45% of the total volume of saliva. As with the parotid gland, control of secretion is by the autonomic nervous system.[95]

Developmental abnormalities

Atresia of one or more major salivary gland ducts—usually the submandibular or sublingual glands—is rare and is associated with xerostomia and possibly the development of a retention cyst.[6,8]

Investigation of the submandibular gland

Clinical evaluation

Most lesions of the submandibular gland are due to obstructive stone disease and only occasionally due to tumour. The gland should be palpated bimanually and any degree of fixity noted. Stones may be palpated in the gland itself or in Wharton's duct on the floor of the mouth, and the duct orifice should be inspected. Cervical lymphadenopathy should be noted and all other salivary glands should be inspected to determine whether the submandibular enlargement is part of a generalised disease.

The diagnosis of a submandibular mass is usually obvious but may easily be mistaken for an enlarged submandibular lymph node mass.

Radiology

The indications for radiological investigation of the submandibular gland are similar to those of the parotid.[37] Submandibular stones are nearly always radio-opaque and therefore plain films are much more useful. Sialography is also more informative and is especially helpful in locating the position of a stone within the duct system. This enables a decision to be made as to whether a stone can be removed from a duct via the floor of the mouth or whether submandibular gland excision is more appropriate. The indications for ultrasonography, CT and MRI are similar to those for the parotid gland.[37]

FNAC

The major problem in evaluating the submandibular region has been in distinguishing between chronic sialodenitis and squamous cell carcinoma.[24] FNAC is valuable, however, in distinguishing metastatic carcinoma from squamous carcinoma of the oral cavity. Primary salivary gland tumours in the submandibular region pose similar diagnostic problems to those in the parotid region, and these have been described above. Lymphoma and tuberculosis are quite common in the submandibular lymph nodes, and FNAC is useful in making a diagnosis. The diagnosis of other benign conditions such as lipoma or neurofibroma are difficult on FNAC. Diagnostic accuracy of submandibular masses is similar to that of parotid masses.[24]

Sialometry

Wharton's duct can be cannulated to assess submandibular gland output and composition and may be helpful in confirming a hyposecretory state.

Infections

Bacterial and viral infections are much less common than in the parotid gland. Even primary tuberculosis of a salivary gland seems to occur less frequently in the submandibular gland compared with the parotid (27% *vs.* 70%).[42] The principles of diagnosis and treatment are the same as those outlined for the parotid gland.

Autoimmune diseases

The submandibular glands are commonly involved in Sjögren's syndrome, and the principles in diagnosis and treatment are the same as for parotid gland involvement.

Obstructive submandibular gland disease

Stricture of Wharton's duct

This may occur due to repeated infection, trauma due to stones or iatrogenic injury, congenital abnormalities or compression by a tumour. Treatment options are similar to those for Stensen's duct.

Sialolithiasis

The most common sites for a salivary gland calculus are within the submandibular gland or its duct. It is almost 50 times more common in the submandibular gland than in the parotid[38] because the saliva is more mucinous. Other predisposing causes are otherwise the same as for the parotid gland.

The clinical features are of recurrent painful swelling of the gland before or during meals. To reproduce the swelling at the time of examination, the patient can be given some fruit juice to sip. The orifices of Wharton's duct are then examined and compared. Saliva will be seen issuing from the unaffected side but not from the side of the swollen gland. If the stone is in Wharton's duct, it can often be palpated in the floor of the mouth. The diagnosis may be confirmed by sialography.

If the stone lies in the duct, it can be removed from the floor of the mouth. If the stone is in the hilum of the gland or is associated with other stones in the gland itself, excision of the gland is curative.

Tumours of the submandibular gland

Classification and staging

These are classified as illustrated in Tables 9.3 and 9.4. It should be emphasised that tumours of the submandibular gland are extremely uncommon. They comprise between 4 and 8% of all salivary tumours and are benign in 57 to 66% of all submandibular neoplasms.[58,71,72] The commonest tumour is a pleomorphic adenoma. Diagnosis is confirmed by FNAC. Imaging of the gland with ultrasonography and MRI may be useful if malignancy is suspected due to local fixity, especially to the mandible.

Treatment

Benign tumours are adequately treated by complete excision of the gland. Malignant tumours should be staged appropriately. Surgery may involve simple excision of the gland if this is sufficient to obtain clear margins. However, fixity to surrounding structures or involved lymph nodes requires a radical excision, radical neck dissection and reconstruction. Early involvement with a reconstructive surgeon and oncologist is mandatory. Radiotherapy is recommended postoperatively in most patients with malignant disease and in those undergoing surgery for recurrent pleomorphic adenoma.[71] It seems that survival is related to the histological type of the cancer and the stage at presentation and is similar to that quoted for parotid cancers.

Surgery of the submandibular gland

Removal of duct calculus

This may be performed under general or local anaesthesia if the stone is near the duct orifice. The tissues immediately behind the stone are grasped with tissue forceps, which steadies the stone, elevates it and prevents inadvertent dislocation proximally down the duct. An incision in the floor of the mouth is made on to the stone in the long axis of the duct and the stone retrieved. Haemostasis is achieved if necessary and the wound left unsutured.

Excision of the submandibular gland

The most common indication for excision of the submandibular gland is recurrent swelling and pain due to stones in the gland or in the proximal portion of

Wharton's duct. Other indications are after acute phlegmonous sialadenitis and recurrent sialectasis. Neoplasia is an absolute indication for excision and may need to be combined with a radical neck dissection for malignant disease.

The patient is positioned in the supine position, with a small sandbag under the shoulders and the head turned in the opposite direction. A horizontal skin incision is made well below the mandible, preferably in a skin crease just above the hyoid bone to avoid the lowest branch of the facial nerve. The incision should overlap the sternomastoid posteriorly and extend to just beyond the limit of the gland anteriorly. The incision is deepened through the fat and platysma to the level of the deep cervical fascia, which is then incised along the anterior border of the sternomastoid and horizontally above the hyoid bone to expose the fascial condensation around the gland. This is incised horizontally at the lower border of the gland.

The upper flap, consisting of skin, subcutaneous fat, platysma, deep cervical fascia and the fascial capsule superficial to the gland, is now elevated by sharp dissection. The dissection proceeds from below upwards and the tissues are retracted. The common facial or anterior facial vein is divided between ligatures, and the lower border of the gland is grasped by suitable traction forceps and lifted up. This reveals the common tendon of the digastric muscle and the hyoglossus muscle. The gland is separated from the muscular floor of the submandibular triangle using sharp dissection, and the hypoglossal nerve with its venae commitantes is identified on the hyoglossus muscle. The anterior segment of the gland is released from the mylohyoid muscle. Traction on the gland is applied forwards and upwards, and the stylohyoid and posterior belly of the digastric is retracted downwards and backwards. The facial artery is identified as it emerges from its position deep between these muscles and divided proximal to the gland between strong ligatures, freeing the gland posteriorly.

The gland is retracted downwards and its superior fascial attachments to the mandible divided. This exposes the facial artery and anterior facial vein, which are divided between ligatures as close to the gland as possible to avoid the mandibular branch of the facial nerve. A blunt retractor is inserted deep to the posterior free border of the mylohyoid, exposing the deep part of the gland. Traction on the gland drags down the lingual nerve, which should be separated from the gland. Traction in a downward and lateral direction exposes the duct, which is ligated and divided. Haemostasis is secured and the wound closed by suturing the platysma and skin. A suction drain may be employed if desired but is often unnecessary.

Postoperative complications

Paralysis of the depressor anguli oris due to damage of the mandibular branch of the facial nerve is the commonest complication. Hypoglossal nerve palsy leads to deviation of the tongue to the affected side and eventually fasciculation and wasting. It is uncommon and requires no action in a unilateral palsy. Lingual nerve damage is very uncommon and results in paraesthesiae or loss of taste in the homolateral half of the tongue. Should this be troublesome, division of the lingual nerve relieves the symptoms but results in loss of taste.

References

1. Langman J. Medical embryology. Baltimore: Williams and Wilkins, 1963; pp. 195–211.

2. Sperber GH. Craniofacial embryology, 4th. London: Wright, 1989; pp. 188–91.

3. Batsakis JG. Tumours of the head and neck: clinical and pathological considerations, 2nd edit. Baltimore: Williams and Wilkins, 1979.

 4. Davis RA, Anson BJ, Budinger JM *et al.* Surgical anatomy of the facial nerve and parotid gland based upon a study of 350 cervico-facial halves. Surg Gynecol Obstet 1956; 102: 385–412.

5. Snyderman NL, Suen JY. Neoplasms. In: Cummings CW, Schuller DE, eds. Otolaryngology—head and neck surgery, Vol 2. St Louis: Mosby Year Book, 1986: 1027–69.

6. Johns ME. The salivary glands: anatomy and embryology. Otolaryngol Clin North Am 1977; 10: 261–71.

7. Kelly BA, Black MJM, Soames JV. Unilateral enlargement of the parotid gland in a patient with sialosis and contralateral parotid aplasia. Br J Oral Maxillofac Surg 1990; 28: 409–12.

8. Mason DK, Chisholm DM. Salivary glands in health and disease. London: WB Saunders, 1975: 37–69.

9. Hobsley M. Salivary tumours. Br J Hosp Med 1973; 10: 555–62.

10. Phillps DE, Jones AS. Reliability of clinical examination in the diagnosis of parotid tumours. J R Coll Surg Edinburgh 1994; 39: 100–2.

11. Yousem DM. Head and neck imaging. Radiol Clin North Am 1998; 36: 941–66.

12. Bryan RN, Miller RH, Ferreyro RI *et al.* Computed tomography of the salivary glands. Am J Roentgenol 1982; 139: 547–54.

13. Parker GD, Harnsberger HR. Clinical-radiologic issues in perineural tumour spread of malignant diseases of the extra-cranial head and neck. Radiographics 1991; 11: 383–99.

14. Chaudhuri R, Bingham JB, Crossman JE *et al.* Magnetic resonance imaging of the parotid gland using the STIR sequence. Clin Otolaryngol 1992; 17: 211–7.

15. McGhee RB Jr, Chakeres DW, Schmalkbrock P *et al.* The extra-cranial facial nerve: high resolution three-dimensional Fourier transform MR imaging. Am J Neuroradiol 1992; 14: 465–72.

16. Ahuja A, Ying M, Yang WT *et al.* The use of sonography in differentiating cervical lymphomatous lymph nodes from cervical metastatic lymph nodes. Clin Radiol 1996; 51: 186–90.

17. Diederich S, Roos N, Bick U *et al.* Diagnostic imaging of the salivary glands in children and adolescents. *Radiologie* 1991; 31: 550–7.

18. Kawamura H, Taniguchi N, Itoh K *et al.* Salivary gland echography in patients with Sjogren's syndrome. Arthritis Rheum 1990; 33: 505–10.

19. Mann W, Wachter W. Ultrasonic diagnosis of the salivary glands. Laryngorhinootologie 1988; 67: 355–61.

20. Brandwein MS, Huvos AG. Oncocytic tumours of major salivary glands: a study of 68 cases with follow-up of 44 patients. Am J Surg Pathol 1991; 15: 514–28.

21. Cogan MI, Gill PS. Value of sialography and scintigraphy in diagnosis of salivary gland disorders. Int J Oral Surg 1981; 10: 216–22.

22. Vogl TJ, Dadashi A, Jassoy A *et al.* The 31-phosphorus spectroscopy of space occupying lesion of the salivary glands. The clinical results and differential diagnosis. Rofo Fortschr Geb Rontgenstr Neuen Bildgeb Verfahr 1993; 158: 31–8.

 23. McGurk M, Hussain K. Role of fine needle aspiration cytology in the management of the discrete parotid lump. Ann R Coll Surg Engl 1997; 79: 198–202.

24. Shaha A, Webber C, DiMaio T *et al.* Needle aspiration biopsy in salivary gland lesions. Am J Surg 1990; 160: 373–6.

25. Rodriguez HP, Silver CE, Moisa II *et al.* Fine needle aspiration of parotid tumours. Am J Surg 1989; 158: 342–3.

26. Lewis DR, Webb AJ, Lott MF *et al.* Improving cytological diagnosis and surgical management of parotid adenolymphoma. Br J Surg 1999; 86: 1275–9.

27. Pitts DB, Hilsinger RL, Karandy E *et al.* Fine needle aspiration in the diagnosis of salivary gland disorders in the community hospital setting. Arch Otolaryngol Head Neck Surg 1992; 118: 479–82.

28. Orell SR, Nettle WJS. Fine needle aspiration biopsy of salivary gland tumours. Problems and pitfalls. Pathology 1988; 20: 332–7.

29. Eneroth CM, Franzen S, Zajicek J. Cytologic diagnosis on aspirate from 1000 salivary gland tumours. Acta Otolaryngol 1967; 1: 168–71.

30. Layfield LJ, Tan P, Glasgow BJ. Fine-needle aspiration of salivary gland lesions. Comparison with frozen sections and histologic findings. Arch Pathol Lab Med 1987; 111: 346–53.

31. Lindberg LG, Akerman M. Aspiration cytology of salivary gland tumours: diagnostic experience from six years of routine laboratory work. Laryngoscope 1976; 86: 584–94.

32. O'Dwyer P, Farrar WB, James AG *et al.* Needle aspiration biopsy of major salivary gland tumours. Its value. Cancer 1986; 57: 554–7.

33. Persson PS, Zettergren L. Cytological diagnosis of salivary gland tumours by aspiration biopsy. Acta Cytol 1973; 17: 351–4.

34. Qizilbash AH, Sianos J, Young JE *et al.* Fine needle aspiration biopsy cytology of major salivary glands. Acta Cytol 1985; 29: 503–12.

35. Filopoulos E, Angeli S, Daskalopoulou D *et al.* Preoperative evaluation of parotid tumours by fine needle biopsy. Eur J Surg Oncol 1998; 24: 180–3.

36. Miglets AW. Infections, Part III. Clinical entities. In: Cummings CW, Fredrickson JM, Harker LA (eds). Otolaryngology—head and neck surgery, Vol 2. St Louis: Mosby Year Book, 1986: 999–1006.

37. Yousem DM. The radiologic clinics of North America; head and neck imaging, Vol 36. Philadelphia: WB Saunders, 1998; 949–50.

38. Harding Rains AJ, Ritchie HD (eds). Bailey and Love's short practice of surgery, 16th edit. London: HK Lewis, 1975: 537–8.

39. Moss-Salentijn L, Moss L. Development and functional anatomy. In: Rankow RM, Polayes IM (eds) Diseases of the salivary glands. Philadelphia: WB Saunders, 1976: 17–31.

40. Al-Deeb SM. Herpes simplex encephalitis mimicking mumps. Clin Neurol Neurosurg 1993; 95: 49–53.

41. Chapnick JS, Noyek AM, Berris B *et al.* Parotid gland enlargement in HIV infection: clinical/imaging findings. J Otolaryngol 1990; 19: 189–94.

42. Rabinov K, Weber AL. Radiology of the salivary glands. Boston: G Hall, 1985: 153–66.

43. Marx RE, Hartman KS, Rethman KV. A prospective study comparing incisional labial to incisional parotid biopsies in the detection and confirmation of sarcoidosis, Sjogren's disease, sialosis and lymphoma. J Rheumatol 1988; 15: 621–9.

44. Work WP, Hecht DW. Inflammatory diseases of the major salivary glands. In: Paparella MM, Shumrick DA (eds). Otolaryngology, Vol 3. Philadelphia: WB Saunders, 1973: 258–65.

45. Hudson NP. Manifestations of systemic disease. In: Cummings CW, Fredrickson JM, Harker LA *et al.* (eds). Head and neck surgery, Vol 2. St Louis: Mosby Year Book, 1986: 1007–13.

46. Bloch KJ. Sjogren's syndrome. In: Stein JH (ed). Internal medicine. Boston: Little Brown, 1983: 1034–6.

47. Daniels TE, Fox PC. Salivary and oral components of Sjogren's syndrome. In: Fox RI (ed). Rheumatic disease clinics of North America, Vol 18. Philadelphia: WB Saunders, 1992; 571–89.

48. Fox RI, Carstens SA, Fong S *et al.* Use of monoclonal antibodies to analyse peripheral blood and salivary gland lymphocyte subsets in Sjögren's syndrome. Arthritis Rheum 1982; 25: 419–26.

49. Drosos AA, Skopouli FN, Costopoulos JS *et al.* Cyclosporin A (CyA) in primary Sjögren's syndrome: a double blind study. Ann Rheum Dis 1986; 45: 732–5.

50. Vasil'ev VI, Simonova MV, Safonova TN *et al.* [Comparative evaluation of the treatment of Sjögren's syndrome with anti-rheumatic preparations]. Ter Arkh 1988; 60: 67–72.

51. Izumi M, Eguchi K, Nakamura H *et al.* Corticosteroid irrigation of parotid gland for treatment of xerostomia in patients with Sjögren's syndrome. Ann Rheum Dis 1998; 57: 464–9.

52. Thackray AC. Sialectasis. Arch Middlesex Hosp 1955; 5: 151.

53. Santonja C, Garcia-Aroca J, Colomar PJ. Castleman's disease and lymphoepithelial cysts of the parotid in childhood. Histopathol 1997; 30: 369–72.

54. Thackray AC, Sobin LH. In: Thackray AC, Sobin LH (eds). Histological typing of salivary tumours. Geneva: World Health Organisation, 1972: 16–25.

55. Hermanek P, Sobin LH. TNM classification of malignant tumours. Berlin: Springer-Verlag, 1987: 30–2.

56. Aigner T, Neureiter D, Völker U *et al.* Epithelial-mesenchymal transdifferentiation and extracellular

matrix gene expression in pleomorphic adenomas of the parotid salivary gland. J Pathol 1998; 186: 178–85.

57. McGurk M. Parotid pleomorphic adenoma. Br J Surg 1997; 84: 1491–2.

58. Renehan A, Gleave FN, Hancock BD *et al.* Long-term follow-up of over 1000 patients with salivary gland tumours treated in a single centre. Br J Surg 1996; 83: 1750–4.

59. Patey DH, Thackray AC. The treatment of parotid tumours in the light of pathological study of parotidectomy material. Br J Surg 1957; 45: 477–87.

60. McGurk M, Renehan A, Gleave EN *et al.* Clinical significance of the tumour capsule in the treatment of parotid pleomorphic adenomas. Br J Surg 1996; 83: 1747–9.

61. Leverstein H, van der Wal JE, Tiwari RM *et al.* Surgical management of 246 previously untreated pleomorphic adenomas of the parotid gland. Br J Surg 1997; 84: 399–403.

62. Renehan A, Gleave EN, McGurk M. An analysis of the treatment of 114 patients with recurrent pleomorphic adenomas of the parotid gland. Am J Surg 1996; 172: 710–4.

63. Stevens KL, Hobsley M. The treatment of pleomorphic adenomas by formal parotidectomy. Br J Surg 1982; 69: 1–3.

64. Buchanan C, Stringer SP, Mendenhall WM *et al.* Pleomorphic adenoma: effect of tumour spill and inadequate resection on tumour recurrence. Laryngoscope 1994; 104: 1231–4.

65. Warthin AS. Papillary cystadenoma lymphomatosum. A rare teratoid of the parotid region. J Cancer Res 1929; 13: 116–25.

66. Kennedy TL. Warthin's tumour: a review indicating no male predominance. Laryngoscope 1983; 93: 889–91.

67. Ebbs SR, Webb AJ. Adenolymphoma of the parotid: aetiology, diagnosis and treatment. Br J Surg 1986; 73: 627–30.

68. Cadier M, Watkin G, Hobsley M. Smoking predisposes to parotid adenolymphoma. Br J Surg 1992; 79: 929–30.

69. Allegra SR. Warthin's tumour: a hypersensitivity disease? Hum Pathol 1971; 2: 403–20.

70. Heller KS, Attie JN. Treatment of Warthin's tumour by enucleation. Am J Surg 1988; 156: 294–6.

71. Gleave EN, Whittaker JS, Nicholson A. Salivary tumours—experience over thirty years. Clin Otolaryngol 1979; 4: 247–57.

72. Spiro RH. Salivary neoplasms: overview of a 35-year experience with 2 807 patients. Head Neck Surg 1986; 8: 177–84.

73. Spiro RH, Huvos AG, Strong EW. Adenoid cystic carcinoma: factors influencing survival. Am J Surg 1979; 138: 579–83.

74. Spiro RH, Huvos AG, Strong EW. Cancer of the parotid gland. Clinicopathological study of 288 primary cases. Am J Surg 1975; 130: 452–9.

75. Spiro RH, Huvos AG. Stage means more than grade in adenoid cystic carcinoma. Am J Surg 1992; 164: 623–8.

76. Perzin KH, Gullane PJ, Clairmont AA. Adenoid cystic carcinoma arising in salivary glands: a correlation of histological features and clinical course. Cancer 1978; 42: 265–82.

77. Maran AGD. The salivary glands. In: Cuschieri A, Giles GR, Moosa AR (eds). Essential surgical practice, 3e. Oxford: Butterworth–Heinemann 1995; 5991–6000.

78. Balm AJM, Delaere P, Hilgers FJM *et al.* Primary lymphoma of mucosa associated lymphoid tissue (MALT) in the parotid gland. Clin Otolaryngol 1993; 18: 528–32.

79. Helmus C. Subtotal parotidectomy: a 10-year review (1985–1994). Laryngoscope 1997; 107: 1024–7.

80. Watkin GT, Hobsley M. Influence of local surgery and radiotherapy on the natural history of pleomorphic adenomas. Br J Surg 1986; 73: 74–6.

81. Ball ABS, Thomas JM. Salivary glands. In: Allen-Mersh TG (ed). Surgical oncology. London: Chapman & Hall Medical, 1996: 93–9.

82. Rosenfeld S, Sessions DG, McSwain B *et al.* Malignant tumours of salivary gland origin: a review of 184 cases. Ann Surg 1966; 163: 726–35.

83. Ball ABS, Rajagopal G, Thomas JM. Malignant epithelial parotid tumours. Ann R Coll Surg Engl 1990; 72: 247–9.

84. Yamashita T, Tomoda K, Kumazawa T. The usefulness of partial parotidectomy for benign parotid gland tumours. Acta Otolaryngol 1993; Suppl 500: 113–6.

85. Chan S, Gunn A. Conservative parotidectomy by the peripheral approach. Br J Surg 1981; 68: 405–7.

86. House JW. Facial nerve grading systems. Laryngoscope 1983; 93: 1056–9.

87. Saeed SR, Ramsden RT. Rehabilitation of the paralysed face: results of facial nerve surgery. J Laryngol Otol 1996; 110: 922–5.

88. Hays LL, Novack AJ, Worsham JC. The Frey syndrome: a simple effective treatment. Otolaryngol Head Neck Surg 1982; 90: 419–25.

89. Dulguerov P, Quinodoz D, Cosendai G *et al.* Prevention of Frey syndrome during parotidectomy. Arch Otolaryngol Head Neck Surg 1999; 125: 833–9.

90. Jianjun Y, Tong T, Wenzhu S *et al.* The use of a parotid fascia flap to prevent postoperative fistula. Oral Surg Oral Med Oral Pathol Oral Radiol Endod 1999; 87: 673–5.

91. Borthne A, Kjellevold K, Kaalhus O *et al.* Salivary gland malignant neoplasms: treatment and prognosis. Int J Radiat Oncol Biol Phys 1986; 12: 747–84.

92. Guillamondegui OM, Byers RM, Luna MA *et al.* Aggressive surgery in treatment for parotid cancer: the role of adjunctive postoperative radiotherapy. J Roentgenol Radium Ther Nucl Med 1975; 123: 49–54.

93. Corcoran MO, Cook HP, Hobsley M. Radical surgery following radiotherapy for advanced parotid carcinomas. Br J Surg 1983; 70: 261–3.

94. Gallegos NC, Watkin G, Cook HP *et al.* Further evaluation of radical surgery following radiotherapy for advanced parotid carcinoma. Br J Surg 1991; 78: 97–100.

95. Wotson S, Mandel ID. The salivary secretions in health and disease. In: Rankow RM, Polayes IM (eds). Diseases of the salivary glands. Philadelphia: WB Saunders, 1976: 32–53.

Index

Pages numbers in italics refer to tables or figures